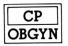

Clinical Perspectives in Obstetrics and Gynecology

Series Editor:

Herbert J. Buchsbaum, M.D.

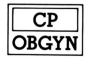 Clinical Perspectives in Obstetrics and Gynecology

perspective *noun:* . . . the capacity to view subjects in their true relations or relative importance.

*Each volume in Clinical Perspectives in Obstetrics and
Gynecology will cover in depth a major clinical area in the
health care of women. The objective is to present to the reader
the pathophysiologic and biochemical basis of the condition
under discussion, and to provide a scientific basis for clinical
management. These volumes are not intended as "how to"
books, but as a ready reference by authorities in the field.*

*Though the obstetrician and gynecologist may be the primary
provider of health care for the female, this role is shared with
family practitioners, pediatricians, medical and surgical
specialists, and geriatricians. It is to all these physicians that
the series is addressed.*

Series Editor: Herbert J. Buchsbaum, M.D.

Forthcoming Volumes:

Aiman: *Infertility*
Galask: *Infectious Disease in the Female Patient*
Lavery and Sanfilippo: *Pediatric and Adolescent Gynecology*
Lifshitz: *Strategies in Surgical Gynecology*

The
Menopause

Edited by

Herbert J. Buchsbaum

Professor of Obstetrics and Gynecology
Director, Division of Gynecologic Oncology
University of Texas Health Science Center at Dallas

With 74 illustrations

Springer-Verlag
New York Berlin Heidelberg Tokyo

Series Editor: Herbert J. Buchsbaum, M.D., Department of Obstetrics and Gynecology, University of Texas Health Science Center at Dallas, 5323 Harry Hines Boulevard, Dallas, Texas 75235.

Library of Congress Cataloging in Publication Data
Main entry under title:

The Menopause.

   (Clinical perspectives in obstetrics and gynecology)
   Includes bibliographical references and index.
   1. Menopause. I. Buchsbaum, Herbert J.
II. Series. [DNLM: 1. Menopause. WP 580 M545]
RG186.M434 1983   618.1′72   83-405
ISBN 0-387-90825-0

Typeset by Bi-Comp., Incorporated
Printed and bound by Halliday Lithograph
Printed in the United States of America.

9 8 7 6 5 4 3 2 1

ISBN 0-387-90825-0
Springer-Verlag New York Berlin Heidelberg Tokyo
ISBN 3-540-90825-0
Springer-Verlag Berlin Heidelberg New York Tokyo

To my family,
Linda, Jon, and Julie

Contributors

Steven G. Bernstein, M.D.
Assistant Professor, Department of Obstetrics and Gynecology, Division of Gynecologic Oncology, Southwestern Medical School, University of Texas Health Science Center at Dallas, Dallas, Texas.

M. Linette Casey, PH.D.
Instructor, Departments of Biochemistry and Obstetrics and Gynecology; The Cecil H. and Ida Green Center for Reproductive Biology Sciences, Southwestern Medical School, University of Texas Health Science Center at Dallas, Dallas, Texas.

Robert C. Corlett, M.D.
Assistant Clinical Professor, Department of Obstetrics and Gynecology, University of Southern California Medical Center, Los Angeles, California.

Clare D. Edman, M.D.
Associate Professor, Department of Obstetrics and Gynecology, Southwestern Medical School; Director, Division of Clinical Endocrinology/Infertility, University of Texas Health Science Center at Dallas, Dallas, Texas.

Marc A. Fritz, M.D.
Fellow, Reproductive Endocrinology, Department of Obstetrics and Gynecology, School of Medicine, Oregon Health Sciences University, Portland, Oregon.

Félix Krauer, M.D.
Professor of Gynecology and Obstetrics, University of Geneva; Head, Department of Gynecology, University Hospital, Geneva, Switzerland.

Samuel Lifshitz, M.D., F.A.C.O.G., F.A.C.S.
Associate Professor, Department of Obstetrics and Gynecology; Associate Director, Division of Gynecologic Oncology, Southwestern Medical School, University of Texas Health Science Center at Dallas, Dallas, Texas.

Marie DuMont Low, M.S., PH.D.
Senior Medical Editor, Springer-Verlag New York, Inc., New York, New York

Paul C. MacDonald, M.D.
Director, Cecil H. and Ida Green Center for Reproductive Biology Sciences; Professor of Obstetrics/Gynecology and Biochemistry, Southwestern Medical School, University of Texas Health Science Center at Dallas, Dallas, Texas.

Douglas J. Marchant, M.D.
Professor of Obstetrics and Gynecology and Professor of Surgery, Tufts University School of Medicine; Director, The Cancer Institute, Tufts-New England Medical Center; Director, The Breast Health Center, Tufts-New England Medical Center, Boston, Massachusetts.

Charles Y.C. Pak, M.D.
Professor, Department of Internal Medicine; Director, General Clinical Research Center, Southwestern Medical School, University of Texas Health Science Center at Dallas, Dallas, Texas.

J. Gerald Quirk, Jr., M.D., PH.D.
Assistant Professor, Department of Obstetrics and Gynecology, Southwestern Medical School, University of Texas Health Science Center at Dallas; Director, Obstetrics and Gynecology Clinic, Parkland Memorial Hospital, Dallas, Texas.

Veronica A. Ravnikar, M.D.
Instructor in Obstetrics and Gynecology, Harvard Medical School; Director of Menopause Unit, Brigham and Women's Hospital, Boston, Massachusetts.

Quentin R. Regestein, M.D.
Associate Professor of Psychiatry, Harvard Medical School; Director, Sleep Clinic, Brigham and Women's Hospital, Boston, Massachusetts.

Isaac Schiff, M.D.
Associate Professor of Obstetrics and Gynecology, Harvard Medical School; Associate Director, Reproductive Endocrine Services, Brigham and Women's Hospital, Boston, Massachusetts.

James P. Semmens, M.D., F.A.C.O.G.
Professor, Department of Obstetrics and Gynecology, Medical University of South Carolina; Medical University Hospital; Charleston Memorial Hospital, Charleston, South Carolina.

Mona M. Shangold, M.D.
Assistant Professor of Obstetrics and Gynecology, Cornell University Medical College; Director, Sports Gynecology Center, The New York Hospital/Cornell Medical Center, New York, New York.

Leon Speroff, M.D.
Professor and Chairman, Department of Obstetrics and Gynecology, School of Medicine, Oregon Health Sciences University, Portland, Oregon.

Meir Steiner, M.D. PH.D., F.R.C.P. (C)
Associate Professor of Psychiatry and Neurosciences, Departments of Psychiatry and Neurosciences, McMaster University,

Faculty of Health Sciences; Head, Clinical Studies Program, Mc-Master Psychiatric Unit, St. Joseph's Hospital, Hamilton, Ontario, Canada.

Richard L. Voet, M.D.
Assistant Professor of Pathology and Obstetrics and Gynecology, Southwestern Medical School, University of Texas Health Science Center at Dallas; Attending Pathologist, Division of Surgical Pathology, Parkland Memorial Hospital, Dallas, Texas.

George D. Wendel, Jr., M.D.
Instructor, Department of Obstetrics and Gynecology, Southwestern Medical School, University of Texas Health Science Center at Dallas, Dallas, Texas.

Contents

Preface

Nearly one-half of an American woman's life is spent after the cessation of reproductive function. A woman of 40 years has an additional life expectancy of nearly 40 years; a woman of 75, over 11 years. This pattern of longevity is likely to continue, so that by the year 2000, it has been estimated, 30 percent of the female population will be postmenopausal.

While it is difficult to separate the results of aging from those of estrogen deprivation, it is important that we try to do so, since the results of the latter are amenable to treatment. The medical infirmities resulting from estrogen deprivation take a high toll among postmenopausal women. Nearly 200,000 hip fractures occur annually in this group, resulting in 15,000 deaths and a high morbidity rate. Sleep disorders, compromised sexuality, psychomotor alterations of the climacterium, and urinary tract disorders all contribute to a lowered quality of life.

Appropriate treatment of these disturbing postmenopausal conditions requires an understanding of the underlying biochemical, endocrinologic, psychologic, and pathophysiologic alterations of estrogen deprivation. Toward this end, the reader will find herein chapters dealing with estrogen metabolism in the postmenopausal female, end-organ response to estrogen deprivation, and bone metabolism and osteoporosis.

Next, the reader will find chapters dealing with specific organs, organ systems, or conditions related to the quality of life; for example, sexuality, urinary tract problems, sleep disorders, the breast, sports and exercise, the climacteric, and the psychobiology of the menopause.

The management of these problems, in part, is estrogen replacement therapy. The "estrogens forever" era closed with a striking rise in the incidence of adenocarcinoma of the endometrium, an issue addressed in the chapter dealing with this neoplasm, now the most common female genital malignancy. The physician must be aware of the benefits and risks of estrogen treatment to choose appropriately.

To aid the clinician in the choice of medications and regimens, there is a chapter dealing with the physiology and metabolism of the natural and synthetic estrogens, as well as two chapters dealing with estrogen replacement regimens: one author advocating estrogens only, the other estrogen with a terminal progestational agent. The reader is also referred to the chapter on sleep disorders to gain information on the therapeutic effects of estrogens and progestagens.

We have not included in this volume a discussion of specific medical diseases, since none are unique to the menopause. Instead, there is a chapter dealing with surgery in the postmenopausal patient. In it the reader will find a description of what constitutes appropriate preoperative evaluation and specifics of postoperative monitoring in postmenopausal women to reduce surgical risks. And finally, there is a delightful presentation of the postmenopausal woman as depicted in literature. This chapter, not directed at quality of care, should help the physician understand society's perception of the postmenopausal woman, and should highlight the fact that our perception has not yet completely caught up with the reality.

The editor has attempted to avoid repetition and duplication, a common problem in multiauthored texts, by discussing the content of chapters with authors prior to submission, and later by editing. Nevertheless, we have allowed authors' presentations to overlap when necessary to develop a thesis.

We received considerable help from the publisher in this, the first volume of *Clinical Perspectives in Obstetrics and Gynecology*, and would like to acknowledge the contributions of Ute Bujard, Manager, Book Production Department, and John Morgan, Production Editor, who ably managed the transfer of manuscript to bound book. Special thanks are also due Joyce Perry, my administrative secretary, who played a vital role in coordinating all aspects of manuscript preparation.

Herbert J. Buchsbaum, M.D.

Origin of Estrogen and Regulation of Its Formation in Postmenopausal Women*

M. Linette Casey and Paul C. MacDonald

In premenopausal, ovulatory women, estrogen arises by two mechanisms. It is believed that the biologically more important of these is the synthesis of 17β-estradiol in the developing follicle. This obtains since 17β-estradiol is a more potent estrogen than that produced by the second mechanism, i.e., the extraglandular formation of estrone from circulating androstenedione. The rate of extraglandular estrone formation does not vary appreciably during the ovarian cycle (Fig. 1–1).[1] On average, about 3 mg of androstenedione are produced each day in young women and 1.5% of plasma androstenedione is aromatized (the process of converting androgen to estrogen) to estrone in extraglandular tissues.[1-4] Thus, approximately 45 μg of estrone arise by this mechanism. At the extremes of the ovarian cycle, this amount of estrone may constitute 50% or more of the total estrogen produced in young women.[1] The rate of secretion of 17β-estradiol by the ovary, however, varies widely during the ovarian cycle (Fig. 1–1). It is estimated that the rate of secretion of 17β-estradiol varies from 20–40 μg/day early and late in the cycle to as much as 600–1000 μg/day just prior to the midcycle LH (luteinizing hormone) surge and ovulation.[1]

Usually there is a decrease in the rate of 17β-estradiol synthesis in the ovary during the perimenopausal period and likely, in consequence, the onset of anovulation. At this time, estrogen still arises by the two mechanisms cited. But after menopause, it is established that estrogen is produced almost singularly by the extraglandular aromatization of plasma androstenedione.[5,6]

Little or no estrogen is secreted by the adrenal glands of any person or by the ovaries of postmenopausal women. On average, the rate of secretion of androstenedione in postmenopausal women is 1.5 mg/day.[5] The lower production rate of androstenedione in postmenopausal women than in premenopausal women is attributable to the decline in androstenedione secretion by the ovaries of postmenopausal women.[1,5,7] Before menopause, the ovaries secrete an amount of androstenedione similar to that of the adrenals, i.e., about 1.5 mg/day.

Insignificant amounts of 17β-estradiol are produced in extraglandular tissues from the aromatization of circulating dehydroisoandrosterone[8] or testosterone.[1,9] In the case of dehydroisoandrosterone, there is little aromatization of this C_{19}-steroid except in trophoblast; and in the case of testosterone, the fractional conversion to 17β-estradiol is less than that of androstenedione to estrone and in women far less testosterone than androstenedione is available for aromatization.

Estrone is converted to 17β-estradiol in extraglandular sites. Indeed, 50% of estrone is metabolized by way of 17β-estradiol.[9,10] The 17β-estradiol formed, however, is metabolized further in the tissue sites of its formation and thus only about 5% of plasma estrone is converted to 17β-estradiol that enters blood.[11] This, however, may not be a completely accurate representation of the availability of 17β-

* Supported in part by USPHS Grant No. 2-P01-AG00306.

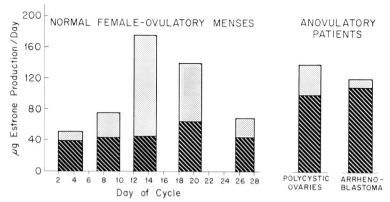

Fig. 1–1. The origin of estrogen in premenopausal ovulatory women as a function of time of the ovarian cycle and in women with polycystic ovarian disease and an endocrine tumor of the ovary. The total height of the bar is indicative of total estrogen, i.e., estrone plus 17β-estradiol production. The hatched portion of each bar is representative of the rate of estrone formation in extraglandular sites from plasma androstenedione. The stippled portion of the bar is the amount of total estrogen production that is attributable to 17β-estradiol secretion by the ovary.

estradiol from estrone to a cell responsive to 17β-estradiol. For example, in endometrium estrone is converted to 17β-estradiol[10] and such 17β-estradiol could be available to interact with the estrogen receptor protein in cytosol. Before leaving the cell, however, the 17β-estradiol formed likely is converted back to estrone.[10] This conversion of estrone to 17β-estradiol, therefore, would not be measured in the blood-to-blood interconversion of the two steroids.

Regulation of Extraglandular Estrogen Biosynthesis

It now is known that the enzymatic capacity for the conversion of androstenedione to estrone is present in a number of human tissues. These include adipose tissue,[12–15] skin,[16] hair follicles,[17] brain,[18] bone,[19] and muscle.[20] It seems probable, however, that the quantitatively most important tissue of extraglandular estrone formation is adipose tissue.

On the other hand, it is exciting to consider extraglandular estrogen formation from another vantage point. Namely, estrogen can be produced in tissue sites of estrogen action, e.g., brain (hypothalamus),[18] hair follicles,[17] breast,[14,21] bone,[19] prostate,[22] and breast cancer.[23] It is conceivable, therefore, that the in situ formation of estrogen in an estrogen-responsive tissue could constitute a mechanism that could give rise to far greater intracellular concentrations of the hormone than could be attained by delivery through blood.

Thus, it is apparent that the mechanism of estrogen biosynthesis in postmenopausal women is a continuation of one of two means by which estrogen is produced in nonpregnant premenopausal women. In postmenopausal women, extraglandular estrone formation from plasma androstenedione of adrenal origin is the nearly singular means of estrogen formation. Nonetheless, this is not necessarily a static process (Fig. 1–2), since there are two determinants of the rate of extraglandular aromatization of plasma androstenedione, i.e., (1) the fractional conversion of plasma androstenedione to estrone and (2) the rate of production of androstenedione. There are a number of metabolic and pathophysiologic processes that give rise to increased conversion of androstenedione to estrone. It is known that extraglandular aromatase activity is not rate-limiting over wide ranges of plasma concentrations of androstenedione.[1,24–26] Thus, the rate of extraglandular estrone formation in a given person is directly proportional to the production rate of androstenedione. Importantly, we believe, the metabolic and pathophysiologic processes that give rise to increased extraglan-

ORIGIN OF ESTROGEN IN
POSTMENOPAUSAL WOMEN

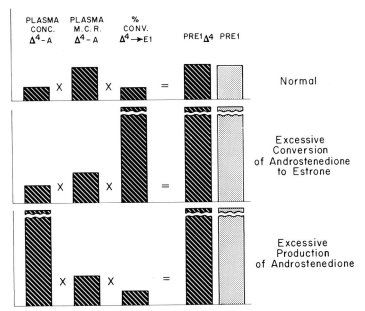

Fig. 1–2. Determinants of the rate of extraglandular estrone formation. The extraglandular formation of estrone is increased when the extent of aromatization is increased or when there is greater availability of androstenedione.

dular estrone formation are those that appear also to give rise to an increased risk of endometrial neoplasia.

Metabolic Processes that Favor Increased Extraglandular Aromatization of Plasma Androstenedione

OBESITY. Intuitively, it seemed reasonable on first consideration that extraglandular aromatization should increase with an increase in adipose tissue mass (Fig. 1–3). It seemed to follow that if there were more adipose tissue there would be greater rates of estrogen formation. On the other hand, this seemed somewhat less plausible on closer scrutiny, since it was known that the development of obesity involved as much an increase in the size of adipocytes as adipocyte cell number.[27,28] Thus, it was not clear how there should be a greater capacity for aromatization in a lipid-laden adipocyte. One might suspect the opposite. This follows because the prehormone, androstenedione, is a nonpolar (non-water soluble) compound that is readily soluble in lipid. This characteristic is one that should deter accessibility of the substrate, i.e., androstenedione, to the site of aromatization, i.e., the endoplasmic reticulum of the adipocyte. Thus a dilemma arose. More-

over, this paradox was complicated further when it was found that the extent of aromatization in morbidly obese subjects was not reduced after massive weight loss.[29] Ackerman and colleagues[30] have obtained data that appear to provide an explanation of these heretofore inexplicable findings. They determined that the aromatase activity in adipose tissue is present principally in the stromal cells of this tissue, not in the adipocytes. It is known that with the development of obesity there is an increase in the number of stromal cells;[27,28] moreover, with weight loss in obese subjects there is no reduction in the number of stromal cells.[29] Interestingly, the stromal cell of human adipose tissue appears to be unique in its capacity for aromatization of C_{19}-steroids. In these cells, the aromatase activity is stimulated strikingly (10–50-fold) by treatment with glucocorticosteroids or cyclic AMP analogs.[31] Thus it can be envisioned that not only the number of stromal cells of fat tissue are important in the control of extraglandular estrogen formation, but hormonal factors as well may contribute to the regulation of estrone biosynthesis. In any event, obesity, one of the primary factors that leads to an increased risk of endometrial carcinoma in women, also is one that causes increased extraglandular estrone formation.

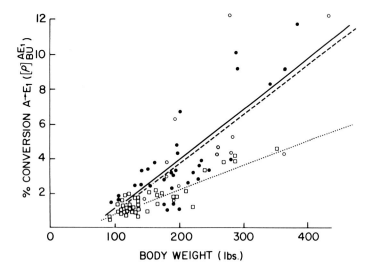

Fig. 1–3. The extent of aromatization of plasma androstenedione as a function of body weight in postmenopausal women with (○) and without (●) endometrial carcinoma and in premenopausal (□) women.

AGING. The transfer constant of conversion of plasma androstenedione to estrone increases as a function of age in men and women (Fig. 1–4).[32] From the data available it is not clear whether the increase in extraglandular aromatization with aging is a progressive phenomenon or rather a sudden one that occurs at or about the age of menopause. Irrespective of the answer to this question, it is clear that the fractional conversion of androstenedione to estrone in postmenopausal women is two to three times greater than in premenopausal women. But more than that, aging and obesity appear to act in concert to increase extraglandular estrone formation.[33] It is important also to note that aging is another risk factor for endometrial carcinoma in women. The highest incidence of this neoplasia is found in women at age 60.[34] Thus, a second factor that gives

rise to an increased risk of endometrial carcinoma also gives rise to increased extraglandular estrone production.

LIVER DISEASE. It is well known that feminization is common in men with cirrhosis of the liver. The pathogenesis of gynecomastia and impotency in such men, however, has not been clear. Some investigators attributed the cause of this disorder to decreased liver clearance of estrogen. The evidence in favor of this proposition, however, was not strong. There also were reasons to believe that cirrhosis of the liver in women gave rise to apparent estrogen excess, i.e., anovulation in young women and uterine bleeding in older women with liver disease are quite common.[35,36] With the recognition that estrogen is formed in extraglandular tissues, it soon was discovered that the ex-

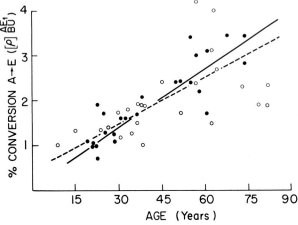

Fig. 1–4. The extent of aromatization of plasma androstenedione as a function of age in men (●) of similar body weight and in women (○) of similar body weight.

tent of aromatization of androstenedione is increased, sometimes strikingly, in men and women with cirrhosis of the liver.[37,38]

The mechanism by which this occurs also appears to have been defined, in part. In normal persons the hepatic extraction of androstenedione, i.e., irreversible clearance by liver, is about 90%;[39] there is little or no conversion of androstenedione to estrone, however, in liver.[38,40] Thus hepatic metabolism of androstenedione precludes aromatization of this C_{19}-steroid as a consequence of conversion to metabolites that are not aromatase substrates. Rather, it is the extrahepatic, extraglandular metabolism of androstenedione that accounts for estrone formation. With cirrhosis, the hepatic extraction of androstenedione is diminished, sometimes strikingly so, and therefore extrahepatic metabolism is favored. As a consequence there is relatively greater extrahepatic than intrahepatic metabolism of androstenedione and thus greater aromatization. It seems probable that this explanation is a correct formulation, but at the same time it is clear that this explanation of the pathophysiology of increased aromatization of C_{19}-steroids in persons with liver disease is incomplete. For example, it can be computed that if liver blood flow were zero and if extrahepatic metabolism of androstenedione did not change, the conversion of plasma androstenedione to estrone would increase only to 4.5%, a value that is three times normal. The conversion of androstendione to estrone in some persons with cirrhosis of the liver, however, is massive. In one postmenopausal woman with cirrhosis, we found that 16% of plasma androstenedione was converted to estrone.[41] She developed carcinoma of the endometrium; indeed, liver disease in women also may be a pathophysiologic process that predisposes to an increased risk of endometrial carcinoma.[41]

OTHER PROCESSES THAT CAUSE INCREASED EXTRAGLANDULAR AROMATIZATION OF PLASMA C_{19}-STEROIDS. Southern and colleagues[42] found that extraglandular aromatase activity in persons with hyperthyroidism was increased compared with that in euthyroid individuals. We observed that extraglandular estrogen formation also was increased in men and women in the postoperative period after abdominal surgery. Finally,

an apparent congenital disorder characterized by feminization of a prepubertal boy that was identified to be due to massive extraglandular aromatization of androstenedione has been described.[43] Interestingly, in this disorder the estrogen produced was principally estrone sulfate.

Increased Production of Androstenedione

As stated, if greater amounts of androstenedione are available, a proportional increase in estrone formation is obliged.

ENDOCRINE TUMORS OF THE OVARY. Androstenedione usually is the principal steroid secreted by certain ovarian tumors. Among these are lipoid cell tumors of the ovary and the luteoma of pregnancy. In such cases, extraglandular estrone production increases as the consequence of increased availability of substrate for the aromatase enzyme system. Importantly, women with endocrine tumors of the ovary are known to be at increased risk for the development of endometrial carcinoma.

NONENDOCRINE TUMORS OF THE OVARY. Feminization as well as virilization may be seen in women with "nonendocrine" tumors of the ovary. Specifically, abnormal endocrine manifestations may accompany tumors of the ovary in which the tumor cells are known not to produce steroid hormones. In such cases, the major steroid secreted is androstenedione; the androstenedione is produced in contiguous nonmalignant stromal cells that undergo hyperplasia.[1,24,25,44] A variety of ovarian tumors incite ovarian stromal cell hyperplasia. Among the more common are Brenner tumors,[45] pseudomucinous cystadenomas,[47] and cystadenocarcinomas[24] as well as serous cystadenocarcinomas.[46] In women with "nonendocrine" tumors of the ovary, the risk of endometrial carcinoma also is increased.[46]

POLYCYSTIC OVARIAN DISEASE. Endometrial carcinoma in young, i.e., premenopausal, women is rare. Many investigators have taken the view that progesterone, produced by the corpus luteum, acts in a manner that is protective against the development of endometrial neoplasia. This may be a correct formulation of the evidence since endometrial neoplasia in young women almost always occurs in those who are anovulatory. Endometrial cancer has been found in (1) women with gonadal dysgenesis who were ingesting estrogen,[47-52] (2) women ingesting the sequential type oral contraceptives,[53] (3) young women with endocrine and "nonendocrine" tumors of the ovary,[46] and (4) young women with anovulation due to polycystic ovarian disease.[54,55]

The pathophysiology of polycystic ovarian disease, in terms of estrogen formation, is similar to that found in women with endocrine and "nonendocrine" tumors of the ovary. Specifically, in such women, the ovarian secretion of 17β-estradiol is attenuated whereas the ovarian secretion of androstenedione is accentuated.[56] Thus estrogen formation in these women is accounted for principally by the extraglandular formation of estrone from circulating androstenedione.

Summary

Estrogen formation in postmenopausal women can be accounted for by the extraglandular aromatization, principally in stromal cells of adipose tissue, of androstenedione that is secreted by the adrenal cortex. Increased extraglandular aromatization is known to occur with obesity, aging, and liver disease, all of which are abnormalities known to be associated with increased risk for endometrial cancer. If androstenedione production is high, as with endocrine and nonendocrine tumors of the ovary, and in polycystic ovarian disease, the risk of endometrial neoplasia also is high. Thus, the pathophysiologic processes that favor increased extraglandular estrone synthesis are the same as those that are known to be associated with an increased risk of endometrial carcinoma.

REFERENCES

1. Siiteri PK, MacDonald PC. Role of extraglandular estrogen in human endocrinology. In: Greep RO, Astwood EB, eds. Handbook of physiology. Washington DC: American Physiology Society, Section 7: Endocrinology, 1963:615–629.

2. VandeWiele RL, MacDonald PC, Gurpide E, et al. Studies on the secretion and interconversion of the androgens. Rec Prog Horm Res. 1963; 19:275–309.

3. MacDonald PC, VandeWiele RL., Lieberman S. Precursors of the urinary 11-desoxy-17-ketosteroids of ovarian origin. Am J Obstet Gynecol. 1963; 86:1–10.

4. MacDonald PC, Grodin JM, Siiteri PC. Dynamics of androgen and oestrogen secretion. In: Baird D, ed. Gonadal steroid secretion. Edinburgh: Ciba Foundation Symposium, 1971:158–174.

5. Grodin JM, Siiteri PK, MacDonald PC. Source of estrogen production in postmenopausal women. J Clin Endocrinol Metab. 1973; 36:207–214.

6. Longcope C. Metabolic clearance and blood production rates of estrogens in postmenopausal women. Am J Obstet Gynecol. 1971; 111:778–781.

7. Judd HL, Judd GE, Lucas WE. Endocrine function of the postmenopausal ovary: Concentration of androgens and estrogens in ovarian and peripheral vein blood. J Clin Endocrinol Metab. 1974; 39:1020–1024.

8. MacDonald PC, Edman CD, Kerber IJ, et al. Plasma precursors of estrogen: III. Conversion of plasma dehydroisoandrosterone to estrogen in young, nonpregnant women. Gynecol Invest. 1976; 7:165–175.

9. MacDonald PC, Madden JD, Brenner PF, et al. Origin of estrogen in normal men and in women with testicular feminization. J Clin Endocrinol Metab. 1979; 49:905–916.

10. Gurpide E. Hormones and gynecologic cancer. Cancer. 1976; 38(suppl 1):503–508.

11. Longcope C, Layne DS, Tait JF. Metabolic clearance rates and interconversions of estrone and 17β-estradiol in normal males and females. J Clin Invest. 1968; 47:93–106.

12. Schindler AE, Ebert A, Friedrich E. Conversion of androstenedione to estrone by human fat tissue. J Clin Endocrinol Metab. 1972; 35:627–630.

13. Bolt HM, Gobel P. Formation of estrogens from androgens by human subcutaneous adipose tissue in vitro. Horm Metab Res. 1972; 4:312–313.

14. Nimrod A, Ryan KJ. Aromatization of androgens by human abdominal and breast fat tissue. J Clin Endocrinol Metab. 1975; 40:367–372.

15. Perel E, Killinger DW. The interconversion and aromatization of androgens by human adipose tissue. J Steroid Biochem. 1979; 10:623–627.

16. Schweikert HU, Milewich L, Wilson JD. Aromatization of androstenedione by cultured hu-

man fibroblasts. J Clin Endocrinol Metab. 1976; 43:785–795.

17. Schweikert HU, Milewich L, Wilson JD. Aromatization of androstenedione by isolated human hairs. J Clin Endocrinol Metab. 1975; 40:413–417.

18. Naftolin F, Ryan K, Petro Z. Aromatization of androstenedione by the diencephalon. J Clin Endocrinol Metab. 1971; 33:368–370.

19. Frisch RE, Canick JA, Tulchinsky D. Human fatty marrow aromatizes androgen to estrogen. J Clin Endocrinol Metab. 1980; 51:394–396.

20. Longcope C, Pratt JH, Schneider SH, et al. Aromatization of androgens by muscle and adipose tissue in vivo. J Clin Endocrinol Metab. 1978; 46:146–152.

21. Perel E, Wilkins D, Killinger DW. The conversion of androstenedione to estrone, estradiol, and testosterone in breast tissue. J Steroid Biochem. 1980; 13:89–94.

22. Schweikert HU. Conversion of androstenedione to estrone in human fibroblasts cultured from prostate, genital and nongenital skin. Horm Metab Res. 1979; 11:635–640.

23. MacIndoe JH. Estradiol formation from testosterone by continuously cultured human breast cancer cells. J Clin Endocrinol Metab. 1979; 49:272–277.

24. MacDonald PC, Grodin JM, Edman CD, et al. Origin of estrogen in a postmenopausal woman with a nonendocrine tumor of the ovary and endometrial hyperplasia. Obstet Gynecol. 1976; 47:644–650.

25. Aiman EJ, Nalick RH, Jacobs A, et al. The origin of androgen and estrogen in a virilized postmenopausal woman with bilateral benign cystic teratomas. Obstet Gynecol. 1977; 49:695–704.

26. Aiman EJ, Edman CD, Worley RJ, et al. Androgen and estrogen formation in women with ovarian hyperthecosis. Obstet Gynecol. 1978; 51:1–9.

27. Klyde BJ, Hirsch J. Increased cellular proliferation in adipose tissue of adult rats fed a high fat diet. J Lipid Res. 1979; 20:705–715.

28. Klyde BJ, Hirsch J. Isotopic labeling of DNA in rat adipose tissue for proliferating cells associated with mature adipocytes. J Lipid Res. 1979; 20:691–704.

29. Siiteri PK, Williams JE, Takaki NK. Steroid abnormalities in endometrial and breast carcinoma: A unifying hypothesis. J Steroid Biochem. 1976; 7:897–903.

30. Ackerman GE, Smith ME, Mendelson CR, et al. Aromatization of androstenedione by human adipose tissue stromal cells in monolayer culture. J Clin Endocrinol Metab. 1981; 412–417.

31. Mendelson CR, Cleland WH, Smith ME, et al. Regulation of aromatase activity of stromal cells derived from human adipose tissue. Endocrinology. 1982; 1077–1085.

32. Hemsell DL, Grodin JM, Brenner PF, et al. Plasma precursors of estrogen. II. Correlation of the extent of conversion of plasma androstenedione to estrone with age. J Clin Endocrinol Metab. 1974; 38:476–479.

33. MacDonald PC, Edman CD, Hemsell DL, et al. Effect of obesity on conversion of plasma androstenedione to estrone in postmenopausal women with and without endometrial cancer. Am J Obstet Gynecol 1978; 130:448–455.

34. Wynder EL, Fisher GC, Mantel N. An epidemiological investigation of cancer of the endometrium. Cancer. 1966; 19:489–520.

35. Speert H. Endometrial cancer and hepatic cirrhosis. Cancer. 1949; 2:597–603.

36. Apperly FL. Endometrial hyperplasia in elderly women with hepatic cirrhosis. Va Med Monthly. 1951; 78:602.

37. Gordon GG, Olivo J, Rafii F, et al. Conversion of androgens to estrogens in cirrhosis of the liver. J Clin Endocrinol Metab. 1975; 40:1018–1026.

38. Edman CD, MacDonald PC, Combes B. Extraglandular production of estrogen in subjects with liver disease. Gastroenterology. 1975; 69:819.

39. Rivarola MA, Singleton RT, Mignon CJ. Splanchnic extraction and interconversion of testosterone and androstenedione in man. J Clin Invest. 1967; 46:2096–2100.

40. Edman CD, MacDonald PC. Extraglandular aromatization—primarily an extrahepatic metabolic process. Gynecol Invest. 1977; 8:50.

41. Edman CD, MacDonald PC. The role of extraglandular estrogen in women in health and disease. In: James VHT, Serio M, Gusti, G, eds. The endocrine function of the human ovary. London: Academic Press, 1976:135–140.

42. Southern AL, Olivo J, Gordon GG, et al. The conversion of androgens to estrogens in hyperthyroidism. J Clin Endocrinol Metab. 1974; 38:207–214.

43. Hemsell DL, Edman CD, Marks JF, et al. Massive extraglandular aromatization of plasma androstenedione resulting in feminization of a prepubertal boy. J Clin Invest. 1977; 60:455–464.

44. MacDonald PC. Determinants of the rate of estrogen formation in postmenopausal women. Eur J Obstet Gynaecol Reprod Biol. 1979; 9/3:187–189.

45. Silverberg SG. Brenner tumor of the ovary. A clinical study of 60 tumors in 54 women. Cancer. 1971; 28:588–596.

46. Wren BG, Frampton J. Oestrogenic activity as-

sociated with nonfeminizing ovarian tumors after the menopause. Br Med J. 1963; 2:842–
844.

47. Wilkinson EJ, Friedrich EG, Mattingly RF.
Turner's syndrome with endometrial adenocarcinoma and stilbestrol therapy. Obstet Gynecol.
1973; 42:193–200.

48. Cutler BS, Forbes AP, Ingersoll FM, et al. Endometrial carcinoma after stilbestrol therapy. N
Engl J Med. 1972; 287:628–631.

49. Dewhurst CJ, deKoos EB, Haines RM. Replacement hormone therapy in gonadal dysgenesis.
Br J Obstet Gynaecol. 1975; 82:412–416.

50. McCarroll AM, Montgomery DAD, Harley
JMG, et al. Endometrial carcinoma after cyclical
oestrogen-progestogen therapy for Turner's
syndrome. Br J Obstet Gynaecol. 1975;
82:421–425.

51. Roberts G, Wells AL: Oestrogen-induced endometrial carcinoma in a patient with gonadal
dysgenesis. Br J Obstet Gynaecol. 1975;
82:417–420.

52. Sirota DK, Marinoff SC. Endometrial carcinoma in Turner's syndrome following prolonged treatment with diethylstilbestrol. Mt Si-
nai J Med. 1975; 42:586–590.

53. Silverberg SG, Makowski EL. Endometrial carcinoma in young women taking oral contraceptive agents. Obstet Gynecol. 1975; 46:503–
506.

54. Fechner RE, Kaufman RH. Endometrial adenocarcinoma in Stein-Leventhal syndrome.
Cancer. 1974; 24:444–452.

55. Jackson RL, Dockerty MB. The Stein-Leventhal
syndrome: Analysis of 43 cases with special reference to association with endometrial carcinoma. Am J Obstet Gynecol. 1957; 73:161–
173.

56. Edman CD, MacDonald PC. Effect of obesity
on conversion of plasma androstenedione to estrone in ovulatory and anovulatory young
women. Am J Obstet Gynecol. 1978; 130:456–
461.

End Organ Response to Estrogen Deprivation

2

Richard L. Voet

The effect of estrogen deprivation upon organs which have a high dependency for circulating estrogen will be considered in this chapter. Although the menopause is the primary reason for estrogen deprivation, there are other situations which provide clinical models for the study of estrogen dependency and the result of its deprivation. The menopause has a significant complicating factor in that the aging process must also be considered when evaluating the effect of estrogens on host tissues. The aging process is a physiologic phenomenon which is currently the subject of many excellent reviews[1–8] and ongoing research. Aging begins at the moment of conception and continues throughout life. However, the aging process is usually referred to the period of life in which our bodies can no longer maintain the equilibrium and literally begin to "wear out."

We will attempt to distinguish between the natural aging process and those features which are the direct result of the withdrawal of estrogen during the menopause. Three areas will be considered: (1) the female reproductive tract, (2) the breast, and (3) nonreproductive organs.

The Female Reproductive Tract

THE VULVA. The vulva responds to hormones both in a systemic fashion, as the rest of the skin, but also in a more unique fashion, as part of the female reproductive system. Changes occur in the vulva and perineal region at the time of puberty.[7] In childhood, the labia minora protrude between the labia ma-

jora and at the time of puberty, under the influence of estrogen, the labia majora begin to develop. The mons and the lateral aspects of the vulva begin to develop pubic hair, and the skin becomes slightly more pigmented. At the menopause, a general atrophy of the skin begins, but on the vulva there is also a reversal of the processes occurring at puberty; the pubic hair decreases and the labia majora become very small. Histologically, the vulvar skin shows atrophy and reduction in the amount of glycogen in the epithelial cells, as compared to the reproductive age (Fig. 2–1A). There are certain skin conditions which are more prevalent in the postmenopausal patient, such as lichen sclerosus (Fig. 2–1B) and hyperplastic dystrophy. The role of hormonal factors in these conditions is currently being studied.

THE VAGINA. The vaginal epithelium is highly responsive to estrogen. At birth, the infant vagina is usually slightly rugated in response to maternal estrogen. After the withdrawal of maternal estrogens, and throughout childhood, the vaginal epithelium becomes thin; at the time of puberty, rugae begin to form. The vaginal epithelium from this point on is thick, nonkeratinized, and contains abundant glycogen. During and after the menopause, the vaginal epithelium loses its rugae and becomes slightly shortened and thinned. Histologically there is loss of glycogen and flattening of the epithelium. This can present problems during intercourse since the vagina will become more irritated and bleeds easily. This condition is known clinically as atrophic

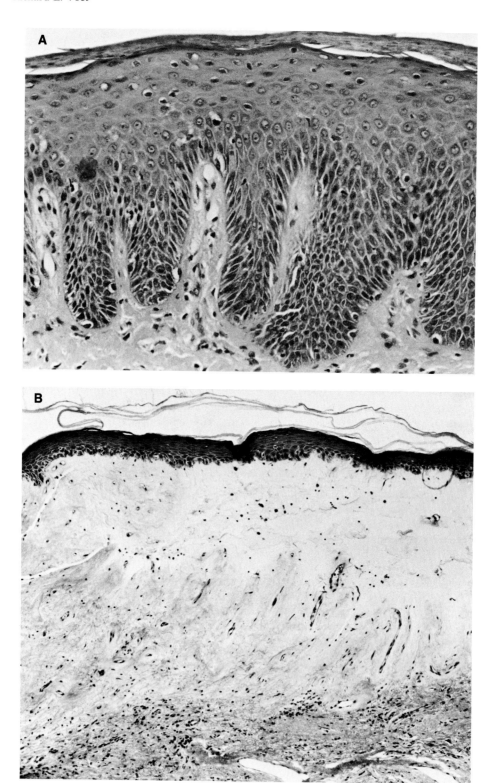

Fig. 2–1. A Normal vulvar skin from a 30-year-old female. There are prominent rete ridges and normal maturation of the acanthocytes giving rise to a keratinized surface. Hematoxylin and eosin (H&E); **B** Lichen sclerosus. Note the thin epithelium with almost complete absence of rete ridges. There is decreased keratin on the surface and a pale lucent zone in the upper dermis. H&E; × 100.

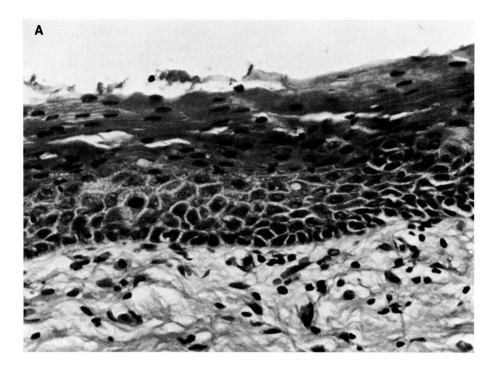

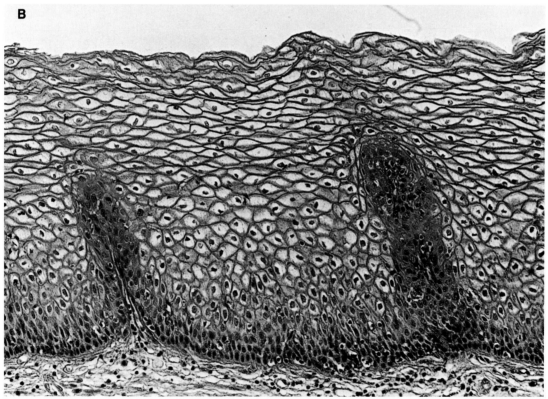

Fig. 2–2. A Postmenopausal cervix showing atrophy. There is thinning of the epithelium with a flattening of the superficial zone showing a parakeratoticlike epithelium. There is prominence of the parabasal zone and lack of maturation in the intermediate area. H&E; × 400. **B** Uterine cervix from a 30-year-old female. There is maturation beginning near the basal layer with a small parabasal zone. The epithelium is thicker than the atrophic cervix, and there are numerous superficial cells with abundant glycogen present. H&E; × 400.

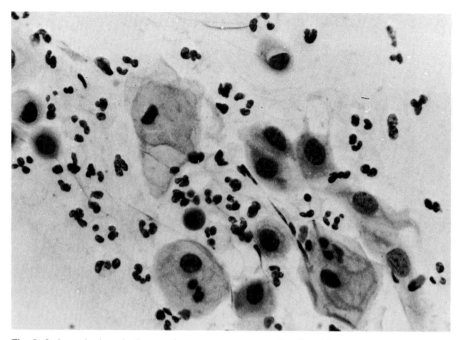

Fig. 2–3. A cervical-vaginal smear from a postmenopausal patient. Note the predominance of parabasal cells and the accompanying inflammation. This is an example of atrophic cervico-vaginitis. Papanicolaou stain; × 400.

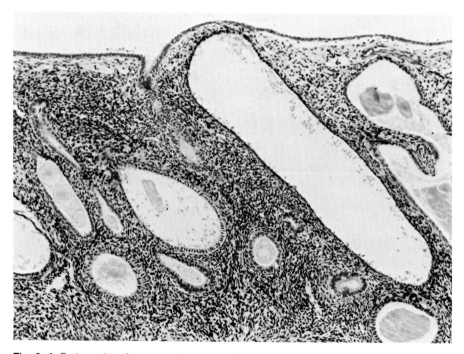

Fig. 2–4. Endometrium from a postmenopausal patient. Section shows cystic atrophy with flattening of the epithelial lining and dilatation of the glands with scattered amorphous material. The adjacent endometrial stroma is scanty and compact and the underlying myometrium shows a high nuclear density and lack of eosinophilic cytoplasm. H&E; × 100.

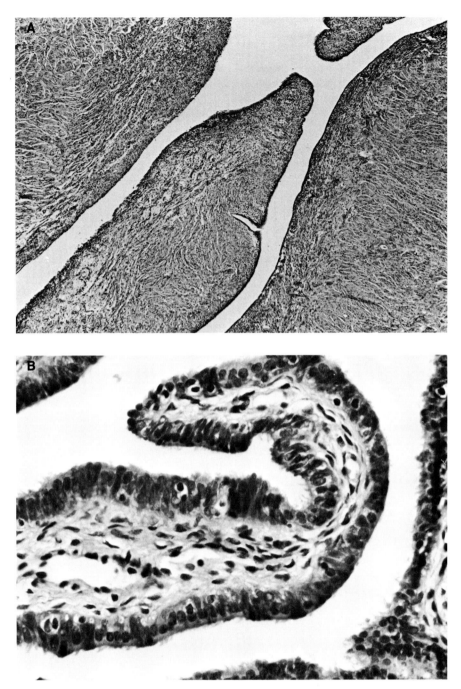

Fig. 2–5. A Fallopian tube from a postmenopausal patient. There is blunting of the villi and flattening of the epithelium. A marked decrease in the number of cilia is evident and the delicate fibrovascular stroma is replaced by a more dense fibromuscular tissue. H&E; × 100. **B** Fallopian tube from a 30-year-old female. There are numerous clear or peg cells, abundant cilia present, and a delicate fibrovascular core in the villi. H&E; × 400.

vaginitis and responds well to either topical or systemic estrogens.

THE CERVIX. During the menopause, the uterine cervix becomes atrophic, with epithelial atrophy and loss of the fibromuscular stroma.[9] As the vagina shortens and the uterine corpus and cervix become atrophic, the cervix often becomes flush with the apex of the vagina and the cervical os is visible as a small opening. The epithelium becomes thinned with a flattened superficial layer (Fig. 2–2A), when compared to the premenopausal state (Fig. 2–2B). The endocervical glandular tissue is much less active and little mucin is produced. The squamocolumnar junction moves up into the canal, which can present problems for colposcopic examination of cervical dysplasia. A considerable problem in the postmenopausal female is the evaluation of cervicovaginal cytologic smears.[10] The atrophic changes resulting from estrogen depletion cause a predominance of parabasal cells (Fig. 2–3). The atrophic vaginitis and the often accompanying inflammation make cytologic smears difficult to interpret. The short-term use of vaginal or systemic estrogen usually allows satisfactory maturation of the epithelium and reduces the inflammatory changes, allowing a more reliable interpretation of the smears.

THE UTERINE CORPUS. In the child the cervix is twice as large as the corpus, a ratio which changes during the reproductive years. The postmenopausal uterus reverts back to the prepubertal ratio: a corpus smaller than the cervix.[11,12] The normal adult uterus during reproductive years weighs approximately 120 g; the postmenopausal uterus may be reduced by as much as 30 to 50%. Both estrogen and progesterone receptors are present in the premenopausal endometrium with larger numbers of progesterone receptors.[13]

Histologically, the changes of estrogen deprivation affect both the endometrium and the myometrium. The endometrium becomes atrophic with residual cystic dilatation of the glands (Fig. 2–4). The columnar epithelium in the glands is flattened to cuboidal with little or no secretions. The endometrial stroma becomes markedly diminished or absent, and the glands appear to intermingle with the underlying muscular fibers. The myometrial fibers are atrophic and the elongated eosinophilic cytoplasm is markedly decreased. This gives the smooth muscle stroma the appearance of high cellularity and can be confused occasionally with stromal neoplasms of the uterus. The cystic atrophy of the endometrium needs to be differentiated from cystic hyperplasia in curettage specimens. Endometrial curettings in the postmenopausal patient are usually scanty and show only superficial fragments of epithelium. The appearance can be similar to curettings from the lower uterine segment and one must be cautious in interpreting curettings from postmenopausal patients. This is particularly a problem when the endometrial cavity is obstructed or occluded either by tumor or by leiomyoma, and curettings reveal only superficial fragments of inactive epithelium from the lower uterine segment. This could give an erroneous impression that the endometrial cavity was sampled showing only atrophy.

In the perimenopausal period, there is temporary unopposed estrogen stimulation of the endometrium which can give confusing patterns, the result of excess estrogen without intervening progesterone production. This pattern has been described as a disordered proliferative pattern.[14] As the proliferation continues to hyperplasia, there may also be accompanying "metaplastic" patterns which can also be confused with adenocarcinoma.[15] For a full discussion of the histopathology of endometrial carcinoma, see Chapter 8.

THE FALLOPIAN TUBES. The fallopian tubes also contain estrogen receptors[16] and the postmenopausal changes parallel the changes in the uterine corpus: epithelial and muscular atrophy.[11] The tube becomes shortened and its diameter decreased. The lumen narrows and, as the epithelium becomes atrophic, the underlying muscular stroma forms blunted villi (Fig. 2–5A). Ciliated and peg cells usually present in the fallopian tube (Fig. 2–5B) are markedly decreased. Tubal secretions and tubal peristalsis are decreased or absent in the postmenopausal fallopian tube.

THE OVARY. The aging ovary[17,18] becomes smaller and there is a striking absence of follicles and germ cells. In the prepubertal ovary, the ovarian cortex is crowded with primordial

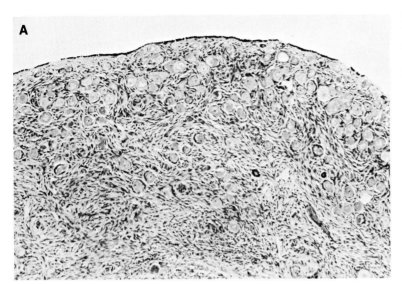

Fig. 2–6. A Section of infant ovary. There is a well-developed overlying germinal epithelium and numerous underlying primordial follicles with prominent germ cells. H&E; × 100.

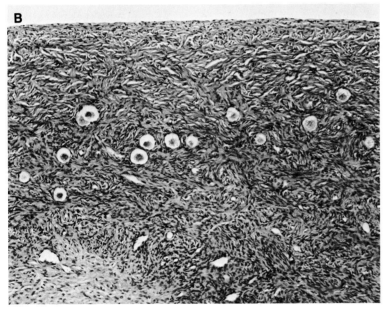

B Section of an ovary of a 30-year-old female. There is lack of a prominent germinal epithelium and the number of germ cells has decreased in density as compared to the prepubertal ovary. H&E; × 100.

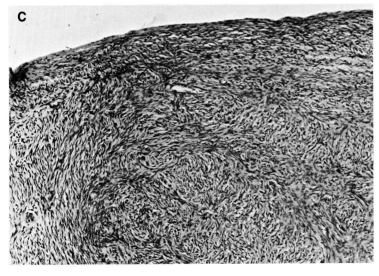

C Postmenopausal ovary. There is virtual absence of germ cells with only dense fibrous tissue. H&E; × 100.

Fig. 2–7. A Section of a postmenopausal ovary showing the deep convolutions, which give rise to the cerebriform convulutions characteristic of postmenopausal ovaries. There are scattered corpora albicantia with preservation of the germinal epithelium in some of the clefts. H&E; × 40.

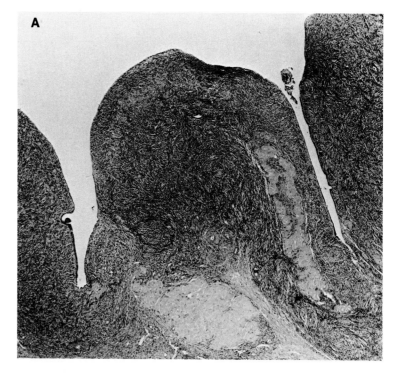

B Section of a postmenopausal ovary demonstrating a germinal inclusion cyst. The convolutions shown in **A** that retain the germinal epithelium can be covered and produce the inclusion cysts from the surface epithelium. H&E; × 100.

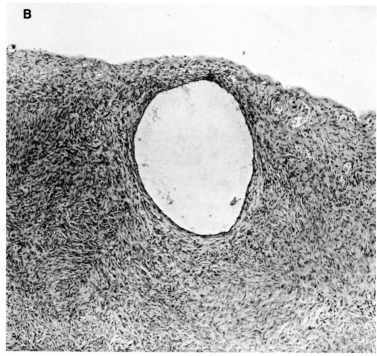

follicles and abundant germ cells (Fig. 2–6A). The number of germ cells is continually declining and, by the time of puberty, and throughout the reproductive years, there is a much more random and even distribution of the fol- licles (Fig. 2–6B). In the postmenopausal ovary, there is virtual absence of these struc- tures (Fig. 2–6C). The surface of the post- menopausal ovary now appears convoluted (Fig. 2–7A), giving rise to numerous inclu-

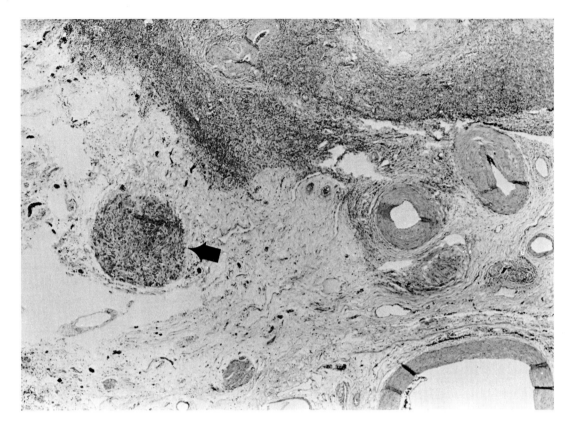

Fig. 2–8. Section of postmenopausal ovary near the hilum showing enlarged, thickened blood vessels and a prominent cluster of hilus cells (*arrow*). H&E; × 40.

sion cysts (Fig. 2–7B). These inclusion cysts may be the precursors of cystadenomas of the ovary. The ovarian stroma becomes more fibrotic with only scattered scars of prior follicular activity evident. The hilum of the ovary shows thickened blood vessels with occasional prominent clusters of hilus cells (Fig. 2–8).

The Breast

The breast is a target organ for estrogen stimulation and serves as an indicator of estrogen activity at puberty. Tanner[19] has developed a grading system of breast response to estrogen stimulation. There is an increase in glandular, fibrous, and adipose tissue as well as development of the nipple and areola under the influence of estrogen. During pregnancy, there is marked stimulation of the lobules (Fig. 2–9A) with secretion, with subsequent postpartum involution. During the menopause, and in the postmenopausal years, the breasts become atrophic with a reduction in the amount of adipose tissue and lobules, with replacement by fibrous tissue (Fig. 2–9B). The skin of the breast does not atrophy in unison with the underlying tissue and the breasts develop a flattened appearance. Diseases of the breast in the postmenopausal female are discussed in Chapter 13.

Nonreproductive Organs

SKIN. Reference has been made both to the vulva and the breast regarding skin changes in the menopause. The remainder of the body also shows changes related to estrogen deprivation. Receptors for estrogen function have been identified in skin.[20] Pigmentation and hypopigmentation are not uncommon findings in aging patients and may relate to hormonal deprivation. Pigmented areas commonly re-

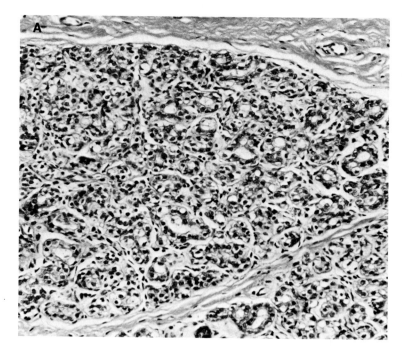

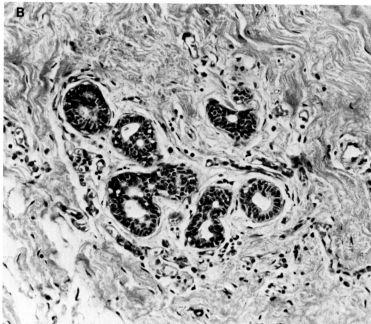

Fig. 2–9. A Breast tissue from 20-year-old pregnant woman. There is significant hyperplasia of the lobules, yielding dense, closely packed structures surrounded by thin fibrous strands. H&E; × 200. **B** Tissue from the breast of a postmenopausal patient showing a residual lobule containing predominantly ductular structures and surrounding fibrosis. H&E; × 200.

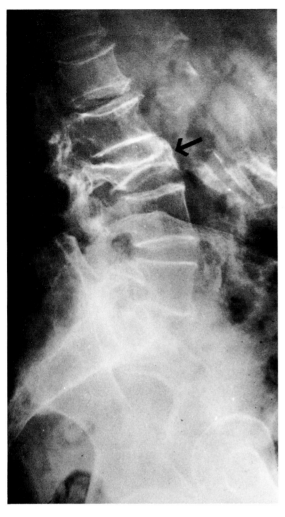

Fig. 2–10. A radiograph of the lumbar vertebrae in a post-menopausal patient showing a compression fracture due to osteoporosis (*arrow*).

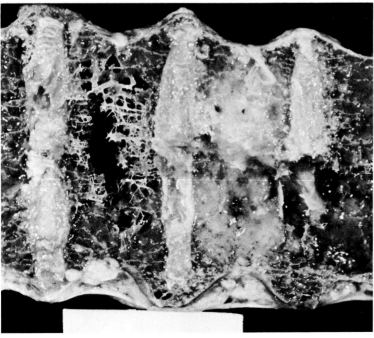

Fig. 2–11. A gross photograph of the vertebral column in a patient with extensive osteoporosis. Note the thin, "moth-eaten" appearance of the bone trabeculae.

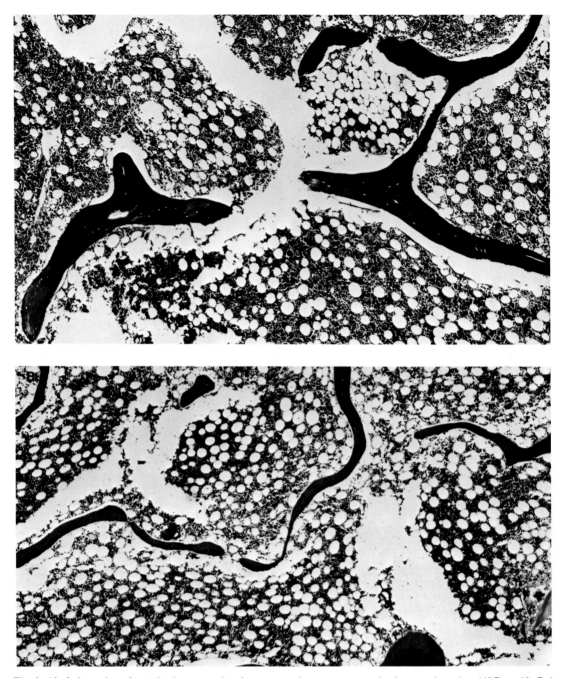

Fig. 2–12. A A section of vertebral marrow showing a normal appearance to the bone trabeculae. H&E; × 40. **B** A section of vertebral marrow from a patient with osteoporosis. Note the hypoplastic, thin trabeculae as compared to the normal bone in **A**. H&E; × 40.

ferred to as "aging spots" are a form of senile lentigo with a benign proliferation of melanocytes. Vitiligo is due to a multifocal loss of pigmentation giving rise to pale "bleached" areas. Histologically they show an absence of melanocytes.

There is a decrease in sebaceous and sweat gland activity as well as atrophy and thinning of the overlying epidermis. This makes the skin more sensitive to temperature and humidity; there is also an increased sensitivity to trauma. The dermis becomes thinner with changes in the collagen, accounting for the loss of resilience and pliability of the skin. Loss of subcutaneous fat gives rise to the wrinkling of the skin associated with aging.

BLADDER AND URETHRA. The distal urethra is affected by similar atrophic changes to those of the vagina.[21] This can allow for irritation and trauma resulting in ascending infections. Relaxation of the pelvic floor and atrophy of the pelvic structures may also lead to problems with incontinence.

The transitional epithelium of the urinary bladder shows a similar response to estrogen as that of the vaginal epithelium.[22] In fact, there is a direct relation so that hormonal profiles can theoretically be determined for the bladder epithelium from the vaginal epithelium. The transitional epithelium in the postmenopausal patient will contain less glycogen and will have a more flattened appearance. Clinical problems related to the genitourinary tract are discussed in Chapter 9.

CARDIOVASCULAR SYSTEM. Changes within the cardiovascular system are extremely difficult to differentiate from the aging process, since arteriosclerosis continues in a linear fashion with age. The vessels of the genital structures, particularly the uterus and ovary, show hypertrophic changes, often with medial calcification. These changes may be the result of disuse atrophy and dystrophic changes. The incidence of coronary artery disease is lower in reproductive age females; however, the protective nature of estrogen still remains controversial.[23]

THE SKELETAL SYSTEM. One of the most pronounced effects of estrogen deprivation is upon the skeletal system, where osteoporosis may result. A common complication is a compression fracture in the vertebral column (Fig. 2–10). The easy friability is due to loss of the bone substance (Fig. 2–11) which histologically shows thin trabeculae (Fig. 2–12). Physiologic aspects are considered in detail in Chapter 4.

REFERENCES

1. Calkins E. Aging of cells and people. Clin Obstet Gynecol. 1981; 24:165–79.
2. Roth GS, Adelman RC. Age-related changes in hormone binding by target cells and tissues; possible role in altered adaptive responsiveness. Exp Geront. 1975: 10:1–11.
3. Talbert GB. Aging of the reproductive system. In: Finch CE, Hayflick L, eds. Handbook of the pathology of aging. New York: Van Nostrand Reinhold, 1977:318–56.
4. Kuppe G, Metzger H, Lugwig H. Aging and structural changes in female reproductive tract. In: Finch CE, Hayflick L, eds. Handbook of the pathology of aging. New York: Van Nostrand Reinhold, 1977:21–34.
5. Lang WR, Aponte GE. Gross and microscopic anatomy of the aged female reproductive organs. Clin Obstet Gynecol. 1967; 10:454–65.
6. Notelovitz M. Gynecologic problems of menopausal women: Part 1. Changes in genital tissue. Geriatrics. 1978, 33:24–30.
7. Krouse TB. Menopausal pathology. In: Eskin BA, ed. The menopause: Comprehensive management. New York: Masson, 1980:1–46.
8. Utian WH: Target tissue response to ovarian failure. In: Menopause in modern perspective: a guide to clinical practice. New York: Appelton-Century-Crofts, 1980.
9. Singer A. The uterine cervix from adolescence to the menopause. Br J Obstet Gynaecol. 1975; 82:81–99.
10. Tweeddale DN. Cytopathology of cervical squamous carcinoma in situ in postmenopausal women. Acta Cytol. 1970; 14:363–369.
11. Soriero AA. The aging uterus and fallopian tubes. In: Schneider EL, ed. The aging reproductive system. New York: Raven Press, 1978:85–126.
12. Woessner JF. Age-related changes of the human uterus and its connective tissue framework. J Gerontol. 1963; 18:220–26.
13. Tsibris JCM, Cazenave CR, Cantor B, et al. Distribution of cytoplasmic estrogen and progesterone receptors in human endometrium. Am J Obstet Gynecol. 1978; 132:449–54.
14. Hendrickson MR, Kempson RL. Surgical pathology of the uterine corpus. Philadelphia: Saunders, 1980.
15. Hendrickson MR, Kempson RL. Endometrial epithelial metaplasias: proliferations frequently misdiagnosed as adenocarcinoma. Am J Surg Pathol. 1980; 4:525–42.
16. Robertson DM, Landgren B-M. Oestradiol receptor levels in the human fallopian tube during the menstrual cycle and after menopause. J Steroid Biochem. 1975; 6:511–3.
17. Talbert GB. Effect of aging of the ovaries and female gametes on reproductive capacity. In: Schneider EL, ed. The aging reproductive system. New York: Raven Press, 1978: 59–83.

18. Chang RJ, Judd HL. The ovary after menopause. Clin Obstet Gynecol. 1981; 24:181–91.
19. Tanner JM. Growth and endocrinology of the adolescent. In: Gradner L, ed. Endocrine and genetic diseases of childhood. Philadelphia: Saunders, 1969:19.
20. Stumpf WE, Sar M, Joshi SG. Estrogen target cells in the skin. Experientia. 1974; 30:196–8.
21. Smith P. Age changes in the female urethra. Br J Urol. 1972; 44:667–76.
22. Youngblood VH, Tomlin EM, Williams JO, et al. Exfoliative cytology of the senile female urethra. J Urol. 1958; 79:110–4.
23. Benditt EP, Gown AM. Atheroma: the artery wall and the environment. In: Richter GW, Epstein MA, eds. International review of experimental pathology, Vol. 21. New York: Academic Press, 1980:55–118.

The Climacteric 3

Clare D. Edman

Until about 30 years ago, the climacteric was regarded as a state of undesirable physiologic changes from which menopausal women could not escape. They were often considered to be psychoneurotic whenever they complained of its annoying discomforts. That view was exemplified in *Diseases of Women,* written in 1850, in which the author stated that since women were "compelled to yield to the power of time, women now cease to exist . . . and henceforward live only for themselves. Their features are stamped with the impress of age, and their genital organs are sealed with the signet of sterility. . . . It is the dictate of prudence to avoid all such circumstances as might tend to awaken any erotic thoughts in the mind and reanimate a sentiment that ought to become extinct . . . to cause regret for charms, that are lost, and enjoyments that are ended forever."[1] Fortunately, such views have changed. Although the menopause is still considered to be primarily an aging event, it is now considered to be a normal, physiologic process rather than a pathologic condition or a disease resulting from defective ovarian function.

During the past 100 years, both the reproductive and total life span of women have increased gradually. Prior to the late nineteenth century, fewer than 30% of females reached the menopausal age of 51 years. Today, nearly 90% of women in the United States will experience menopause; almost 60% will live to age 75. In fact, recent census figures indicate that of the 113 million women living in the United States, nearly 40 million are over 50 years of age and have a life expectancy of 78 years. Thus, most women can expect to live a considerable portion of their lives in the postmenopausal years.

Although the length of the reproductive era is expanding, the average age of menopause, 50 to 51 years, has not changed since medieval times. The expanding reproductive years are due primarily to the earlier appearance of menarche which is correlated with a critical body weight and percentage of body fat. The critical body weight can be attributed to improved nutrition and general health as well as better socioeconomic conditions. The age of menopause does not appear to be related to the age of menarche, socioeconomic factors, race, parity, weight, or height. The only factor that may influence the earlier onset of menopause is cigarette smoking.[2]

Many authors have referred to the perimenopausal years, the menopause, and the postmenopausal years, collectively as the "climacteric." In this chapter, the term "menopause" refers to the last episode of menstrual bleeding and signifies the end of the reproductive era. The terms "climacteric" and "perimenopause" refer to the transitional period between the reproductive years and the actual menopause and "postmenopause" to that period starting 1 year after cessation of menstruation.

Endocrine Changes

During the reproductive years, two sources of estrogen production exist. The major source is the secretion of 17β-estradiol by granulosa cells of ovarian follicles. The second source involves extraglandular aromatization of plasma androstenedione (Fig. 3–1).

The endocrine changes associated with the female climacteric are due mainly to the loss of

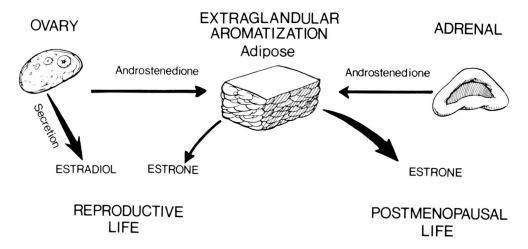

Fig. 3–1. Sources of estrogen during reproductive and postmenopausal life. Reproduced with permission from Carr BR, MacDonald PC. Estrogen treatment of postmenopausal women. In Stollerman GH, et al., eds. *Advances in internal medicine*, Vol. 28. Copyright © 1983 by Year Book Medical Publishers, Chicago: (in press).

cyclic secretion of 17β-estradiol. Cessation of 17β-estradiol secretion is attributed to loss of follicular granulosa cells and to a decreased responsiveness of these cells to follicle-stimulating hormone (FSH).[3] These alterations cause the menstrual cycle initially to shorten and then gradually to lengthen as anovulation occurs, and eventually to cease completely.

In postmenopausal women, estrogen production occurs almost exclusively by a mechanism known as "peripheral or extraglandular aromatization."[4] This mechanism utilizes circulating androstenedione, secreted primarily by the adrenals, and converts it to estrone in stromal tissue of fat, bone, muscle, hair, and brain. Little, if any, estrogen is derived from ovarian or adrenal secretion in menopausal women. In fact, plasma levels of estrogen do not change if the ovaries are removed after menopause. The estrogen production in postmenopausal women is characterized by the extraglandular formation of a biologically weaker estrogen, estrone, rather than by the ovarian secretion of the potent estrogen, 17β-estradiol.

Estrogen production in postmenopausal women is not a static process. Indeed, as described in Chapter 1, estrone production is increased significantly as the capacity of aromatase enzyme increases with aging, obesity, liver

disease, hyperthyroidism, compensated congestive heart failure, or starvation.[5] Estrone production also increases whenever the amount of circulating androstenedione increases, such as may occur with nonendocrine tumors of the ovary. Nonobese postmenopausal women produce about 40 μg of estrone per day. It should be noted that while estrogen production is decreased in most postmenopausal women, it may be equal to or greater in some obese postmenopausal women than that in premenopausal women. In fact, when the daily production rate of estrone exceeds 70–75 μg/day, uterine bleeding occurs in nearly all women (Fig. 3–2).[6] The preponderance of circulating estradiol found in postmenopausal women is derived from the peripheral conversion of estrone.[7]

In premenopausal women, androstenedione is derived from both ovaries and adrenals, but in postmenopausal women, androstenedione is derived almost exclusively from the adrenal cortex. Several investigators have found that androstenedione levels decrease by 45–50% after the menopause from levels of 1500 to 800–900 pg/ml, and remain constant even if ovaries are removed.[8] Circulating levels of the adrenal androgens, dehydroisoandrosterone and its sulfate (DS), decrease by 20–40% with age; by the seventh decade, mean concentra-

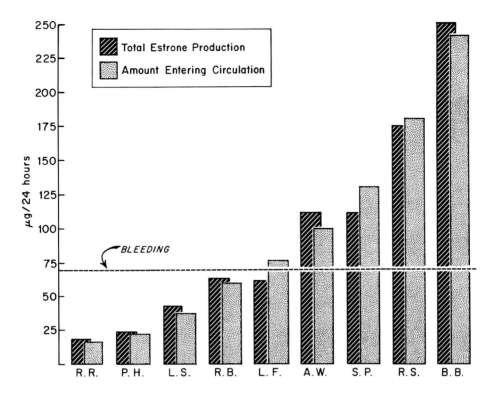

Fig. 3–2. Uterine bleeding in relationship to the total amount of estrone produced and the amount of estrone entering the circulation in postmenopausal women. From MacDonald PC, Grodin JM, Siiteri PK.[6]

tions are 1.8 and 300 ng/ml, respectively. DS levels often double during estrogen therapy after the menopause.[9]

Although the quantity of testosterone secreted by the menopausal ovary does not change from previous levels, testosterone becomes the principal steroidal hormone secreted by ovarian stroma. The growth of hair on the upper lip and chin of many elderly women may be due to diminished estrogen levels and unopposed action of testosterone in these women. Pubic, axillary, and scalp hair are partially lost; residual hair becomes coarser, mainly due to degeneration of skin and loss of skin appendages rather than to hormonal alterations. There is generalized thinning of the skin and wrinkling due to loss of elasticity and rete pegs.

In perimenopausal women, circulating levels of FSH rise gradually for several years before the actual menopause or menstrual irregularity occurs.[3] With the onset of menopause, serum levels of FSH may rise 20-fold to ranges of 75–200 mIU/ml, whereas levels of luteinizing

hormone (LH) only rise three- to fivefold to ranges of 60–90 mIU/ml.[10] The discordant rise in FSH is presumably due to a slower clearance of FSH from the circulation. These high circulating levels of FSH in menopausal women are due presumably to the loss of the negative feedback of 17β-estradiol at the hypothalamic-pituitary level. Some investigators find that plasma levels of gonadotropins are relatively constant after age 60,[11] whereas others find a persistent downward trend during the latter decades of life.[12]

The actual levels of FSH and LH oscillate at varying frequencies in postmenopausal women as in young women. These pulsating bursts occur every 1 to 2 h (similar to those seen in the follicular phase of ovulatory women); and although the frequency is similar, the amplitude is much greater. The increased amplitude is believed to be secondary to increased release of the hypothalamic hormone, gonadotropin-releasing hormone (GnRH). The finding of high urinary levels of GnRH in postmenopausal women is consistent with enhanced hypothalamic activity after ovarian failure.[13] Administration of GnRH to postemenopausal women results in a greater rise in LH than in FSH.[11]

Menopausal Symptoms

Several factors may influence the development of menopausal symptoms. An important factor appears to be the rate at which tissue levels of estrogen decline. A second factor involves the inherited or acquired propensity to withstand or succumb to the aging process. A third factor is the woman's ability to cope with major alterations in her interpersonal relationships, especially with family members. For example, severe emotional distress may occur with the loss of one or both parents, or children to college or marriage. She may have to cope with a husband who has become severely ill or who is seeking a younger mate. She is bombarded constantly by reminders that she is growing older in a youth-oriented culture. Her ability to cope with these stresses successfully will depend, in large part, upon her educational, socioeconomic, racial, and cultural background. The common menopausal complaints are listed in Table 3–1.

Vasomotor Symptoms

Vasomotor instability is characterized by a rise in skin temperature, peripheral vasodilation, a transient increase in heart rate, and changes in skin impedance.[14,15] The hot flush is described as a sudden onset of warmth in the face and neck that progresses to the chest. This sensation generally lasts several minutes and is often accompanied by a visible red flush. The hands become warm and the skin of the face and neck become moist. These episodes may last for several minutes, be exceedingly uncomfortable, and are frequently associated with dizziness, nausea, headaches, palpitations, diaphoresis, and "night sweats." These unpleasant symptoms can also be triggered by emotional stress, excitement, fear, or anxiety and disappear as quickly as they appeared.

It is estimated that 85% of peri- and postmenopausal women experience hot flushes. Eighty percent of women who experience hot flushes have symptoms for more than 1 year, but less than 25% have symptoms for more

TABLE 3–1. Frequency of Complaints in Menopausal Women, Ages 45–54 Years.

COMPLAINT	%
Irritability	92
Lethargy/Fatigue	88
Depression	78
Headaches	71
Hot flushes	68
Forgetfulness	64
Weight gain	61
Insomnia	51
Joint pain/backache	48
Palpitations	44
Crying spells	42
Constipation	37
Dysuria	20
Decreased libido	20

Data from Neugarten BL, Kraines RJ. "Menopausal symptoms" in women of various ages. Psychosom Med. 1965; 27:270.

than 5 years. In general, there is no correlation between the absolute levels of estrogen or gonadotropic concentrations and the occurrence of vasomotor symptoms. For example, women with gonadal dysgenesis have a hormonal milieu similar to that of postmenopausal women, but do not experience vasomotor flushes until after estrogen therapy has been given and discontinued. Flushes frequently occur during danazol administration or clomiphene citrate therapy (gonadotropin levels are low or normal—estrogen levels are low). Women may experience vasomotor flushing after hypophysectomy despite the disruption of the hypothalamic-pituitary axis and resultant low gonadotropins. Not all postmenopausal women experience vasomotor symptoms, perhaps because of alterations in metabolism of catecholamine or catecholestrogen within the brain or because extraglandular formation of estrone was sufficient in these women to suppress the symptoms. Thus, it appears that hot flushes are triggered by "estrogen withdrawal" rather than by a lack of estrogen. If hot flushes are left untreated, the hypothalamus and autonomic nervous system adjust gradually, and symptoms abate.

The mechanism(s) responsible for the vasomotor flush is unknown. Although the flush is synchronous with a pulsatile release of LH from the pituitary, LH levels per se do not activate the vasomotor centers. As was pointed out earlier, the hypothalamus is the likely site of origin of the vasomotor flush. It is known that the preoptic portion of the anterior hypothalamus contains both thermoregulatory centers and high concentrations of GnRH neurons.[16]

It has been suggested that alterations in the metabolism of catecholamines coupled with decreased estrogen production may result in menopausal symptoms.[17] Catecholamines, particularly dopamine and norepinephrine, act as neurotransmitters. These agents appear to serve a significant role in modulating mood, behavior, motor activity, and hypothalamic-pituitary function. The conversion of L-tyrosine to L-dopa by dopamine hydroxylase action decreases with aging; monoamine oxidase (MAO) and catechol-o-methyl transferase (COMT) activities increase, and neuronal uptake of catecholamines decreases, as a function of aging.[18] The concentrations of dopamine fall and norepinephrine increase in the hypothalamus following castration.[19] Moreover, the activity of tyrosine hydroxylase (the rate-limiting enzyme of catecholamine synthesis in the brain) and the turnover rate of norepinephrine increase in the hypothalamus following castration.[20] These changes are reversed by estrogen treatment. Taken together, these observations suggest that aging and decreased estrogen levels may alter dopamine-norepinephrine metabolism in the brain sufficiently to result in an instability of the autonomic nervous system.

Prostaglandins may also serve an important role in the pathogenesis of the menopausal syndrome.[21] These compounds are present in high concentrations in the hypothalamus and are known to act on smooth muscle of vessel walls. Since many cerebral vessels particularly those in the hypothalamus, are innervated by noradrenergic neurons, it is not unreasonable to speculate that stimulation of these neurons by either norepinephrine or prostaglandin could produce central vasospasm and result in nervousness, anxiety, irritability, depression, and loss of memory.[22]

Urogenital Atrophy

During the reproductive years, maturation of the vaginal epithelium follows the hormonal patterns of the ovarian cycle. The production of glycogen-rich superficial cells supports the presence of Döderlein's bacilli and maintains the vaginal pH between 4.0 and 5.5. As ovarian function begins to wane, this maturational process is lost, Döderlein's bacilli are lost, and the vaginal pH increases to a range between 6.0 and 8.0. These changes lead to a higher incidence of vaginitis.

Atrophy of the vaginal epithelium ultimately results in senile vaginitis with symptoms of irritation, burning, pruritis, leukorrhea, dyspareunia, and occasionally vaginal bleeding. The loss of the vaginal epithelium correlates with the extent of estrogen deprivation and tends to worsen with time. The loss of vaginal rugae and reduction of lubrication during intercourse are due mainly to a decrease in vaginal fluids, blood flow, and glycogen production. The atrophic vagina is easily traumatized; loss of elasticity results in a decrease in depth and diameter of the vagina. Maintenance of sexual intercourse at regular intervals during climacteric and postmenopausal years may slow these changes and delay development of vaginal and introital constrictions and dyspareunia. Atrophic vaginitis accounts for approximately 15% of cases of postmenopausal bleeding.[23]

In general, atrophy of the urethra parallels similar changes in the vagina since these tissues are derived from a common embryonic anlage. The urethra and trigone areas of the bladder are rich in estrogen receptors and, therefore, are responsive to estrogen. Atrophy of these structures may result in complaints of dysuria, urinary frequency, and cystitis with sterile urine cultures. Urethral caruncles and noninflammatory urethritis are common findings in elderly postmenopausal women.

The vulvar epithelium also becomes thin and often irritated as aging advances. Vulvar dystrophies are common in menopausal women, but there are insufficient data to implicate estrogen deprivation as the primary cause of these disorders. For example, the loss of subcutaneous fat and elasticity after the menopause is not responsive to estrogen therapy.

The relationship between estrogen deprivation and pelvic relaxation is poorly defined. Although it is true that the degree of pelvic relaxation may be age-related and due to a loss of tissue elasticity and a slowing of cell division and repair, clinicians have found that pelvic relaxation correlates more closely with parity, birth trauma, racial background, obesity, constipation, and chronic lung disease than with estrogen deprivation. The incidence of stress-related urinary incontinence in postmenopausal women (15%) is similar to that in premenopausal women.[24]

Psychiatric Symptoms

Although the menopause was considered previously to be synonymous with psychoneurotic disorders, there is little evidence now to support this concept.[25] Most investigators have not found an increased incidence of depression during the menopause. There does appear to be an increase in paranoid psychoses in postmenopausal women which is not hormone-dependent. It is often difficult to ascertain which symptoms are due to hormonal changes and which are due to the normal aging process or to psychologic readjustments that are normally required at this time of life. The female climacteric may be quite stressful. Many menopausal women experience *nervousness* (easy excitability, mental and physical unrest), *anxiety* (feelings of apprehension, uncertainty, fear, and loss of self-image), *irritability* (uncontrollable crying, frequent rage or anger), and *depression* (inability to make decisions, apathy, psychomotor retardation, loss of libido, or loss of emotional reaction). Most investigators agree that depression is not hormone-dependent.[26] The diagnosis of "involutional melancholia," previously used to describe menopausal depression, has been deleted from the list of acceptable diagnostic codes.

The menopausal headache may have many causes, most of which do not relate to estrogen deprivation.[27] Hormonal therapy is frequently associated with headaches in premenopausal women. Estrogen therapy may improve headaches in some individuals, but does not relieve headaches predictably in most menopausal women.

Estrogen therapy does alter rapid eye movement (REM) sleep and the number of waking episodes associated with hot flushes in symptomatic menopausal women.[28] In one study, estrogen therapy resulted in restful sleep and less irritability, anxiety, and fatigue.[29] However, when these observations were reexamined using double-blind crossover studies, there was no significant difference between the effectiveness of estrogen or placebo in relieving insomnia, depression or headaches.[30,31]

Musculoskeletal Symptoms

Osteoporosis may produce a variety of musculoskeletal complaints in menopausal women, especially low back pain. In this disorder, the mineral-to-matrix ratio of bone is normal, but total bone mass is reduced. Normally, the amount of new bone formed is equal to or greater than that resorbed. In osteoporosis, bone resorption is greater than bone formation and affects trabecular bone more severely than cortical bone before age 60. After age 60, loss of trabecular bone appears to be self-limiting, but loss of cortical bone continues until death.

Loss of bone density is a serious consequence of the aging process—not because of the net loss of bone structure per se, but because bone fractures resulting from osteoporosis are associated with increased morbidity and mortality.[30] The maximum density of bone is reached between the ages of 25 and 36 years. By age 45 to 50, the rate of bone resorption is greater in women than in men and more prevalent in Caucasians than in blacks. A common site of fracture in young postmenopausal women is the vertebral body; it is estimated that by age 60, 25% of all white women have compression fractures of the spinal column, commonly in the lumbar area. By age 75, 50% of women will suffer vertebral fractures.

Although demineralization of the bony skeleton occurs in central bones earlier than in peripheral bones, it will ultimately affect the entire skeleton. Fractures in the distal forearm increase so dramatically in women that by age 60, the incidence of forearm fractures is ten times higher than in men of comparable age.[32] Moreover, the incidence of fractures of the proximal femur doubles every 10 years in women over the age of 60 (Fig. 3–3). In 1979, it was estimated that 125,000 hip fractures occurred in elderly American women. Fifteen percent of these women died of complications resulting from the fractures. The medical cost of treating fractures is currently exceeding $2 billion annually.[33]

Although Albright and colleagues are credited with recognizing an association between estrogen deprivation and progressive loss of bone mass in 1940,[34] the role of estrogen in the pathogenesis of postmenopausal osteoporosis is still unclear and thus controversial. The dy-

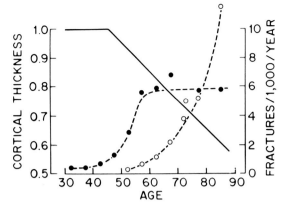

Fig. 3–3. Decrease in thickness of metacarpal bone (—) and frequency of fractures of the forearm (● ●) and femur (○ ○) as a function of age in women. From Worley RJ. Age, estrogen, and bone density. Clin Obstet Gynecol. 1981; 24(1):204. Data adapted from Morgan B. Osteomalacia, renal osteodystrophy and osteoporosis. Springfield, Ill.: Thomas, 1973.

namic equilibrium between the rate of bone formation and resorption is complex and involves a sensitive relationship between dietary calcium intake and absorption, serum concentrations of calcium and phosphorus, and secretion of parathyroid hormone (PTH), calcitonin, and 1,25-dihydroxy-vitamin D. There are no specific estrogen receptors in bone, and estrogen per se does not stimulate osteoblastic activity. However, estrogen therapy does reduce urinary calcium excretion, presumably by increasing calcium absorption in the renal tubules. Estrogen appears to inhibit bone resorption, perhaps by diminishing the response of bone to circulating parathyroid hormones or by altering PTH levels directly. The plasma calcitonin level decreases progressively with age and more so in women than in men of similar age.[35] Since calcitonin is known to inhibit bone resorption, the progressive loss of calcitonin may contribute to the accelerated bone loss of aging women.

Although considerable evidence has accrued which lends credibility to the existence of a causal relationship between estrogen deprivation and osteoporosis, the issue of whether estrogen deprivation is the primary cause of osteoporosis has not been resolved. Those investigators who favor this view cite evidence that the rate of bone loss accelerates alarmingly after cessation of ovarian function. In general, bone loss in white menopausal women is 1–2%

per year after age 50 and results in a 30–60% reduction in bone mass by age 80.[36] Moreover, in estrogen-deficient young *premenopausal* women (those with gonadal dysgenesis or who were castrated early in life), bone loss is accelerated but corresponds more to the time of ovarian loss rather than to chronologic age. Furthermore, women who are menstruating after age 50 have a slower rate of bone loss than do menopausal women of similar age. On the other hand, those investigators who disagree with the concept that estrogen deficiency is a principal cause of osteoporosis cite the fact that loss of bone mass begins normally during the fourth decade of life, i.e., prior to menopause. The rate of osteoporosis actually declines with advancing age and is greatest during the first 5 years after menopause. Young persons who are hospitalized or immobilized for prolonged periods of time lose bone mass and develop bone fragility and fractures at a rate similar to that seen in older postmenopausal women. Moreover, there are no differences in plasma levels of estrogen in postmenopausal women with osteoporotic fractures and in age-matched women without fractures. Thus, it would seem that many factors influence the rate of bone resorption in menopausal women[37] (Table 3–2); therefore, to select one variable as the controlling factor of the osteoporotic process is probably fortuitous.

Several investigators have proposed that estrogen deficiency impairs adaptation to low calcium diets by increasing bone sensitivity to

TABLE 3–2. Factors Associated with Increased Bone Resorption in Menopausal Women

Aging
Alcohol consumption
Cigarette smoking
Decreased physical activity
Diet (insufficient calcium and vitamin D intake)
Elevated fasting urinary calcium/creatinine ratio
Elevated fasting urinary hydroxyproline/creatine ratio
  (over 0.012)
Elevated plasma levels of parathyroid hormone
Genetic variables
  Low bone mass
  Race (Oriental or Caucasian)
Low plasma calcitonin levels
Low estrogen/progesterone status
Malabsorption of calcium

Modified from data presented in Upton GV.[37]

parathyroid hormone.[36] If true, it is not surprising that urinary hydroxyproline/creatinine values are high in postmenopausal women with confirmed osteoporosis. Estrogen does increase intestinal absorption of calcium and the circulating levels of 1,25-dihydroxy vitamin D and slows the rate of bone resorption, thus reducing hydroxyproline excretion.[38]

The problem for most physicians is how to identify individuals at high risk of developing osteoporosis (e.g., low hormonal status, deficient calcium intake, and so on), so that therapy can be initiated before extensive bone loss occurs. Unfortunately, most studies do not provide useful information to the physician since they describe, rather than predict, rapid bone turnover. Most of the tests currently available to assess bone mass are too sophisticated for routine monitoring; therefore, many clinicians generally use risk factors outlined in Table 3–2 to decide whether to initiate therapy. (Therapy is discussed in Chapter 6.)

Atherosclerosis

Several epidemiologic studies have demonstrated that the incidence of coronary heart disease (CHD) and hypertension increases steadily in women after age 50.[39–42] In the Framingham study,[39] the incidence of death from CHD was 2.4 times greater in postmenopausal women, aged 45 to 54 years, than in premenopausal women. In fact, there were no CHD deaths among the premenopausal women in that population during the observation period. Since death from CHD is rare in premenopausal women and relatively high in men less than 50 years of age, it was assumed that estrogens protect premenopausal women from the risks of arteriosclerotic cardiovascular heart disease (ASCVD). The incidence of ASCVD appears to increase disproportionately in women following the menopause because the ratio of male/female deaths from CHD decreases progressively from an 8 : 1 ratio at age 45 to 1 : 1 at age 85. However, that shift in age-related deaths from CHD between the sexes is not due to a rapid acceleration of CHD deaths in women after the menopause, but rather to a decreased acceleration in the CHD mortality rate in men as age advances. The latter observation may be due to the high incidence of early deaths in males who are predisposed genetically to fatal CHD.

It appears that factors other than the decline of estrogen levels at the menopause may be responsible for the progressive increase in ASCVD deaths in postmenopausal women. For example, during the 1950s, while the ratio of male/female deaths from CHD was observed to be 5 : 1 in the United States, it was 2 : 1 in Italy and 1 : 1 in Japan in individuals 45 to 54 years of age. These observations suggest that factors such as diet, smoking, hypertension, and diabetes may have a major impact on the incidence rate of coronary deaths, especially since the sex ratio among blacks in the United States was much lower than among whites. Moreover, when hypertension or diabetes were present, the sex ratio was narrowed to 2 : 1 among whites and was similar (1 : 1) among blacks regardless of age.

Advanced atherosclerosis was prevalent in more autopsy studies of oophorectomized women not treated with estrogen than in estrogen-treated subjects. It was commonly believed that the incidence of angina and CHD was higher in oophorectomized than in non-oophorectomized women as the consequence of estrogen deprivation. These studies all had major deficiencies which cast considerable doubt upon the validity of the conclusions.[30,31] For example, none of the studies had adequate controls. There was no attempt to correct for known risk factors associated with CHD deaths or to define the criteria used to determine the association between CHD and estrogen deprivation. When carefully controlled studies were reviewed, it was concluded that estrogen treatment does not provide protection against the development of ischemic CHD in postmenopausal women, castrated premenopausal women, or premenopausal women taking oral contraceptives.[40–42] Moreover, several investigators have found that low-dose estrogen treatment neither causes nor provides protection from cerebrovascular disease in postmenopausal women.[43] The recent use of estrogen/progestin combination therapy in postmenopausal women to prevent endometrial neoplasia rekindles the issue of increased risk of cardiovascular complications, particularly myocardial infarction and thromboembolic problems, in menopausal women. From previous experience with oral contraceptives, it

TABLE 3–3. Lipoprotein Profiles in an Adult Population. Ages 50–59 Years.

SEX	TAKING HORMONES	HDL	LDL (μg/dl)	VLDL
Women	No	14	20	61
Women	Yes	20	24	90
Men	No	12	22	85

From Wahl PW, et al.[44]

is well known that the risk of these complications increases markedly after age 35 in women who smoke, are obese, and/or are hypertensive.

Atherosclerosis appears to be associated, in part, with particular types of plasma lipoproteins. High-density lipoproteins (HDL) contain predominantly phospholipids, low-density lipoproteins (LDL) contain predominantly esterified cholesterol, and very-low-density lipoproteins (VLDL) contain predominantly triglycerides. The LDL and VLDL fractions are associated with a high incidence of ASCVD, whereas HDL-cholesterol appears to offer some protection against the development of atherosclerosis.

Postmenopausal women have increased plasma levels of all lipoprotein fractions, especially LDL, which may account, in part, for the high incidence of CHD following the menopause (Table 3–3). Although there is a gradual rise in HDL-cholesterol levels in women until about age 60, there is a moderate increase in LDL levels about age 40 (Table 3–4).[44] Krauss[45] presented evidence that the elevated HDL-cholesterol levels may be associated with the high gonadotropin levels of postmenopausal women.

Unfortunately, although estrogen therapy

TABLE 3–4. Effect of Estrogen on Low-density Lipoprotein as a Function of Age in Women.

AGE	LCL (mg/dl) No Estrogen	Estrogen
20–29	15	24
30–39	15	27
40–49	20	26
50–59	20	24

From Wahl PW, et al.[44]

increases HDL-cholesterol in menopausal women, it also increases LDL and VLDL plasma concentrations, both of which are associated with CHD (Table 3–3). The HDL_2 fraction, which is specifically elevated during estrogen therapy, is associated with a reduced risk of ASCVD. The HDL (phospholipids) and VLDL (triglycerides) levels increase during estrogen therapy and become constant, but levels of LDL (esterified cholesterol) may be quite variable. For instance, 50 μg of ethinyl estradiol increases HDL, LDL, and VLDL fractions, whereas 20 μg of the same estrogen increases HDL and VLDL fractions but not the LDL fraction. Moreover, when a progestogen is added with the estrogen, an atherogenic pattern results, i.e., increased LDL, decreased HDL, and a marked increase in cholesterol esters. It now appears that certain combinations of estrogen/progestins may potentiate cardiovascular risks in postmenopausal women.[46] Presently, there is no direct evidence that estrogen induces any specific changes in lipoprotein patterns which attenuate atherosclerosis. Thus, it would appear that the decreased production of estrogen in menopausal women does not affect the development of ASCVD significantly nor does estrogen therapy reduce the incidence of CHD in postmenopausal women.

REFERENCES

1. Utian WH. Scientific basis for post-menopausal estrogen therapy: the management of specific symptoms and the rationale for long-term replacement. In: Beard RJ, ed. The menopause, a guide to current research and practice. Baltimore: University Park Press, 1976:175–201.
2. Frie JF. Aging, natural death, and the compression of morbidity. N Engl J Med. 1980; 303:130–135.
3. Sherman BM, West JH, Korenman SG. The menopausal transition: analysis of LH, FSH, estradiol, and progesterone concentrations during menstrual cycles of older women. J Clin Endocrinol Metab. 1976; 42:629–636.
4. Grodin JM, Siiteri PK, MacDonald PC. Source of estrogen production in postmenopausal women. J Clin Endocrinol Metab. 1973; 36:207–214.
5. Siiteri PK, MacDonald PC. Role of extraglandular estrogen in human endocrinology. In: Greep R, Astwood E, eds. Handbook of physi-

ology. Endocrinology, Vol. 2, Part 1. Washington, DC: American Physiological Society, 1973:615–629.

6. MacDonald PC, Grodin JM, Siiteri PK. The utilization of plasma androstenedione for estrone production in women. In: Progress in endocrinology. Proceedings of the Third International Congress of Endocrinology. Amsterdam Excerpta Medica Int Cong Series 184. 1969:770–776.

7. Judd HL, Shamonki JM, Furmar AM, et al. Origin of serum estradiol in postmenopausal women. Obstet Gynecol. 1982; 59:680–686.

8. Chang RJ, Judd HL. The ovary after menopause. Clin Obstet Gynecol. 1981; 24:181–191.

9. Abraham GE, Maroulis GB. Effect of exogenous estrogen on serum pregnenolone, cortisol, and androgens in postmenopausal women. Obstet Gynecol. 1975; 45:271–274.

10. Wide L, Nillus JS, Gemzell C, et al. Radioimmunosorbent assay of follicle-stimulating hormone and luteinizing hormone in serum and urine from men and women. Acta Endocrinol (Kbh). 1973; 174(suppl):7–58.

11. Scaglin HM, Medina M, Pinto-Ferreira AL, et al. Pituitary LH and FSH secretion and responsiveness in women of old age. Acta Endocrinol (Kbh). 1976; 81:673–679.

12. Chakravarti S, Collins WP, Forecast JD, et al. Hormonal profiles after the menopause. Br Med J. 1976; 2:784–787.

13. Bourguigamon J, Hoyoux C, Reuten A, et al. Urinary excretion of immunoreactive luteinizing hormone-releasing hormone-like material and gonadotropins at different stages of life. J Clin Endocrinol Metab. 1979; 48:78–84.

14. Tataryn IV, Meldrum DR, Lu KH, et al. LH, FSH, and skin temperature during the menopausal hot flush. J Clin Endocrinol Metab. 1979; 49:152–154.

15. Meldrum DR, Shamonki IM, Frumar M, et al. Elevations of skin temperature of the finger as an objective index of postmenopausal hot flashes: standardization of the technique. Am J Obstet Gynecol. 1979; 135:713–717.

16. Casper RF, Yen SSC, Wilkes MM. Menopausal flushes: a neuroendocrine link with pulsatile luteinizing hormone secretion. Science. 1979; 205:823–825.

17. Axelrod J. Relationship between catecholamines and other hormones. Recent Prog Horm Res. 1975; 31:1–50.

18. Yen SSC. The biology of menopause. J Reprod Med. 1977; 18:287–296.

19. Donoso AL, Stefano IJE, Biscardi AM, et al. Effects of castration on hypothalamic catecholamines. Am J Physiol. 1967; 212:737–739.

20. Fuxe K, Hochfelt T, Nilsson O. Castration, sex hormones, and tuberoinfundibular dopamine neurons. Neuroendocrinology. 1969; 5:107–120.

21. Brody MJ, Kadowitz PJ. Prostaglandins as modulators of the autonomic nervous system. Fed Proc. 1974; 33:48–60.

22. Finch CE. Neuroendocrinology of aging: a view of an emerging area. Biol Sci. 1975; 25:645–647.

23. Notelovitz M. Gynecologic problems of menopausal women. Part 3. Changes in extragenital tissues and sexuality. Geriatrics. 1978; 33:51–58.

24. Hammond CB, Maxson WS. Current studies of estrogen therapy for the menopause. Fertil Steril. 1982; 37:5–25.

25. Diagnostic and Statistical Manual of Mental Disorders, 2nd ed. Washington, DC: American Psychiatric Association, 1968:36.

26. Winokur G. Depression in the menopause. Am J Psychiatry. 1973; 130:92–93.

27. Dennenstein L, Laby B, Burrows GD, et al. Headaches and sex hormone therapy. Headache. 1978; 18:146–153.

28. Erlik T, Tataryn IV, Meldrum DR, et al. Association of waking episodes with menopausal hot flushes. JAMA. 1981; 245:1741–1744.

29. Thomson J, Oswald I. Effect of estrogen on sleep, mood, and anxiety of menopausal women. Br Med J. 1977; 2:1317–1319.

30. National Institutes of Health. Estrogen use and postmenopausal women: summary report. Washington, DC: US Government Printing Office, 1979.

31. Research on the menopause. WHO Techn Rep Ser 1981; 670:1–120.

32. Morgan B. Osteomalacia, renal osteodystrophy and osteoporosis. Springfield: Thomas, 1973:241–338.

33. Knowelden J, Buhr AJ, Dunbar O. Incidence of fractures in persons over 35 years of age. Br J Prev Soc Med. 1964; 18:130–141.

34. Albright F, Smith PH, Richardson HM. Postmenopausal osteoporosis: its clinical features. JAMA. 1941; 116:2465–2468.

35. Deftos LJ, Weisman MH, Williams GW, et al. Influence of age and sex on plasma calcitonin in human beings. N Engl J Med. 1980; 302:1351–1353.

36. Gallagher JC, Aaron J, Horsman A, et al. The crush fracture syndrome in postmenopausal women. Clin Endocrinol Metab. 1973; 2:293–298.

37. Upton GV. The perimenopause: physiologic correlates and clinical management. J Reprod Med. 1982; 27:1–28.

38. Gallagher JC, Riggs BL, DeLuca HF. Effect of estrogen on calcium absorption and serum vita-

min D metabolites in postmenopausal osteoporosis. J Clin Endocrinol Metab. 1980; 51:1359–1364.

39. Gordon, T, Kannell WB, Hjortland MC, et al. Menopausal and coronary artery disease: the Framingham study. Ann Int Med. 1978; 89:157–162.

40. Furman RH. Coronary heart disease and the menopause. In: Ryan KJ, Gibson DC, eds. Menopause and aging. Washington, DC: US Government Printing Office, 1971:39–55.

41. Pfeffer RI, Whipple GH, Kurosaki TT, et al. Coronary risk and estrogen use in postmenopausal women. Am J Epidemiol. 1978; 107:479–487.

42. Ross RK, Paganini-Hill A, Mack TM, et al. Menopausal estrogen therapy and protection from death from ischemic heart disease. Lancet. 1981; 1:858–860.

43. Shoemaker ESS, Forney JP, MacDonald, PC. Estrogen treatment of postmenopausal women. JAMA. 1977; 238:1524–1530.

44. Wahl PW, Warnick GR, Albers JJ, et al. Distribution of lipoproteins, triglycerides, and lipoprotein cholesterol in an adult population by age, sex, and hormone use. Atherosclerosis. 1981; 39:111–124.

45. Krauss RM. Regulation of high density lipoprotein levels. Med Clin North Am. 1982; 66:403–430.

46. Hirvonen E, Malkonen M, Manninen V. Effects of different progestogens on lipoproteins during postmenopausal replacement therapy. N Engl J Med. 1981; 304:560–563.

Postmenopausal Osteoporosis 4

Charles Y.C. Pak

Osteoporosis is a common skeletal disorder in the postmenopausal state. The primary abnormality is the reduced amount of bone mass (osteopenia) resulting from bone resorption which is proportionately greater than formation. The loss of bone affects bone mineral and matrix equally. The remaining bone is grossly normal. When the bone mass has decreased to a point where it is insufficient to maintain the normal structural integrity of the skeleton, fractures and skeletal symptoms appear. The term osteoporosis describes this disease state.

Osteoporosis arises from different pathogenetic mechanisms. Moreover, this form of bone disease differs clinically and pathogenetically from two other forms of metabolic bone disease, i.e., osteitis fibrosa and osteomalacia. It is clear that bone cell metabolism in bone remodeling units ultimately dictates events in the whole skeleton. This chapter will first review normal bone cell metabolism, and consider hormonal influences on that metabolism. The development of osteoporosis, as well as that of osteitis fibrosa and osteomalacia, will then be described from the perspective of disturbances in bone cell metabolism.

The remainder of the chapter will be devoted to the discussion of postmenopausal osteoporosis with respect to its unique pathogenetic mechanisms, clinical presentation, and management.

Normal Bone Cell Metabolism

Bone tissue may be depicted schematically as a block, composed of osteoid (nonmineralized matrix) and calcified bone (Fig. 4–1). It is a dynamic tissue undergoing continuous remodeling. The remodeling entails three processes: (1) *matrix* (collagen) *synthesis* by osteoblasts, (2) *mineralization* of collagen (or deposition principally of calcium phosphate) to form calcified bone, and (3) *bone resorption,* or destruction of calcified bone by osteoclasts. In its customary usage, bone formation refers to matrix synthesis. The formation of calcified bone is therefore the sum of bone formation and mineralization.

These processes occur principally at bone surfaces—*endosteal* surface covering trabecular (cancellous) bone, *periosteal* surface, and *Haversian* system within the cortical bone (Fig. 4–2).[1] Each surface, called cell envelope, is covered by mesenchymal cells, thought to be precursor cells for osteoclasts, osteoblasts, and osteocytes.

At the cellular level, bone undergoes continual breakdown and repair in discrete areas called "bone remodeling units" or basic multicellular units.[2] In periosteum and in trabecular bone, these units are spread out over the surface, and are supplied by blood from the periosteal and medullary vessels. In cortical bone, the remodeling units are parallel to the long

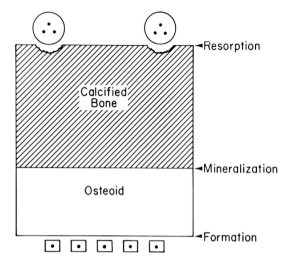

Fig. 4–1. A simplified diagram of bone depicting formation of osteoid by osteoblasts, mineralization of osteoid to form calcified bone, and resorption of calcified bone by osteoclasts.

axis of the Haversian system; they are supplied by Haversian vessels.

Each unit has areas of resorption and formation. The resorption is initiated by osteoblasts that resorb calcified bone, forming a cavity of about 50–250 μm in diameter. The osteoclasts in the areas of resorption are followed by osteoblasts which form osteoid. After the osteoid grows to a thickness of 10–15 μm, it becomes mineralized. Thus, the creation of a new basic multicellular unit, normally occurring over 4 months, is represented as follows:

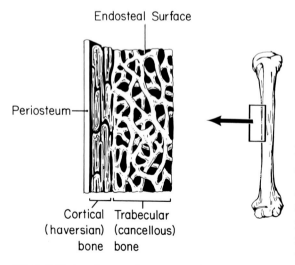

Fig. 4–2. Various bone surfaces or envelopes.

Appearance of   → Resorption →
osteoclasts

Appearance of   → Formation
osteoblasts

Central to the remodeling process is the concept of "coupling" between bone resorption and bone formation. To explain how osteoblastic matrix synthesis quickly follows osteoclastic resorption, Rasmussen and Bordier introduced the hypothesis of cellular continuity, where osteoclasts derive their origin from osteoprogenitor cells, and osteoblasts form by transformation of osteoclasts.[3] However, the validity of this hypothesis has been questioned by recent studies suggesting separate cellular origins for osteoclasts and osteoblasts, osteoclasts derived from monocytes and macrophages and osteoblasts from fibroblasts.[4]

There may be internal remodeling as well. After osteoblasts form collagen, they are incorporated into matrix and become osteoid osteocytes. These cells are believed to be responsible for the mineralization of the matrix by an elaboration of matrix vesicles.[5] When mineralization is completed, the cells become enclosed within calcified bone as mature osteocytes. These osteocytes are connected to each other and with surface osteocytes (cell envelope) by protoplasmic extensions passing through canaliculi (Fig. 4–3). This system, comprising the minicirculation of bone, provides a functional boundary between blood and bone. There is some evidence that mature osteocytes may participate in bone remodeling, being involved in "osteocytic osteolysis" which allows a rapid skeletal mobilization of calcium.

In Fig. 4–4, the functional roles of four principal cell types are schematically presented.[6] As previously described, osteoclasts resorb calcified bone and osteoblasts synthesize the matrix. Osteoid osteocytes, located over osteoid lamellae, may be responsible for the initiation of mineralization by elaborating membrane-bound extracellular matrix vesicles.[7] These vesicles are rich in alkaline phosphatase and are believed to be the initial site of mineralization. A sharp line of calcification separating the osteoid and calcified bone is called the mineralization front. Osteoid width represents the thickness of nonmineralized matrix. Osteocytes located in calcified bone may play a cru-

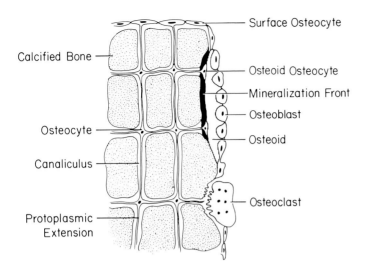

Fig. 4–3. Cellular processes in a bone remodeling unit. Osteoblasts elaborate matrix and eventually become enclosed in it to become osteoid osteocytes. Osteoid osteocytes initiate calcification and are transformed to osteocytes upon formation of calcified bone. Osteoclasts resorb calcified bone.

cial role in mediating rapid mobilization of calcium and phosphate into the circulation under appropriate stimuli.

Hormonal Influences on Bone Cell Metabolism

Certain substances influence bone cell metabolism, e.g., parathyroid hormone, estrogen, and vitamin D.

Parathyroid hormone (PTH) activates osteoclasts, augments the skeletal content of cyclic AMP, and promotes osteoclastic bone resorption (by probably increasing the number and activity of osteoclasts).[8] Whether PTH influences bone formation has not been fully deter-

mined, although there is some evidence that it may directly decrease osteoblastic activity.[9] Although a continuous administration of low doses of PTH has been shown to increase bone formation,[10] this action may represent an osteoblastic activation coupled to the primary osteoclastic stimulation. There is no evidence that PTH directly affects mineralization. The PTH excess may cause marrow fibrosis by fibrocytic proliferation.

Estrogen has been reported to inhibit PTH-induced bone resorption in vitro.[11] Although this observation is supported by extensive clinical data,[12–14] it was not confirmed in another in vitro study.[15] Estrogen has been shown to stimulate collagen synthesis in vitro.[16–19] However, there is limited substantive evidence that it

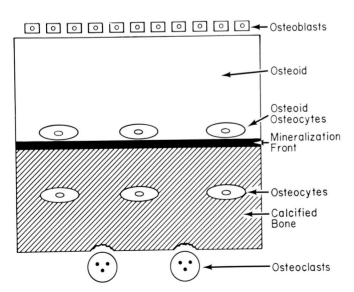

Fig. 4–4. A simplified diagram of cellular processes in bone.

augments bone formation clinically (in vivo). It probably exerts no direct effect on mineralization. Estrogen may be necessary for the maintenance of adequate osteoblast function.

The functional role of vitamin D in bone cell metabolism may be specific or unique for each vitamin D metabolite. Three active metabolites of vitamin D are 25-hydroxyvitamin D (25-OHD), 1,25-dihydroxyvitamin D (1,25-(OH)₂D), and 24,25-dihydroxyvitamin D (24,25-(OH)₂D). It is apparent that they differ with respect to biologic actions and effects on bone.

Effects of vitamin D metabolites on extraskeletal tissues will be considered first. In the kidney, 25-OHD has been shown to augment renal tubular reabsorption of Ca and P. The action of 1,25-$(OH)_2$D is much less prominent in this regard,[20] and that of 24,25-$(OH)_2$D is not known. The most potent metabolite with respect to the stimulation of intestinal Ca absorption is 1,25-$(OH)_2$D. However, both 25-OHD and 24,25-$(OH)_2$D[21] are capable of increasing Ca absorption. Vitamin D metabolites may also influence PTH secretion. Although accumulated data are conflicting, a recent study suggests that 24,25-$(OH)_2$D inhibits whereas 1,25-$(OH)_2$D may stimulate the release of PTH by parathyroid gland.[22]

In bone, 1,25-$(OH)_2$D is believed to stimulate the resorptive capacity of performed osteoclasts and potentiate the PTH-induced osteoclastic resorption.[6] It may be responsible for osteocytic osteolysis,[6] although such a role for osteocytes has been questioned. The 1,25-$(OH)_2$D alone is probably capable of promoting the formation of new osteoclasts. The action of 25-OHD in bone resorption is much less prominent whereas that of 24,25-$(OH)_2$D may be negligible.[23] However, 24,25-$(OH)_2$D may mainly account for the stimulation of osteoblastic matrix synthesis and mineralization.[6] Although 25-OHD may share this action with 24,25-$(OH)_2$D, it is not known whether 25-OHD itself, or its metabolic transformation, possibly to 24,25-$(OH)_2$D, accounts for the effects on bone formation and mineralization.[6]

Disturbed Bone Cell Metabolism in Metabolic Bone Diseases

The pathogenesis of metabolic bone diseases may be ascribed to disturbances in hormonal regulation of bone cell metabolism. As prescribed by the traditional view of metabolic bone diseases, PTH excess, vitamin D deficiency, or estrogen lack could lead to the development of osteitis fibrosa, osteomalacia, or osteoporosis, respectively.

The disturbances in bone cell metabolism found in the classic presentations of osteitis fibrosa, osteomalacia, and osteoporosis are compared in Fig. 4–5. They may reflect direct and indirect consequences of hormonal derangements discussed previously.

The PTH excess is characterized by a high turnover rate of bone (an increased number of active remodeling units). Osteoclastic resorp-

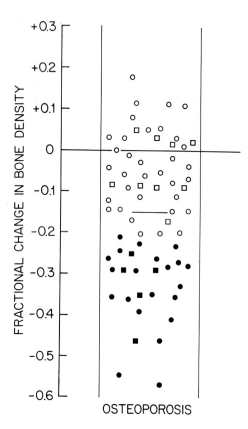

Fig. 4–5. Bone density (bone mineral/bone width) in the distal third of the radius determined by ¹²⁵I-photon absorptiometry in patients with osteoporosis. Values in patients are presented as the fractional change from control age- and sex-matched values. The mean fractional change of −0.152, indicated by the bar, was significantly different from the control mean by one-sample t-test ($p < 0.001$). Closed symbols indicate those patients whose values were below the lower limit of 95% prediction interval for control values. Squares represent male patients; circles represent female patients.

tion is primarily increased, but osteoblastic formation is also high (probably reflecting coupling). Thus, the percentage of bone surface showing either active resorption or formation is increased (high turnover). Since mineralization is not altered, the mineralization front and lag time are normal. Mineralization keeps pace with the accelerated matrix synthesis; the osteoid width is normal. Since bone formation generally lags behind resorption, the total amount of bone may become reduced. When PTH excess is marked, marrow fibrosis may develop (osteitis fibrosa). The hyperparathyroid state affects all three bone cell envelopes. Thus, subperiosteal resorption may develop, and the volume of cortical and trabecular bone is reduced, although the latter is less involved.

In osteomalacia of vitamin D deficiency,[1] bone matrix synthesis is impaired. Osteoblasts appear flat and show a histologic appearance which indicates reduced protein synthesis. The mineralization is even more markedly delayed. The lag time in mineralization (duration between matrix synthesis and mineral deposition) is considerably prolonged and the rate of mineral apposition is substantially reduced. Thus, the osteoid width and osteoid volume (indicative of nonmineralized matrix) are increased and the mineralization front is reduced. The resorption is only slightly increased; thus, the total volume of bone is normal, but the proportion of nonmineralized matrix is substantially elevated. Both cortical and trabecular bone are affected.

The deficiency of $1,25\text{-}(OH)_2D$ probably causes osteomalacia largely indirectly by reducing the availability of calcium and phosphorus at sites of bone formation, because of impaired intestinal calcium absorption and reduced skeletal calcium mobilization. The deficiency of $24,25\text{-}(OH)_2D$ may result in osteomalacia mainly because of the lack of direct action on matrix mineralization. Osteomalacia may result from 25-OHD deficiency via both factors enumerated above.

There is considerable histologic heterogeneity in osteoporosis. In one-third of patients, there is evidence for low remodeling, with normal resorption and apposition surfaces and low osteoblastic appositional rate.[24] The results are compatible with the suggestion of Albright and Reifenstein that the matrix synthesis is impaired because of estrogen lack.[25] In modern terms, the coupling of osteoblastic activity to osteoclastic resorption may be defective because of estrogen deficiency and presumed effect of aging.[26]

One-tenth of patients with osteoporosis exhibit high remodeling, with active remodeling surfaces.[24] Some of them have high serum PTH and urinary hydroxyproline. The results indicate a separate etiology for the osteoporosis. Despite increased remodeling activity, it is presumed that bone formation is inappropriately lower than resorption (indicative of defective coupling) in order for bone disease to have developed. The remainder of patients show no evidence of increased remodeling or defective osteoblastic apposition.

The endosteal cell envelope (trabecular bone) is particularly affected by the osteoblastic process.

Osteoporosis: General Considerations

DIFFERENTIATION FROM OSTEOMALACIA. The basic abnormality in osteomalacia is the defective matrix synthesis and impaired mineralization, whereas that in osteoporosis is the reduced bone mass resulting from an inappropriately elevated bone resorption. Clinically, symptoms of bone tenderness and muscle weakness are common in osteomalacia; they are encountered much more frequently than in osteoporosis. The tenderness of bone can best be elicited in the rib cage and iliac crest. The muscle weakness may be the result of an impaired synthesis of high energy phosphates associated with a defective phosphate transport.[27–30] Roentgenologically, pseudofracture is the hallmark of osteomalacia; it is not found in osteoporosis. Biochemically, severe hypophosphatemia is more typical for osteomalacia than osteoporosis. However, serum phosphorus may be elevated in osteomalacia of chronic renal failure and diphosphonate therapy. Serum alkaline phosphatase of skeletal origin is commonly elevated in osteomalacia, and infrequently high in osteoporosis.

CAUSES OF OSTEOPOROSIS. Different etiologies for osteoporosis are recognized (Table 4–1). They include various hormonal derangements, nutritional or gastrointestinal disturbances, immobilization, aging process, and

TABLE 4-1. Causes of Osteoporosis.

Hormonal
    Lack of estrogens or androgens
    PTH excess: primary or secondary
    Excess of adrenocorticosteroids
    Thyrotoxicosis
    Acromegaly
Nutritional or gastrointestinal
    Diet: low Ca, high P, high acid ash, malnutrition,
        alcohol abuse
    Gastrectomy, gastrojejunostomy, malabsorption,
        cirrhosis
Immobilization
Aging
Other
    Multiple myeloma
    Ehlers-Danlos syndrome
    Mastocytosis

miscellaneous causes. We shall consider here chiefly the most common cause—postmenopausal osteoporosis.

Postmenopausal Osteoporosis

GENERAL COMMENTS. Postmenopausal osteoporosis symptomatically affects 4 million women in the United States. It begins 4–5 years after menopause and increases in frequency thereafter. It is estimated that 25% of Caucasian women over 60 years of age suffer from osteoporosis. It is responsible for 700,000 new fractures yearly. The annual cost of hip fractures alone is approximately $1 billion.[32]

As discussed before, the primary abnormality is the reduced amount of bone mass (osteopenia), resulting from bone resorption which is proportionately greater than formation. When the bone mass has decreased to a point where it is insufficient to maintain structural integrity of the skeleton, fractures and skeletal symptoms develop. Trabecular bone is more severely affected than cortical bone. Thus, bones that are rich in trabecular bone and/or responsible for weight bearing are prime targets for fractures. Thus, common sites of fractures are the vertebrae, ribs, proximal femur, pelvis, and distal radius.

PATHOGENESIS. Since the original description of postmenopausal osteoporosis by Albright et al. in 1941,[31] little progress had been

made concerning the pathogenesis of this condition until the past decade. The recent application of more sophisticated techniques and approaches for the study of skeletal metabolism has disclosed a multifactorial etiology for this condition, including genetic, nutritional, and hormonal factors.

Genetic Factors. Genetic factors include presumed "senile atrophy" of bone cells,[32] involving particularly osteoblasts. The consequent impairment in osteoblastic matrix synthesis could lead to bone loss even in the absence of primary increase in bone resorption, and could explain defective coupling in the bone cell metabolism previously discussed.[26]

It has also been suggested that certain persons may be predisposed to develop postmenopausal osteoporosis because their total bone mass is reduced to begin with.[33] In such persons, the amount of bone loss that occurs normally with aging may be sufficient to cause bone disease. That the initial bone mass may be genetically determined[34] is supported by the finding of higher bone density in black women in whom osteoporosis is uncommon, and lower bone density in Asiatic women in whom osteoporosis is believed to be more prevalent.

Unlike the above view,[33,34] several reports suggest that bone loss in patients with osteoporosis is greater than in matched control subjects,[31,35,36] indicating an interplay of nongenetic factors. The disproportionately greater reduction in vertebral bone density than the decline in appendicular bone density supports this view.[37] The two models are not mutually exclusive, since both genetic and environmental factors are probably important pathogenetically.

Nutritional Factors. An important nutritional factor is the amount of calcium intake required to maintain balance. There is evidence that this requirement for calcium increases with advancing age.[39] This finding may reflect the continued decline in intestinal calcium absorption reported with aging,[38] and the apparent loss of intestinal adaptation to varying calcium intake in older women.[40] Calcium intake is lower in women than in men. Reduced calcium intake has been associated with a higher fracture rate.[41] Intestinal lactase deficiency has been reported to be more common in osteoporosis.[42] The consequent avoidance of calcium-rich dairy products has been implicated in the development of bone disease.

Other nutritional influences include protein intake and body weight. A high protein intake may provide an acid load and cause hypercalciuria and negative calcium balance.[43] Slenderness of many osteoporotic women may predispose them to bone disease.[44] Obese women have higher circulating estrogen levels,[45] greater bone mass,[46] and are less likely to develop symptomatic osteoporosis.

Hormonal Factors. There are several hormonal disturbances in postmenopausal osteoporosis which could profoundly influence bone cell metabolism. They include estrogen lack, as well as altered metabolism of PTH and vitamin D metabolites.

ESTROGEN LACK. This theory, which has been recently popularized by Riggs et al.,[32,40] considers that bone disease may be a direct consequence of estrogen lack ensuing from menopause. Both qualitative and quantitative changes in estrogen production ensue from menopause.[47–50] During the premenopausal state the predominant estrogen is estradiol secreted from the ovarian follicle. Presumed to be of less physiologic importance in the premenopausal years is estrone derived from "extraglandular" aromatization of adrenal androstenedione. During the postmenopausal state, estrogen production can be totally accounted for by estrone produced from circulating androstenedione; essentially no estradiol is secreted. Besides the qualitative difference in the type of estrogen produced, the total amount of estrogen produced is substantially reduced in the postmenopausal state.[47,50] Although the extent of conversion of estrone from androstenedione is increased twofold,[48] the total amount of estrogen produced in the postmenopausal state only approximates that of the extremes of the menstrual cycle of the premenopausal state, and is substantially lower than that of the late follicular and luteal phases of the menstrual cycle.[47,50] Serum concentrations of estrone and estradiol have been shown to be reduced in menopause.[51]

This theory assumes that estrogen plays a critical role in bone metabolism. There is considerable evidence which suggests that estrogen might modify the PTH-induced bone re-

sorption. The PTH-induced loss of bone, as measured from decreases in bone content of calcium and hydroxyproline, is accentuated by oophorectomy.[52] In postmenopausal women with hypoparathyroidism, the age-related loss of bone does not develop.[53] In our experience, the bone density, as measured by ^{125}I-photon absorption of the distal third of the radius,[54] is significantly reduced in the majority of white postmenopausal women with primary hyperthyroidism, unlike in male patients of comparable age with this condition.

When estrogens are given to patients with postmenopausal osteoporosis or primary hyperparathyroidism, the following changes are usually found:[55–61] retention of calcium and phosphorus; decreases in serum and urinary calcium and phosphorus, urinary hydroxyproline, fasting urinary calcium, and bone resorption (by histomorphometry); and an increase in serum immunoreactive PTH. Thus, despite stimulation of parathyroid function (presumably from the decline in serum calcium), bone resorption is inhibited. These findings support the concept that estrogens decrease the responsiveness of bone to endogenous PTH. Indeed, estrogen has been shown to inhibit the PTH-induced release of calcium from mouse calvaria in vitro,[11] although this action of estrogen has not been confirmed.[15] Thus, the development of bone disease in the postmenopausal state may be associated at least in part with the loss of the protective effect of estrogens against parathyroid hormone action.

Because of enhanced mobilization of calcium from bone, parathyroid function may be suppressed in postmenopausal osteoporosis. Reduced serum PTH has been reported in the majority of patients with this disease.[24,62] Further, since PTH may be involved in the mediation of 1,25-(OH)$_2$D synthesis,[63,64] a low serum concentration of 1,25-(OH)$_2$D might be expected, and could explain reduced intestinal calcium absorption found in some patients with postmenopausal osteoporosis.[40]

The following pathogenetic scheme may therefore be constructed (Fig. 4–6): estrogen lack → PTH-induced bone resorption → skeletal calcium mobilization → PTH secretion → 1,25-(OH)$_2$D synthesis → intestinal calcium absorption. Two other factors may contribute to impaired 1,25-(OH)$_2$D production during estrogen lack. Although controversial, estrogen

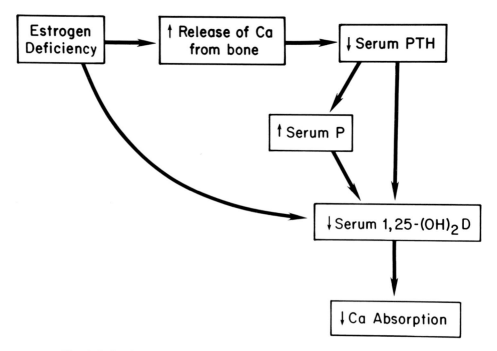

Fig. 4–6. A scheme for the development for low intestinal calcium absorption during estrogen deficiency.

is believed to stimulate renal 1α-hydroxylase activity.[65] Estrogen lack could then cause a reduced $1,25\text{-}(OH)_2D$ synthesis. Moreover, serum phosphorus may rise from an increased mobilization from bone and from reduced renal excretion of phosphorus (associated with parathyroid suppression). This rise may then inhibit $1,25\text{-}(OH)_2D$ synthesis.[66] The validity of this scheme has been supported by the findings of reduced circulating concentrations of PTH and $1,25\text{-}(OH)_2D$ and low intestinal calcium absorption.[40] Moreover, a short-term treatment with estrogen was found to restore these values toward normal.[14]

The pathogenetic role of estrogen lack in osteoporosis is further supported by the finding of accelerated bone loss with the onset of menopause.[67,68] Such a temporal relationship has been shown for "cortical" bone[37,54,68] as well as trabecular bone,[24] although a recent densitometric analysis of the axial skeleton has disclosed a linear decline in bone density occurring before menopause.[24]

Despite its attractiveness, the estrogen lack theory has certain drawbacks. First, although the increased sensitivity of bone to PTH could explain bone loss, it cannot adequately explain the defective coupling[26] and the frequent occurrence of low bone remodeling[24] previously

discussed. Thus, a disturbance in osteoblastic function from estrogen lack or aging is necessary. Secondly, despite a few reports to the contrary,[69,70] it has not been possible to document that the estrogen deficiency was more severe in patients with bone disease than in comparable women without bone disease.[35,51,71] Third, an impaired responsiveness of target tissues to estrogen action is unlikely, since the concentration of estrogen receptors in the cytosolic fraction of cervical tissue was not found to be different.[72] Finally, no estrogen receptors have been demonstrated in bone.[73]

PTH EXCESS. Serum PTH has been reported to be increased in a minority of patients with postmenopausal osteoporosis.[24,62] The low intestinal calcium absorption[38–40] and reduced calcium intake[74] probably contributed to secondary hyperparathyroidism. Our preliminary studies indicate that certain patients with postmenopausal osteoporosis may present with renal hypercalciuria (impaired renal tubular reabsorption of calcium) with secondary hyperparathyroidism. However, unlike patients with renal stones,[75] patients with osteoporosis suffering from renal hypercalciuria do not have a compensatory intestinal hyperabsorption of calcium.

The pathogenetic importance of PTH excess

in osteoporosis is shown by the failure of the development of immobilization osteoporosis in parathyroid deficiency,[76] lack of osteoporosis in hypoparathyroidism, and the frequent occurrence of osteoporosis in primary hyperparathyroidism.[77]

Although PTH excess could explain the development of high remodeling osteoporosis,[24] a recent study disclosed a poor correlation between serum PTH level and parameters of bone cell metabolism.[78]

VITAMIN D DEFICIENCY. Serum 1,25-$(OH)_2D$ has been shown to be reduced in osteoporosis.[40,79] Slovik et al. found that patients with postmenopausal osteoporosis had an impaired 1,25-$(OH)_2D$ synthesis following stimulation by exogenous PTH, compared to young (< 45 years) men and women.[80] However, Riggs et al. were unable to find any difference in the responsiveness of osteoporotic patients from that of postmenopausal control women matched for age.[81] Although our preliminary report had indicated the ability of patients with postmenopausal osteoporosis to increase serum 1,25-$(OH)_2D$ following 25-OHD therapy,[79] a further study disclosed failure of such a response in some patients. The role of estrogen lack in inhibiting 1,25-$(OH)_2D$ synthesis was previously discussed.[40] These results indicate that 1,25-$(OH)_2D$ synthesis is reduced in the postmenopausal state. Nevertheless, it has not been clearly demonstrated that this impairment is more severe in osteoporotic women than in postmenopausal women without bone disease.

Our preliminary study indicates that some patients with postmenopausal osteoporosis may have a reduced circulating concentration of 25-OHD and 24,25-$(OH)_2D$. However, another group found a high serum concentration of 25-OHD.[82]

Vitamin D deficiency probably contributes to the development of osteoporosis by impairing intestinal absorption of calcium and causing negative calcium balance. Whether it contributes to the defect in osteoblast function is not clearly known.

OTHER HORMONES. Low circulating concentration of calcitonin and reduced calcitonin response to calcium infusion have been reported in the postmenopausal state.[83] The defective response in serum calcitonin to calcium infusion was found to be more severe in osteoporotic women than in control subjects,[84]

although no difference in basal serum calcitonin level was detected.[85] That estrogen lack may contribute to calcitonin deficiency was shown by the ability of estrogen therapy to improve calcitonin response to calcium.[86]

Other hormonal factors implicated include growth hormone[87] and cortisol.[88] It is noteworthy that the bone histomorphometric picture in steroid excess resembles that of low remodeling osteoporosis.[24]

CLINICAL PRESENTATION. "Spontaneous" fractures, the hallmark of osteoporosis, represent fractures occurring from minimal trauma which could normally be sustained without incurring damage. Common sites of involvement are the vertebrae, ribs, proximal femur, and distal radius and ulna. Fractures may occur from a minor fall (from ground level) or bending to pick up an object.

Pain is the most common symptomatology of vertebral fracture. It is generally localized to the area of involvement, but may radiate laterally. It may be associated with paravertebral muscle spasm and localized tenderness. The severity and duration of pain vary considerably among patients. It may last for 1–2 months.

Skeletal deformity may develop from anterior wedging and collapse of vertebrae. "Dowager's hump" may occur from fractures of thoracic and lumbar vertebrae. Loss of height is common. Patients often complain of chronic back pain, occurring probably on a mechanical basis. When the spine becomes severely contracted by fractures, abdominal and pulmonary function may be embarrassed.

LABORATORY EXAMINATION. Serum concentrations of calcium, phosphorus, and alkaline phosphatase are normal in patients with postmenopausal osteoporosis. The serum concentration of PTH is usually normal, but it may be high in a minority of patients.[62] Serum 1,25-$(OH)_2D$ and intestinal calcium absorption are generally reduced. Urinary calcium is normal or low in most patients; it may be elevated in a minority of patients, particularly if they suffer from renal hypercalciuria.

Radiologically, early signs include loss of the trabecular pattern on vertebrae and the femoral neck. The trabecular bone which is not parallel to the line of weight bearing is lost first by the osteoporotic process; this accounts for the prominence of vertical striations in the vertebrae, and serves as the basis for the trabecular pattern index for staging of osteoporosis.[89] The cortical thickness of metacarpal bone or the radius may be reduced in osteoporosis.[90] In the long bones there is an accelerated bone loss endosteally with menopause; however, the bone continues to be deposited externally (periosteally) although at a slower rate. Thus, the total width of bone may be greater, but the cortical bone thickness may be less than in the premenopausal state. Other roentgenologic signs include prominence of vertebral endplates, Schmorl's nodes, vertebral collapse, fractures of rib and femoral neck, and kyphoscoliosis.

The skeletal roentgenologic examination is inadequate to measure the extent of bone loss in osteoporosis because up to 40% of bone mineral may be lost before it can be detected roentgenologically. A more sensitive measure of bone density may be obtained from photon absorptiometric analysis. Such an analysis of the shaft of the radius has revealed low bone density in some patients with osteoporosis[91] (Fig. 4–7). Measurement of bone density in the axial skeleton by dual photon absorptiometry may provide a better discrimination.[37]

Bone histologic examination has revealed morphologic heterogeneity, including low and high remodeling activity.[24,78] Unfortunately, the exact histomorphometric picture cannot be accurately predicted from biochemical presentation.[78]

THERAPEUTIC CONSIDERATIONS. In assessing any treatment, it is important to recognize that osteoporosis results from a long-term process. The illness is largely a manifestation of loss of bone mass which has occurred over many years, and not consequent to an acute derangement involving bone. An effective treatment, which averts the acute process, is not likely to produce an immediate clinical improvement. Even if it were capable of creating "new" bone, the treatment would probably have to be continued for several years before the total bone mass would be sufficiently increased to reduce the risk of fractures. There has been a prevailing view that once bone mass is reduced by an osteoporotic process, restoration is difficult. This concept is supported by the failure of most treatment programs to augment total bone mass, despite retardation of the rate of bone loss.

The ultimate goal of therapy is to augment mineralized bone volume, rather than simply to retard the rate of bone loss. To do so, it may be necessary to (1) increase bone turnover, thereby raising the number of active bone remodeling units; and (2) augment osteoblastic matrix synthesis, so that formation would outweigh resorption. This goal may have been partly achieved, since there is some evidence, albeit preliminary, that certain treatment programs may cause a small but significant increment in bone mass.

Available treatment measures may be categorized into those which arrest further bone loss and those which are designed to augment bone mass (Table 4–2).

Therapies Designed to Arrest Further Bone Loss. This treatment approach assumes that various identified physiologic-hormonal dis-

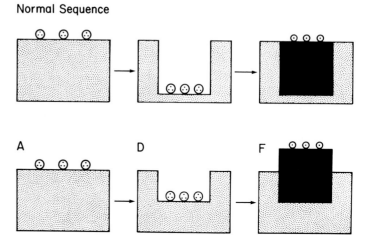

Fig. 4–7. Depiction of coherence treatment in an individual basic multicellular unit. Without ADFR sequence (*top*), the amount of bone destroyed (*top middle*) by osteoclasts is considered to be equal to the amount formed (*top right*) by osteoblasts. During depression phase (*D*) of coherence treatment (*bottom middle*), less bone is destroyed by osteoclasts than without depression (*top middle*). Thus, the total amount of bone left is larger following ADFR sequence than without ADFR (compare *bottom right* with *top right*), assuming an equal amount of new bone formation (*shaded areas*).

Normal Sequence

TABLE 4–2. Treatment Modalities for Osteoporosis.

Therapies designed to arrest further bone loss
  By inhibiting bone resorption
    Oral calcium
    Thiazide
    Calcitonin
    Vitamin D substances
  By stimulating bone formation
    Sex hormones
  Both
    Estrogens
Therapies designed to augment bone mass
  Stimulation of osteoblasts
    Fluoride
  Activation of osteoclasts
    PTH
    Coherence treatment

---

turbances are pathogenetically important in osteoporosis and that the correction of such abnormalities should be efficacious. Examples include oral calcium supplements for intestinal malabsorption and reduced dietary intake of calcium, thiazide for the excessive renal loss of calcium, calcitonin for this hormonal deficiency, vitamin D substances for vitamin D deficiency and the correction of PTH excess, and sex hormones for the defective synthesis of these steroids.

The principal effects of these agents on bone cell metabolism are inhibition of bone resorption, stimulation of bone formation, or both (Table 4–2). Since osteoclasts are not activated to form new bone remodeling units, the total mass of bone is not usually increased although its decline may be prevented.

ORAL CALCIUM. The rationale for oral calcium supplementation is to overcome inadequate calcium absorption resulting from low calcium intake and defective intestinal calcium transport. The total amount of calcium absorbed may be increased substantially by higher calcium intake (probably by the operation of passive absorption), even though the fractional calcium absorption remains subnormal.[92] By enhancing calcium absorption, oral calcium supplements may inhibit parathyroid function and thereby suppress PTH-dependent bone resorption. The rate of bone remodeling or the birth rate of new basic multicellular units is therefore reduced. Thus, this form of therapy may retard loss but is not expected to augment bone mass.

Available studies indicate that oral calcium supplements may improve calcium balance[39] and prevent further loss of bone.[36,93,94] Calcium supplements have been provided as calcium gluconate, calcium carbonate, or calcium lactate, at a dosage of 500–1500 mg calcium/day. A total calcium intake (supplemental and dietary) of 1.5 g/day is often recommended for patients with postmenopausal osteoporosis.

THIAZIDE. The use of thiazide in osteoporosis is based on the ability of this diuretic to reduce renal calcium excretion. This action has been ascribed to the direct stimulation of calcium reabsorption in the distal tubule,[95] and to the enhancement of proximal tubular reabsorption by causing extracellular volume depletion.[96]

In patients with renal hypercalciuria and nephrolithiasis, thiazide has been shown to correct the "renal leak" of calcium and restore normal parathyroid function. However, the state of calcium balance probably did not change since the ensuing suppression of 1,25-$(OH)_2D$ caused a decline in intestinal calcium absorption.[75] Thus, thiazide is expected to reduce bone resorption by inhibition of PTH secretion and thereby prevent further loss of bone. However, this effect is not likely to be sustained because of a compensatory fall in calcium absorption. It may be indicated in the minority of patients with postmenopausal osteoporosis presenting with renal hypercalciuria and secondary hyperparathyroidism. An adequate hypocalciuric response may be obtained with hydrochlorothiazide, 25–50 mg twice daily, or trichlormethiazide, 2–4 mg/day.

The suggested use of thiazide in osteoporosis would seem paradoxical and contraindicated, since thiazide has been believed to accentuate PTH-dependent bone resorption,[97] cause parathyroid glandular enlargement,[98] and induce or accentuate hypercalcemia in primary hyperparathyroidism[99] and secondary hyperparathyroidism of chronic renal failure.[100] However, the finding of parathyroid stimulation by thiazide in the dog could not be confirmed in the rat.[101] In patients with renal hypercalciuria and secondary hyperparathyroidism (and probably in normal subjects), thiazide suppresses parathyroid function via reduction of calcium excretion, and does not cause true hypercalcemia (reflected by increased ionized calcium).[102] Thiazide may potentiate osteocytic resorption.[103] This action could explain the development of true hypercalcemia during thiazide therapy of primary hyperparathyroidism and vitamin D-treated hypoparathyroidism, conditions in which osteocytic activity may already have been stimulated. There is no conclusive evidence that thiazide stimulates osteoclastic resorption. Thiazide has been shown to reduce hydroxyproline excretion[104] and V_{0-} (radiocalcium efflux from bone),[105] and to retard the decline in bone density (in primary hyperparathyroidism).[106]

The effect of long-term thiazide treatment in postmenopausal women was evaluated in a randomized controlled study.[107] Thiazide was shown to prevent a decline in bone density (of the midshaft of forearm bones) during the first 6 months of treatment. Thereafter, the bone density declined at the same rate as in the control group. The transient effect observed probably reflects the time required for the compensatory fall in intestinal calcium absorption to take place.

CALCITONIN. The rationale for the use of calcitonin is based on the finding that the secretory response of calcitonin to calcium infusion may be impaired in patients with postmenopausal osteoporosis[84] and on the knowledge that calcitonin is a well-recognized inhibitor of PTH-induced bone resorption.[108] Unfortunately, calcitonin given alone may cause secondary hyperparathyroidism by decreasing serum calcium concentration. The ensuing stimulation of PTH secretion may negate the inhibition of bone resorption by calcitonin.[109] Moreover, even if calcitonin inhibits bone resorption, this treatment probably will not increase the mass of bone because of the commensurate decline in bone formation.

The above view is supported by available studies which indicate variable effects of calcitonin therapy on bone resorption, formation, calcium balance, and total body calcium.[109,110] The concurrent administration of calcium averted the development of secondary hyperparathyroidism and caused a reduction in bone formation.[111] However, no increment in bone mass was found. Moreover, the effect of calcitonin and calcium was found to be qualitatively the same as that of calcium or calcium plus vitamin D.

VITAMIN D SUBSTANCES. The use of vitamin D substances in postmenopausal osteoporosis would seem logical because of evidence for vitamin D deficiency and low calcium absorption previously enumerated.[40,79] The treatment should increase intestinal calcium absorption, suppress PTH secretion, and inhibit bone resorption. Certain vitamin D metabolites (25-OHD and 24,25-$(OH)_2$D) may stimulate bone formation by affecting osteoblast function, as previously discussed. If 1,25-$(OH)_2$D is capable of activating osteoclasts, the birth rate of new bone remodeling units may be accelerated.

Treatment with vitamin D or 1,25-$(OH)_2$D in osteoporosis has been shown to lower serum PTH and bone resorption.[111–113] However, bone formation declined following vitamin D treatment, probably because of the coupling response to the decline in bone resorption.[112] During 1,25-$(OH)_2$D therapy no improvement in calcium balance occurred despite stimulation of calcium absorption, because of a rise in urinary calcium.[113] Moreover, 1,25-$(OH)_2$D treatment was ineffective in preventing the decline in bone density of appendicular bone occurring in patients with postmenopausal osteoporosis.[114] Similarly, long-term trials with vitamin D indicated no effect on bone loss or the occurrence of new fractures.[36,115]

Although 25-OHD is capable of stimulating the synthesis of 24,25-$(OH)_2$D and 1,25-$(OH)_2$D,[79] our preliminary study indicates that this treatment does not always stimulate intestinal calcium absorption in postmenopausal osteoporosis. As with 1,25-$(OH)_2$D therapy, increased calcium absorption is negated by the rise in urinary calcium excretion. It is noteworthy that the rise in urinary calcium occurring from vitamin D therapy is much more marked than that resulting from increased calcium intake (at comparable values of absorbed calcium),[116] a finding attesting to the direct skeletal action of vitamin D substances.

The above results indicate that vitamin D substances may stimulate skeletal mobilization of calcium despite inhibition of PTH secretion, that they do not accelerate the birth rate of new bone remodeling units, and that their potential stimulation of osteoblast function may be overwhelmed by the decline in bone formation occurring in response to the fall in bone resorption. Thus, there would seem to be little value in the use of vitamin D substances alone

in the management of postmenopausal osteoporosis.

ESTROGEN. Estrogen replacement would
seem rational in postmenopausal osteoporosis
since it should inhibit PTH-induced bone resorption[11] and it may restore normal osteoblast
function.

Indeed, estrogen therapy has been shown to
restore much of the biochemical abnormalities[40] encountered in many patients with postmenopausal osteoporosis. Thus, it has been reported that estrogen treatment decreased
serum calcium, increased serum PTH and
1,25-$(OH)_2$D, and augmented intestinal calcium absorption.[14] Moreover, it has been
shown to inhibit bone resorption.[60] During
short-term therapy (< 6 months), no change in
bone formation was found.[60,61] However, with
continued therapy, bone formation declined
probably as a result of the coupling response to
decreased bone resorption.[61] Thus, in patients
with established bone disease with fractures,
estrogen therapy does not create new bone,[93]
even though it may inhibit the rate of bone
loss.[36]

In healthy postmenopausal and oophorectomized women, the institution of estrogen
therapy shortly after the onset of estrogen lack
has been shown to prevent bone loss.[117] When
the treatment was given 2–6 years after menopause or oophorectomy, a significant rise in
bone density in the appendicular skeleton of
1–3% per year occurred.[117–119] The rise was
observed only during the first 3 years of therapy; no further change occurred thereafter.[117]
Moreover, estrogen therapy was shown to prevent the occurrence of spinal[120] and hip fractures.[121] Thus, there is emerging evidence that
estrogen may have a prophylactic value in the
prevention of age-related bone loss and fractures.

In considering estrogen therapy, potential
side effects should be carefully evaluated.[122]
The usual effective dose is equine estrogen
0.625 mg/day or ethinyl estradiol 0.05–0.1 mg/
day given intermittently (on treatment for 3
weeks and withdrawal for 1 week). A careful
gynecologic examination is mandatory.

ANDROGENS. The mode of action of androgen therapy for osteoporosis is not known. Androgens probably promote bone matrix synthesis. Such a treatment has been shown to
increase total body calcium.[123,124]

***Therapies Designed to Augment Bone
Mass.*** This approach is designed to increase the
total mass of bone by interventions which may
not be considered "physiologic." On the one
hand, an unnatural compound (fluoride) may
be administered to provide marked stimulation of osteoblastic activity. On the other hand,
bone-resorbing agents (e.g., PTH) may be
given to activate the osteoclasts and to accelerate the birth rate of new bone remodeling
units.

FLUORIDE. Fluoride has been recommended for osteoporosis because of its ability
to stimulate osteoblastic matrix synthesis.[125,126]
When it is given alone an abundance of poorly
mineralized osteoid may be found, indicating
that the newly formed osteoid does not undergo adequate calcification.[125,127] Moreover,
there may be an increased resorption as well.
However, the addition of vitamin D and calcium to fluoride has been shown to augment
the amount of mineralized bone, reduce osteoid volume, and prevent increased resorption.[125,128,129] An increased total bone mass has
been reported during long-term treatment
with this combined regimen.[32,129,130]

The available evidence suggests that fluoride
therapy may increase the mass of bone by
markedly stimulating matrix synthesis. Even if
fluoride were to exert this effect, this action
must be short-lived, since the osteoblastic activity becomes markedly reduced after 2 years of
therapy.[129]

It has been argued that the new bone forming under the influence of fluoride may not
confer much benefit, since it is abnormal in
chemical composition and morphology. The
"fluoridic" bone is rich in fluoroapatite which
has a higher crystallinity and reduced solubility
than normally occurring hydroxyapatite.[131]
Moreover, it is composed of mosaic rather than
lamellar bone with decreased elasticity.[132]
Thus, the increase in bone mass occurring after fluoride therapy may not indicate that the
bone has been strengthened.

However, fluoride therapy appears to satisfy
the most important requirement of osteoporosis therapy—inhibition of skeletal fractures.
Earlier reports indicated that fluoride reduced
the rate of new fractures after 1 year of treatment, although these studies did not include a
placebo group.[129,133] A recent randomized
study demonstrated a significant reduction in

the fracture rate during fluoride therapy.[134]

Unfortunately, fluoride therapy has been associated with substantial adverse side effects (in up to 40% of patients), including synovitis, periarticular fasciitis, gastrointestinal bleeding, nausea, pain, and diarrhea.[129,133] The recommended dose of sodium fluoride is 25 mg twice daily, with oral calcium supplements (600–1500 mg calcium/day), with or without vitamin D (50,000 units weekly or twice weekly).

PARATHYROID HORMONE. The use of a potent bone-resorbing agent such as PTH in the treatment of a bone-wasting disease such as osteoporosis would seem paradoxical. However, there is a sound theoretical basis for the assertion that judicious use of PTH may augment the mass of bone. First, PTH is the only substance which has been shown to activate osteoclasts, accelerate the birth rate of new bone remodeling units, and stimulate osteoblasts.[135] Second, the active life of osteoblasts is several times longer than that of osteoclasts.[136]

The above contention is supported by substantial experimental animal and clinical data, particularly when small amounts of PTH involving minor changes in calcium fluxes were used. In young rats, repeated injections of PTH have been shown to augment trabecular bone mass.[137] In human subjects with mild primary hyperparathyroidism or with secondary hyperparathyroidism of renal failure, osteosclerosis may develop.[138–140]

Encouraging results have already emerged from treatment of patients with postmenopausal osteoporosis with daily injections of human parathyroid hormone (1–34 fragment) at subhypercalcemic dosage.[10,141–144] A marked increase in bone turnover was observed by radiocalcium kinetic analysis and bone histology. Both bone formation and resorption increased; however, the increment in formation exceeded the change in resorption. These changes affected principally the trabecular bone. Thus, the most notable change in bone histology was a marked increase in trabecular bone volume (a mean of 92% from base line). The intestinal calcium absorption rose, probably consequent to the PTH-dependent stimulation of $1,25\text{-}(OH)_2D$ synthesis.

Unfortunately, calcium balance for the whole group did not change. Moreover, there was a reduction in cortical bone mass.[144] Although the above results are provocative, the necessity for continued daily injections of PTH may be questioned. If the object of this treatment approach is to activate osteoclasts, a short-term intermittent administration of PTH may be more advantageous (discussed below).[136]

COHERENCE TREATMENT. Coherence treatment[136,145] is an innovative approach which obviates some of the negative effects of treatment with fluoride (reduced bone formation with prolonged treatment)[129] or with PTH (sustained destruction of bone from continued administration).[144] This formulation is based on the following observations.

1) Bone remodeling occurring in basic multicellular units follows the sequence of activation followed by resorption and then formation. Since this sequence appears to be invariant, no new bone remodeling units may be formed without activation. The remodeling process in these units accounts for most of the lamellar bone turnover in adults. Thus, the skeletal balance of the whole body ultimately depends on activation.

2) The activities of individual bone remodeling units are normally out of phase with each other, some undergoing resorption and others formation. In other words, there is temporal incoherence among basic multicellular units.

3) The activities of bone remodeling units may be synchronized or made coherent by intermittent "activation pulses" by purposeful short-term administration of an agent capable of stimulating osteoclasts.

4) Once an activation pulse has been given, the depression of osteoclastic activity by certain inhibitors of bone resorption should not interfere with the stimulation of osteoblasts.

5) Since the active life of osteoblasts is much longer than that of osteoclasts,[136] osteoblastic bone formation should be sustained for some period following withdrawal of suppressive influence (i.e., during the free period).

6) The bone remodeling units should be responsive to repeated pulsing of activation and depression. Thus, the birth rate of new remodeling units may be accelerated and

Normal

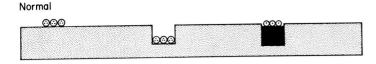

ADFR

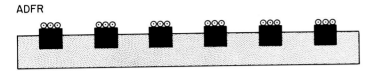

Fig. 4–8. Effect of coherence treatment on total bone. Normally, various basic multicellular units are out of phase (*top*), some undergoing activation or resorption, and others formation. Following a successful ADFR treatment (*bottom*), more basic multicellular units are in phase, all of them completing formation.

the duration of the life of bone remodeling units could be manipulated.

The actual mode of coherence therapy, as recommended by Frost,[136,145] entails a timed sequence of activation, depression, free, and repeat (ADFR) treatment. (Figs. 4–7 and 4–8). Initially, an activating pulse is given for approximately 5 days, e.g., with PTH or a vitamin D metabolite. A drug is then given to depress the osteoclasts (e.g., oral calcium or diphosphonate) over a 1-month period corresponding to the duration of active osteoclastic resorption. During the subsequent 2–3 months, when no drug is given, the osteoblasts stimulated by activation would be allowed to form new bone. The cycle is repeated by reactivation.

This treatment should increase the whole skeletal mass, because more bone remodeling units would have been created (Fig. 4–8), and since bone formation should exceed the resorption in each unit (Fig. 4–7). The latter condition prevails because of the depression phase during which osteoclastic resorption is reduced. This treatment approach is therefore potentially superior to the continuous PTH therapy outlined above where osteoclastic resorption is allowed to proceed unimpeded.

No published report of the use of ADFR treatment in postmenopausal osteoporosis is available. However, Frost noted in his review[145] that promising results are being obtained, using a vitamin D metabolite for activation and oral calcium for depression.

REFERENCES

1. Frame B, Parfitt AM. Osteomalacia: current concepts. Ann Intern Med. 1978; 89:966.

2. Frost HM. Bone remodelling and its relation to metabolic bone disease. Springfield, Ill.: Thomas, 1973.

3. Rasmussen H, Bordier PJ. The physiological and cellular basis of metabolic bone disease. Baltimore: Williams & Wilkins, 1974.

4. Jaworski ZFG. Physiology and pathology of bone remodelling. Orthop Clin North Am. 1981; 12:485–512.

5. Anderson HC. Introduction to the 2nd Conference on Matrix Vesicle Calcification. Metab Bone Dis Rel Res. 1978; 1:83.

6. Rasmussen H, Bordier P. Vitamin D and bone. Metab Bone Dis Rel Res 1978; 1:7.

7. Howell D, Pita JC, Alvarez J. Possible role of extracellular matrix vesicles in initial calcification of healing rachitic cartilage. Fed Proc. 1976; 35:122.

8. Raisz LG. Bone resorption in tissue culture. Factors influencing the response to parathyroid hormone. J Clin Invest. 1965; 44:103.

9. Flanagan B, Nichols G. Metabolic studies of human bone in vitro. II. Changes in hyperparathyroidism. J Clin Invest. 1965; 44:1795–1804.

10. Reeve J, Williams D, Hesp R, et al. Anabolic effect of low doses of a fragment of human parathyroid hormone on the skeleton in postmenopausal osteoporosis. Lancet. 1976; 1:1035.

11. Atkins D, Zanelli JM, Peacock M, Nordin BEC. The effect of oestrogens on the response of bone to parathyroid hormone in vitro. J Endocrinol. 1972; 54:107.

12. Gallagher JC, Nordin BEC. Treatment with oestrogens of primary hyperparathyroidism in postmenopausal women. Lancet. 1972; 1:503.

13. Gallagher JC, Wilkinson R. The effect of ethinyl oestradiol on calcium and phosphorus metabolism of post-menopausal women with primary hyperparathyroidism. Clin Sci. 1973; 45:785.

14. Gallagher JC, Riggs BL, DeLuca HF. Effect of

estrogen on calcium absorption and serum vitamin D metabolites in postmenopausal osteoporosis. J Clin Endocrinol Metab. 1980; 51:1359.

15. Caputo CB, Meadows D, Raisz L. Failure of estrogen and androgen to inhibit bone resorption in tissue culture. Endocrinology. 1976; 98:1065.

16. Henneman DH. Effect of estrogen on in vivo and in vitro collagen biosynthesis and maturation in old and young female guinea pigs. Endocrinology. 1968; 83:678.

17. Henneman DH. Effect of estrogen and growth hormone on collagen. Fourth Int. Congr. Endocrinology Washington, D.C. 1972:1109.

18. Henneman DH. Inhibition of the effect of D-penicillamine on collagen solubility in skin by 1-β-estradiol cypionate. Endocrinology. 1970; 87:456.

19. Henneman DH. Inhibition by estradiol-17 of the lathyritic effect of β-aminopropionitrile (BAPN) on skin and bone collagen. Clin. Orthop. 1972; 83:245.

20. Puschett JB, Fernandez PC, Boyle IT, et al. The acute renal tubular effects of 1,25-dihydroxycholecalciferol (36781). Proc Soc Exp Biol Med. 1972; 141:379.

21. Szymendera J, Gallus K. Effect of 24,25-dihydroxycholecalciferol on calcium absorption in proximal small intestine in uraemia. Br Med J. 1978; 2:1465.

22. Canterbury JM, Lerman S, Claflin J, Henery H. Inhibition of parathyroid hormone secretion by 25-hydroxycholecalciferol and 24,25-dihydroxycholecalciferol in the dog. J Clin Invest. 1978; 21:1375.

23. Stern PH. A monolog on analogs: in vitro effects of vitamin D metabolites and consideration of the mineralization question. Calcif Tissue Int. 1981; 33:1.

24. Meunier PJ, Courpron P, Edouard C, et al. Bone histomorphometry in osteoporotic states. In: Barzel US, ed. Osteoporosis II. New York: Grune & Stratton, 1979:27.

25. Albright F, Reifenstein EC. The Parathyroid Glands and Metabolic Bone Disease: Selected Studies. Baltimore, Williams & Wilkins, 1948.

26. Ivey JL, Baylink DJ. Postmenopausal osteoporosis: proposed roles of defective coupling and estrogen deficiency. Metab Bone Res. 1981; 3:3.

27. Schott GD, Wills MR. Muscle weakness in osteomalacia. Lancet. 1976; 1:626.

28. Mathews C, Heinberg KW, Ritz E, et al. Effect of 1,25-dihydroxycholecalciferol in impaired calcium transport by sarcoplasmic reticulum

in experimental uremia. Kidney Int. 1977; 11:227.

29. Henderson RG, Russell RGG, Ledingham, JGG, et al. Effects of 1,25-dihydroxycholecalciferol on calcium absorption, muscle weakness, and bone disease in chronic renal failure. Lancet. 1974; 1:379.

30. Birge SJ, Haddad JG. 25-hydroxycholecalciferol stimulation of muscle metabolism. J Clin Invest. 1975; 56:1100.

31. Albright F, Smith PH, Richardson AM. Postmenopausal osteoporosis: its clinical features. JAMA. 1941; 116:2465.

32. Riggs BL. Postmenopausal and senile osteoporosis: current concepts of etiology and treatment. Endocrin Jpn. 1979; 1:31.

33. Newton-John HF, Morgan DB. Osteoporosis: disease or senescence? Lancet 1968; 1:232.

34. Smith DM, Nance WE, Kang KW, et al. Genetic factors in determining bone mass. J Clin Invest. 1973; 52:2800.

35. Avioli LV. Postmenopausal osteoporosis: prevention versus cure. Fed Proc. 1981; 40:2418.

36. Nordin BEC, Horsman A, Crilly RG, et al. Treatment of spinal osteoporosis in postmenopausal women. Br Med J. 1980; 280:451.

37. Riggs BL, Wahner HW, Dunn WL, et al. Differential changes in bone mineral density of the appendicular and axial skeleton with aging. J Clin Invest. 1981; 67:328.

38. Ireland P, Fordtran JS. Effect of dietary calcium and age on jejunal calcium absorption in humans studied by intestinal perfusion. J Clin Invest. 1973; 52:2672.

39. Heaney RP, Recker RR, Saville PD. Menopausal changes in calcium balance performance. J Lab Clin Med. 1978; 92:953.

40. Gallagher JC, Riggs BL, Eisman J, et al. Intestinal calcium absorption and serum vitamin D metabolites in normal subjects and osteoporotic patients. J Clin Invest. 1979; 64:729.

41. Matkovic V, Kostial K, Simonovic I. Bone status and fracture rates in two regions of Yugoslavia. Am J Clin Nutr. 1979; 32:540.

42. Birge SJ, Keutmann HT, Cuatrecasas P, Whedon GC. Osteoporosis, intestinal lactase deficiency and low dietary calcium intake. N Engl J Med. 1967; 276:445.

43. Licata AA, Bon E, Bartter FC, West F. Acute effects of dietary protein on calcium metabolism in patients with osteoporosis. J Gerontol. 1981; 36:14.

44. Daniell HW. Osteoporosis of the slender smoker—vertebral compression fractures and loss of metacarpal cortex in relation to postmenopausal cigarette smoking and lack of obesity. Arch Intern Med. 1976; 136:298.

45. Frumar AM, Meldrum DR, Geola F, et al. Relationship of fasting urinary calcium to circulating estrogen and body weight in postmenopausal women. J Clin Endocrinol Metab. 1980; 50:70.

46. Dalen N, Hallberg D, Lamke B. Bone mass in obese subjects. Acta Med Scand. 1975; 197:353.

47. MacDonald PC, Grodin JM, Siiteri PK. The utilization of plasma androstenedione for estrone production in women. Progress in endocrinology. Mexico City: Proc. Third Int Congr Endocrinology 1968: 770.

48. Hemsell DL, Grodin JM, Brenner PF, et al. Plasma precursors of estrogen. II. Correlation of the extent of conversion of plasma androstenedione to estrone with age. J Clin Endocrinol Metab. 1974; 38:476.

49. Grodin JM, Siiteri PK, MacDonald PC. Source of estrogen production in postmenopausal women. J Clin Endocrinol Metab. 1973; 36:207.

50. Siiteri PK, MacDonald PC: Role of extraglandular estrogen in human endocrinology. In: Greep RO, Astwood EB, eds. Handbook of physiology-endocrinology II, Part 1. Washington, D.C.: Am. Physiol. Soc., 1973: 615.

51. Riggs BL, Ryan RJ, Wahner HW, et al. Serum concentrations of estrogen, testosterone and gonadotropins in osteoporotic and nonosteoporotic postmenopausal women. J Clin Endocrinol Metab. 1973; 36:1097.

52. Orimo H, Fujita T, Yoshikawa M. Increased sensitivity of bone to parathyroid hormone in ovariectomized rats. Endocrinology. 1972; 90:760.

53. Hossain M, Smith DA, Nordin BEC. Parathyroid activity and postmenopausal osteoporosis. Lancet. 1970; 1:809.

54. Pak CYC, Stewart A, Kaplan R, et al. Photon absorptiometric analysis of bone density in primary hyperparathyroidism. Lancet 1975; 2:7.

55. Reifenstein EC Jr, Albrigt F. Metabolic effects of steroid hormone in osteoporosis. J. Clin. Invest. 1947; 26:24.

56. Wallach S, Henneman PH. Prolonged estrogen therapy in postmenopausal women. JAMA. 1959; 171:1637.

57. Canniggia A, Gennari C. Sites and modes of action of an estrogen-gestagen combination of calcium and phosphate metabolism in postmenopausal osteoporosis. Clin Orthop. 1972; 85:187.

58. Aitken JM, Hart DM, Smith DA. The effect of long-term mestranol administration on calcium and phosphorus homeostasis in oophorectomized women. Clin Sci. 1971; 41:233.

59. Young MM, Jasani C, Smith DA, Nordin BEC. Some effects of ethinyl oestradiol on calcium and phosphorus metabolism in osteoporosis. Clin Sci. 1968; 34:411.

60. Riggs BL, Jowsey J, Kelly PJ, et al. Effect of sex hormones on bone in primary osteoporosis. J Clin Invest. 1969; 48:1065.

61. Riggs BL, Jowsey J, Goldsmith RS, et al., Short- and long-term effects of estrogen and synthetic anabolic hormone in postmenopausal osteoporosis. J Clin Invest. 1972; 51:1659.

62. Riggs, BL, Arnaud CD, Jowsey J, et al. Parathyroid function in primary osteoporosis. J Clin Invest. 1973; 52:181.

63. Kaplan RA, Haussler MR, Deftos LJ, et al. The role of 1α,25-dihydroxy vitamin D in the mediation of intestinal hyperabsorption of calcium in primary hyperparathyroidism and absorptive hypercalciuria. J Clin Invest. 1977; 59:756.

64. Garabedian M, Holick MF, DeLuca HF, Boyle IT. Control of 25-hydroxycholecalciferol metabolism by parathyroid glands. Proc Natl Acad Sci. 1972; 69:1673.

65. Tanaka Y, Castillo L, DeLuca HF. Control of renal vitamin D hydroxylases in birds by sex hormones. Proc Natl Acad Sci. 1976; 73:2701.

66. Hughes MR, Brumbaugh PR, Haussler MR, et al. Regulation of serum 1α,25-dihydroxyvitamin D_3 by calcium and phosphate in the rat. Science 1975; 190:578.

67. Cohn SH, Vaswani A, Zanzi I, Ellis K. Effect of aging on bone mass in adult women. Am J Physiol. 1976; 230:143.

68. Smith DM, Khairi MRA, Norton J, Age and activity effects on rate of bone mineral loss. J Clin Invest. 1976; 58:716.

69. Lindsey R, Coutts JRT, Hart DM. The effect of endogenous oestrogen on plasma and urinary calcium and phosphate in oophorectomized women. Clin Endocrinol. 1977; 6:87.

70. Marshall DH, Crilly RG, Nordin BEC. Plasma androstenedione and oestrone levels in normal and osteoporotic postmenopausal women. Br Med J. 1977; 2:1177.

71. Adlin EV, Korenman SG. Endocrine aspects of aging. Ann Intern Med. 1980; 92:429.

72. Davidson BJ, Riggs BL, Conlam CB, Toft DO. Concentration of cytosolic estrogen receptors in patients with postmenopausal osteoporosis. Clin Res. 1978; 26:678A.

73. Van Paassen HC, Poortman J, Borgart-Creutzburg IMC, Thijssen JHH, Duursma SA. Oestrogen binding proteins in bone cell cytosol. Calc Tissue Res. 1978; 25:249–254.

74. Insogna KL, Lewis AM, Lipinski BA, et al. Effect of age on serum immunoreactive parathyroid hormone and its biological effects. J Clin Endocrinol Metab. 1981; 53: 1072.

75. Zerwekh JE, Pak CYC. Selective effect of thiazide therapy on serum 1α,25-dihydroxyvitamin D and intestinal calcium absorption in renal and absorptive hypercalciurias. Metabolism, 1980; 29:13.

76. Burkhart JM, Jowsey J. Parathyroid and thyroid hormones in the development of immobilization osteoporosis. Endocrinology. 1967; 81:1053.

77. Bone HG III, Snyder WH, Pak CYC. Diagnosis of hyperparathyroidism. Ann Rev Med. 1977; 28:111.

78. Whyte MP, Bergfeld MA, Murphy WA, et al. Postmenopausal osteoporosis. A heterogeneous disorder as assessed by histomorphometric analysis of iliac crest bone from untreated patients. Am J Med. 1982; 72:193.

79. Lawoyin S, Zerwekh JE, Glass K, Pak CYC. Ability of 25-OH-vitamin D_3 therapy to augment serum 1,25-$(OH)_2$D and 24,25-$(OH)_2$ vitamin D in postmenopausal osteoporosis. J Clin Endocrinol Metab. 1980; 50:593.

80. Slovik DM, Adams JS, Neer RM, et al. Deficient production of 1,25-dihydroxyvitamin D in elderly osteoporotic patients. N Engl J Med. 1981; 305:372.

81. Riggs BL, Hamstra A, DeLuca HF. Assessment of 25-hydroxyvitamin D 1α-hydroxylase reserve in postmenopausal osteoporosis by administration of parathyroid extract. J Clin Endocrinol Metab. 1981; 53:833.

82. Lore F, DiCairaro G, Signorini AM, Caniggia A. Serum levels of 25-hydroxyvitamin D in postmenopausal osteoporosis. Calc Tissue Res. 1981; 33:467.

83. Deftos LJ, Weisman MH, Williams GW, et al. Influence of age and sex on plasma calcitonin in human beings. N Engl J Med. 1980; 302:1351.

84. Taggart HM, Ivey JL, Sisom K, et al. Deficient calcitonin response to calcium stimulation in postmenopausal osteoporosis. Lancet. 1982; 1:475.

85. Chestnut CH, Baylink DJ, Nelp WB, Roos BA. Basal plasma immunoreactive calcitonin in postmenopausal osteoporosis. Metabolism. 1980; 29:559.

86. Morimoto S, Tsuji M, Okada Y, The effect of oestrogens on human calcitonin secretion after calcium infusion in elderly female subjects. Clin Endocrinol. 1980; 13:135.

87. Rico H, Del Rio A, Vila T, et al. The role of growth hormone in the pathogenesis of postmenopausal osteoporosis. Arch Intern Med. 1979; 139:1263.

88. Manolagas SC, Anderson DC. Adrenal steroids and the development of osteoporosis in oophorectomized women. Lancet. 1979; 2:597.

89. Singh M, Riggs BL, Beabout JW, Jowsey J. Femoral trabecular pattern index for evaluation of spinal osteoporosis. Mayo Clin Proc. 1973; 48:184.

90. Meema S, Meema HE. Age trends of bone mineral mass, muscle width, and subcutaneous fat in normals and osteoporotics. Calc Tissue Res. 1973; 12:101.

91. Lawoyin S, Sismilich S, Browne R, Pak CYC. Bone mineral content in patients with primary hyperparathyroidism, osteoporosis, and calcium urolithiasis. Metabolism. 1979; 28:1250.

92. Vergne-Marini P, Parker TF, Pak CYC, et al. Jejunal and ileal calcium absorption in patients with chronic renal disease. Effect of 1α-hydroxycholecalciferol. J Clin Invest. 1976; 57:861.

93. Recker RR, Saville PD, Heaney RP. Effect of estrogens and calcium carbonate on bone loss in postmenopausal women. Ann Intern Med. 1977; 87:649.

94. Riggs BL, Kelly PJ, Kinney VR, et al. Calcium deficiency and osteoporosis. J Bone Joint Surg. 1967; 49A:915.

95. Sutton RAL, Dirks JH. Renal handling of calcium: overview. In: Massry SG, Ritz E, eds. Phosphate metabolism, Adv Exp Med Biol, New York: Plenum, 1977;81:15.

96. Porter RH, Cox BG, Heaney D, et al. Treatment of hypoparathyroid patients with chlorthalidone. N Engl J Med. 1978; 298:577.

97. Parfitt AM. Chlorothiazide-induced hypercalcemia in juvenile osteoporosis and hyperparathyroidism. N Engl J Med. 1969; 281:55.

98. Pickleman JR, Straus FH II, Forland M, Paloyan E. Thiazide-induced parathyroid stimulation. Metabolism. 1969; 18:867.

99. Brickman AS, Massry SG, Coburn JW. Changes in serum and urinary calcium during treatment with hydrochlorothiazide: Studies on mechanisms. J Clin Invest. 1972; 51:945.

100. Koppel MH, Massry SG, Shinaberger JH, et al. Thiazide-induced rise in serum calcium and magnesium in patients on maintenance hemodialysis. Ann Intern Med. 1970; 72:895.

101. Hahn TJ, Avioli LV. Effects of parenteral thiazide administration on parathyroid function. Clin Res. 1970; 18:31A.

102. Yendt ER, Cohanim M. Prevention of calcium stones with thiazides. Kidney Int. 1978; 13:397.

103. Malluche HH, Meyer WA, Singer FR, Massry SG. Thiazide-induced increased density of osteocytes: a mechanism for the rise in serum calcium by thiazides. Am Soc Nephrol 12th Annual Meeting. 1979; December:57A.

104. Yendt ER. Renal calculi. Can Med Assoc J. 1970; 102:479.

105. Gursel E. Effects of diuretics on renal and intestinal handling of calcium. NY State J Med. 1970; 70:399.

106. Paloyan E, Forland M, Pickleman JR. 1969. Hyperparathyroidism coexisting with hypertension and prolonged thiazide administration. JAMA. 1969; 210:1243.

107. Transbol I, Christensen MS, Jensen GF, Christiansen C, McNair P. Thiazide for the postponement of postmenopausal bone loss. Metabolism. 1982; 31:383.

108. Aliapoulios MA, Goldhaber P, Munson PL. Thyrocalcitonin inhibition of bone resorption induced by parathyroid hormone in tissue culture. Science. 1966; 151:330.

109. Jowsey J, Riggs BL, Goldsmith RS, et al. Effects of prolonged administration of porcine calcitonin in postmenopausal osteoporosis. J Clin Endocrinol Metab. 1971; 33:752.

110. Wallach S, Cohn SH, Atkins HL, Effect of salmon calcitonin on skeletal mass in osteoporosis. Curr Ther Res. 1977; 22:556.

111. Jowsey J, Riggs BL, Kelly PJ, Hoffman DL. Calcium and salmon calcitonin in treatment of osteoporosis. J Clin Endocrinol Metab. 1978; 47:633.

112. Riggs BL, Jowsey J, Kelly PJ, et al. Effects of oral therapy with calcium and vitamin D in primary osteoporosis. J Clin Endocrinol Metab. 1976; 42:1139.

113. Davies M, Mawer EB, Adams PH: Vitamin D metabolism and the response to 1,25-dihydroxycholecalciferol in osteoporosis. J Clin Endocrinol Metab. 1977; 45:199.

114. Christiansen C, Christensen MS, Rodbro P, Hagen C, Transbol I. Effect of 1,25-dihydroxyvitamin D in itself or combined with hormone treatment in preventing postmenopausal osteoporosis. Europ J Clin Invest. 1981; 11:305.

115. Wandless I, Jarvis S, Evans JG. Vitamin D_3 in osteoporosis. Br Med J. 1980; 280:1320.

116. Pak CYC, Fordtran JS. 1978. Disorders of mineral metabolism. In: Sleisenger MH, Fordtran JS, Ingelfinger FS, eds. Gastrointestinal disease. Philadelphia: Saunders, 1978:251.

117. Lindsay R, Aitken JM, Anderson JB, et al. Long-term prevention of postmenopausal osteoporosis by oestrogen. Lancet. 1976; 1:1038.

118. Christiansen C, Christensen MS, Transbol I. Bone mass in postmenopausal women after withdrawal of oestrogen/gestagen replacement therapy. Lancet. 1981; 1:459.

119. Christiansen C, Mazess RB, Transbol I, Jensen GF. Factors in response to treatment of early postmenopausal bone loss. Calc Tissue Int. 1981; 33:575.

120. Lindsay R, Hart DM, Forrest C, Baird C. Prevention of spinal osteoporosis in oophorectomised women. Lancet. 1980; 2:1151.

121. Hutchinson TA, Polansky JM, Feinstein AR. Postmenopausal oestrogens protect against fractures of hip and distal radius. Lancet. 1979; 2:705.

122. Weinstein MC. Estrogen use in postmenopausal women—costs, risks, and benefits. N Engl J Med. 1980; 303:308.

123. Aloia JF, Kapoor A, Vaswani A, Cohn SH. Changes in body composition following therapy of osteoporosis with methandrostenolone. Metabolism. 1981; 30:1076.

124. Chestnut CH III, Nelp NB, Baylink DJ, Denney JD. Effect of methandrosteneolone on postmenopausal bone wasting as assessed by changes in total bone mineral mass. Metabolism. 1977; 26:267.

125. Jowsey J, Schenk RK, Reutter FW. Some results of the effect of fluoride on bone tissue in osteoporosis. J Clin Endocrinol Metab. 1968; 28:869.

126. Rich C, Ensinck J. Effect of sodium fluoride on calcium metabolism of human beings. Nature. 1961; 191:184.

127. Cass RM, Croft JD Jr, Perkins P, et al. New bone formation in osteoporosis following treatment with sodium fluoride. Arch Intern Med. 1966; 118:111.

128. Jowsey J, Riggs BL, Kelly PJ, Hoffman DL. Effect of combined therapy with sodium fluoride, vitamin D and calcium in osteoporosis. Am J Med 1972; 53:43.

129. Briancon D, Meunier PJ. Treatment of osteoporosis with fluoride, calcium, and vitamin D. Orthop Clin North Am. 1981; 12:629.

130. Harrison JE, McNeill KG, Sturtridge WC, et al. Three-year changes in bone mineral mass of postmenopausal osteoporotic patients based on neutron activation analysis of the central third of the skeleton. J Clin Endocrinol Metab. 1981; 52:751.

131. McCann HG. The solubility of fluorapatite and its relationship to that of calcium fluoride. Arch Oral Biol. 1968; 13:987.

132. Wolinsky I, Simkin A, Gugqenheim K. Effects of fluoride on metabolism and mechanical properties of rat bone. Am J Physiol. 1972; 223:46.

133. Riggs BL, Hodgson SF, Hoffman DL, et al.

Treatment of primary osteoporosis with fluoride and calcium. Clinical tolerance and fracture occurrence. JAMA. 1980; 243:446.

134. Riggs BL, Seeman E, Hodgson SF, et al. Effect of the fluoride/calcium regimen on vertebral fracture occurrence in postmenopausal osteoporosis. N Engl J Med. 1982; 306:446.

135. Ashton BA, Owen MR, Eagleson CC, Parsons JA. In: Cohn DV, Talmage RV, eds. Endocrinology of calcium regulating hormones. Amsterdam: Excerpta Medica, 1981.

136. Frost HM. Treatment of osteoporosis by manipulation of coherent bone cell populations. Clin Orthop. 1979; 143:227.

137. Kalu DN, Pennock J, Doyle FH, Foster GV. Parathyroid hormone and experimental osteosclerosis. Lancet. 1970; 1:1363.

138. Genant HK, Baron JM, Paloyan E, Jowsey J. Osteosclerosis in primary hyperparathyroidism. Am J Med. 1975; 59:104.

139. Kaye M, Pritchard JE, Halpenny G, Wright W. Bone disease in chronic renal failure with particular reference to osteosclerosis. Medicine (Balt), 1960; 39:157.

140. Teitelbaum SL, Bergfeld MA, Freitag J, et al. Do parathyroid hormone and 1,25-dihydroxyvitamin D modulate bone formation in uremia? J Clin Endocrinol Metab. 1980; 51:247.

141. Slovik DM, Neer RM, Poots JT. Short-term effects of synthetic human parathyroid hormone (1-34) administration on bone mineral metabolism in osteoporotic patients. J Clin Invest. 1981; 68:1261.

142. Parsons JA, Meunier P, Podbesek R, et al. Pathological and therapeutic implications of the cellular and humoral response to parathyroin. Biochem Soc Trans. 1981; 9:383.

143. Reeve J, Arlot M, Bernat M, et al. Calcium-47 kinetic measurements of bone turnover compared to bone histomorphometry in osteoporosis: the influence of human parathyroid fragment (hPTH 1-34) therapy. Metab Bone Dis Rel Res. 1981; 3:23.

144. Reeve J, Meunier P, Parsons JA, et al. Anabolic effect of human parathyroid hormone fragment on trabecular bone in involutional osteoporosis: a multicenter trial. Br Med J. 1980; 2:1340.

145. Frost HM Coherence treatment of osteoporosis. Orthop Clin North Am. 1981; 12:649.

Biologic Effects of Natural and Synthetic Estrogens

5

J. Gerald Quirk, Jr. and George D. Wendel, Jr.

The word estrogen has a heterogenous origin much like the group of compounds it encompasses. It is derived from the Greek "oistros" or Latin "oestrus" (gadfly, frenzy, sexual heat, animal rut, desire) and the Greek suffix "-gen" (born, generate). The Oxford English Dictionary defines estrogens as "sex hormones produced in the ovary usually characterized by ability to produce estrus and secondary sex characteristics in females."[1] They are a diverse group of compounds including both naturally occurring hormones and synthetic compounds with similar biologic properties.

In recent years the concept of estrogenic biologic affect has undergone changes with respect to the traditional definition given above. A greater awareness of the spectrum of effects exerted by these compounds on organs and systems has broadened the previous notions concerning the role of estrogens. It is now known that these steroids may have diverse organ-specific effects outside the genital system. Bioactivity has been attributed to compounds previously felt to be inactive metabolic end-products. Target organs possess the ability to alter the estrogen presented to them, playing a qualitative as well as quantitative role in determining tissue-specific responses. In order to under the present concepts concerning the purported functions and possible therapeutic benefits of estrogen therapy, one must have a basic knowledge of the chemistry and biomechanics involved in the expression of estrogen effects in the body.

History

Our knowledge of the estrogens as sex hormones is intimately related to our understanding of the ovary and its functions. Although the ovary was called the female testis in the sixteenth century, the term ovarium was in use by 1680.[2] The follicles were subsequently discovered by van Horne in 1707,[3] and the first ovum was described by von Baer in 1827.[4]

From a clinical perspective, the first description of the effects of castration is attributed to Percival Scott who in 1750 noted progressive weight loss, breast atrophy, and amenorrhea in a 23-year-old woman following surgical removal of her ovaries.[5] Over 100 years later Hegar noted that development of genitalia, secondary sex characteristics, and menstruation were dependent on functional ovarian tissue.[6] In 1889, Brown-Séquard popularized the concept of rejuvenation with injections of preparations from whole canine testicles.[7] His personal experience was not duplicated by others, but nevertheless spawned the idea of gonadotherapy to reverse the effects of aging. With his empiric results based on the erroneous assumption that the gonads stored hormones rather than synthesizing and secreting them, Brown-Séquard's thesis deflected the efforts of endocrinologists toward whole-gland preparations for several years.[8]

By the turn of the century, ovotherapy became popular for clinical use, although plagued by empiricism and commercialism. In

1896, the Landau Clinic in Berlin reported the use of fresh animal ovarian preparations to relieve severe vasomotor symptoms.[9] Morris in the United States used ovarian transplantation to avoid similar vasomotor symptoms in a young girl.[10] Later experiments were designed to assess the potential of the various components of the ovary: the corpus luteum, follicular cells/fluid, and interstitial cells. By 1904, Fraenkel[11] and Burnam[12] had shown favorable results in treating various gynecologic disorders, including "hot and cold flushing and nervousness," with corpus luteum preparations.

The role of the ovary as an organ of internal secretion was confirmed by experimental evidence from ovarian transplants. In 1896, Knauer showed that the effects of castration could be avoided by ovarian transplantation in rabbits.[13,14] Despite sectioning the nerve and blood supply to the ovary, transplanted ovarian tissue demonstrated peripheral manifestations of ovarian function. Almost simultaneously, Halban showed that castrated, immature female guinea pigs had pubertal development if ovarian tissue was transplanted subcutaneously.[15]

Investigations concerning the site and nature of ovarian internal secretion followed, but were delayed somewhat by World War I. Adler in 1912 showed that aqueous extracts of ovarian and corpus luteum tissue had estrus-producing properties.[16] In the same year, Iscovesco separated an active component from the lipid extract of ovarian tissue preparations.[17] Subsequently, Fellner confirmed these findings and isolated an active estrogenic component from placental tissue.[18] It was not until 1922 that Frank suggested the follicular fluid as a source of material with potent estruslike effects.[19]

Allen and Doisy in 1923 developed a method of detection and assay for estrogenic activity in experimental animals[20] employing Stockard and Papanicolaou's correlation of vaginal cytology with the phases of the reproductive cycle in guinea pigs.[21] By injecting follicular extracts into rats, cytologic changes typical of estrus were produced in vaginal smears which were verified by histologic examination of the uterus and endometrium. This gave investigators the first rapid, inexpensive bioassay for estrogens and was a great impetus to the search for the active principle in ovarian ex-

tracts. Equally important was the discovery of significant concentrations of estrogenic substances in the urine of pregnant women by Aschheim and Zondek[22] in 1927 and in mares by Zondek[23] in 1930.

Aided by a plentiful source from which to work, Doisy et al.[24] and Butenandt[25] in 1929 simultaneously, but independently, isolated the first pure crystalline estrogen, estrone. The next year, Marrian identified a second estrogenic substance in urine, estriol,[26] whose structure he later elucidated. Butenandt later established the structure of estrone and its conversion to estriol through dehydration.[27] Finally, estradiol was identified as the nonketonic estrogen in follicular extracts by MacCorquodale et al.[28] in 1935. They later extracted 6 mg of what proved to be estradiol-17β from one ton of sow ovaries.[28] During the 1930s numerous other natural estrogens of equine origin such as equilin, hippulin, and equilenin were isolated; but discussion of their development is beyond the scope of this chapter.

The same decade also heralded the discovery of the synthetic estrogens. The earliest such compound was isolated by Dodds et al. in 1938; it was diethylstilbestrol, a nonsteroidal, stilbene derivative.[29] In the same year, Inhoffen and Hohlweg reported a synthetic steroidal estrogen, ethinyl estradiol, which differs from its parent compounds, estradiol, by the addition of a 17α-ethinyl group.[30] Thereafter, structural alterations of synthetic compounds already described produced diethylstilbestrol dipropionate, dienestrol, and chlorotrianisene from the stilbene parent structure and mestranol and quinestrol from ethinyl estradiol.

Structure

The naturally occurring estrogens all share a common parental steroid structure and nomenclature. The basic steroid skeleton is cholestane with a tetracyclic structure containing 27 carbons (Fig. 5–1). By convention the four rings are designated A, B, C, and D; the carbons have designated numbers based on their positions in the compound cholesterol. While cholestane is a 27-carbon structure (C_{27}), the estrogen nucleus, estrane, is an 18-carbon skeleton (C_{18}) (Fig. 5–1). The various intermediate structures that are formed in estrogen synthesis are also denoted systematically by the num-

ous steroid precursors is absent. C-16 and invariably C-17 are the main positions for hydroxyl groups and ketones in the three main naturally occurring estrogens, i.e., estradiol, estrone, and estriol (Fig. 5–1). Estradiol is active predominantly in the 17β-hydroxy form; in our discussion the term, estradiol, will be used synonymously with this conformation.

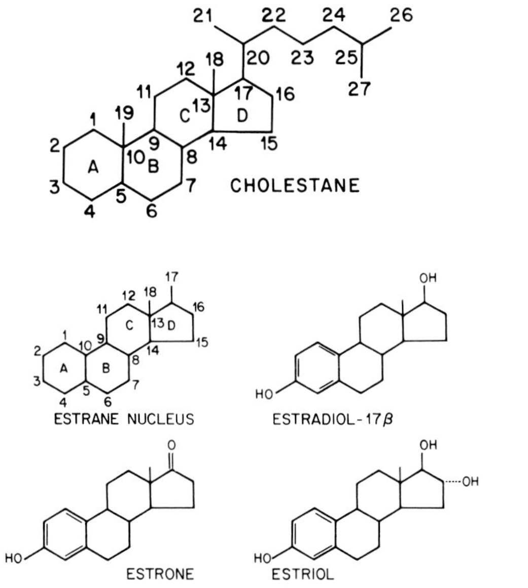

The synthetic estrogens are a heterogenous array of compounds which can be segregated into two groups based on their mode of synthesis. The first group is comprised of steroidal compounds derived from the estrane nucleus through specific structural alterations. Best known are ethinyl estradiol (estradiol + 17α-ethinyl group), mestranol (estradiol + 17α-ethinyl + 3-methyl ether groups), and quinestrol (estradiol + 17α-ethinyl + 3-cyclopentyl ether groups) (Fig. 5–2). Although these compounds are similar to 17β-estradiol, they are classified as synthetic estrogens; they are not found in any natural biologic system and must be synthesized artificially. The second group is made up of nonsteroidal compounds that have estrogenic properties. The coal tar stilbene, comprised of two benzene rings separated by

Fig. 5–1. Structures of the steroidal parent compounds and the natural estrogens. The numbers denote carbon atoms in the formation of cholesterol, here represented by its C_{27} nucleus, cholestane. The nomenclature of the steroidal estrogens is based on this standard numbering system, shown above for the saturated hydrocarbon nucleus, estrane. Notice the designation of the rings with letters A through D and the configuration of side-chain substituents as α (dotted line) or β (straight line).

ber of carbon atoms in their molecules: cholane, C_{24}; pregnane, C_{21}; and androstane, C_{19}. The particular compounds are then given chemical names based on the number of carbons in the steroid nucleus and the standard terminations denoting the positions of unsaturations and substituents. Most structures also are known by common names which will be used predominantly in this discussion. By convention, side-chain group configuration will be designated α (dashed line) or β (straight line) with reference to C_{18} for the estrogens. Those that project behind the plane of the structure will be in α configuration whereas those projecting forward will be in β configuration. Further information concerning structure, stoichiometry, and nomenclature can be found in most texts of biochemistry or endocrinology.

The naturally occurring estrogens share several unique structural features. As previously noted, they are derivatives of the C_{18} saturated hydrocarbon, estrane, a cyclopentanophenanthrene skeleton (Fig. 5–1). They possess an aromatic A ring with a C-3 hydroxyl group which makes the ring phenolic. The C-10 methyl group (C-19 by position) common to the vari-

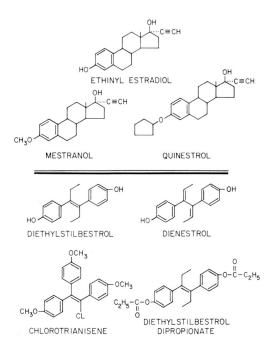

Fig. 5–2. Synthetic steroidal (above) and nonsteroidal (below) estrogens. The steroidal compounds are derivatives of the estrane nucleus, whereas the nonsteroidal compounds, as depicted, can be envisioned to be steroidal analogs.

an unsaturated ethylene chain, serves as the parent compound for the majority of these estrogens. In the active form, many of these substituted compounds are essentially steroidal analogs.[31] The oldest and most potent of this class of drugs is diethylstilbestrol (DES); others are dienestrol (DES diethyldiene derivative), DES dipropionate, and chlorotrianisene (DES with an aromatic ring replacing the ethyl group, a chloride molecule substituting for the second ethyl radical, and methoxy groups on all three rings) (Fig. 5–2).[32]

Synthesis

Since the naturally occurring estrogens have been described previously as steroids, a discussion of their biosynthesis must include the pathways shared with the corticoids, progestins, and androgens. The three main steroid-producing organs, the ovary, adrenal, and testis, all possess enzymes capable of producing any type of steroid de novo from acetate. Each

organ then has a predominant pathway toward its characteristic end-products, mainly due to trophic hormone stimulation and target organ specificity. Ryan has described these shared pathways as the *unified concept* of steroid formation.[33] Although each endocrine organ has its usual end-product, alterations occur with enzymatic defects, neoplasms, and various disease states.

Central to the synthesis of the estrogens are three main steps: (1) biosynthesis of cholesterol from acetate followed by side-chain cleavage of the C-27 molecule and hydroxylation to form the C-21 pregnenolone; (2) conversion of pregnenolone to androstenedione or testosterone; and (3) A-ring aromatization of the androgens androstenedione and testosterone to form estrone or estradiol (Fig. 5–3). The conversion of pregnenolone to its androgenic products proceeds via one of two routes: (1) Δ^4-3-ketone pathway via progesterone and 17-hydroxyprogesterone or (2) Δ^5-3β-hydroxy pathway via 17-hydroxypregnenolone and dehydroepiandrosterone. Attempts to assign a location, cell

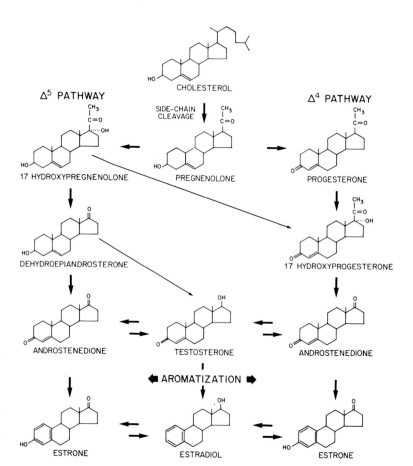

Fig. 5–3. Biosynthetic pathways for the natural estrogens. Step 1: Side-chain cleavage of cholesterol to form pregnenolone. Step 2: Conversion of pregnenolone to the androgens, androstenedione and testosterone, via either the Δ^5-3β-hydroxy or Δ^4-3-ketone pathways. Step 3: A-Ring aromatization of androgenic compounds to form estrone and estradiol.

type, or particular pathway for the synthesis of the various ovarian steroids have resulted in much confusion and conflicting experimental evidence.

Early studies suggested that the predominant biosynthetic pathway in luteinized tissue was the Δ^4 pathway, while synthesis in follicular tissue proceeded via the Δ^5 route. This was thought to be due to a deficiency in 17-hydroxylation and C-20/C-21 side-chain cleavage in luteal cells. Short called this the "two-cell type" theory of ovarian steroid synthesis.[34] He hypothesized that luteinized granulosa cells function like a corpus luteum, secreting progesterone, whereas the theca interna cells function like a follicle, producing estrogen. Subsequent work has shown this difference in steroid production to be more quantitative than qualitative, demonstrative of a unique interdependence between the two cell types, mediated by the gonadotropins FSH and LH.[35] Granulosa cells have little ability to synthesize steroids de novo from acetate,[36] but have high aromatase activity.[37] These cells rapidly convert progesterone precursors into estrogens. Theca interna cells produce large amounts of androstenedione, and thereby enhance estrogen production by granulosa cells.[37] In concert with these biochemical investigations, electron microscopic studies of the ovary throughout its cycle show that theca interna cells have features typical of steroid secretion (lipid droplets, smooth endoplasmic reticulum, and mitochondrial tubular cristae), whereas follicular granulosa cells lack such features, developing them only after luteinization.[38] In addition, the follicular granulosa layer is isolated from the theca interna by an avascular basal lamina while the ovarian stroma, including the specialized theca interna cells, is richly supplied with blood vessels. With corpus luteum formation, the newly luteinized granulosa cells lose their separating basal lamina and are invaded by vascular channels.[39]

Considering the above biochemical and histologic evidence it is tempting to hypothesize roles and a sequence of events in the ovarian cycle. In the preovulatory follicle, the theca interna synthesizes and secretes androstenedione de novo under the influence of LH. Androstenedione is then released into the peripheral circulation and diffuses into the avascular granulosa layers. The follicular granulosa cells, stimulated by FSH, perform aromatization on this androgenic precursor producing estradiol, which then accumulates in the follicular antrum and diffuses back across the basal lamina into the peripheral circulation. After ovulation, the functional difference between the two luteinized cell types is less distinct with both de novo synthesis of progesterone and estradiol and conversion of newly available blood-borne cholesterol precursors into progesterone and estradiol. Thus, the "two cell" theory of ovarian steroid synthesis involves a synergism between the granulosa and luteal cells mediated by the two gonadotropins FSH and LH.[35]

Biologic Effect

As noted previously, the estrogens form a heterogenous group of compounds that differ both by structure (steroidal vs. nonsteroidal) and parent compound (naturally occurring vs. synthetic). Despite their differences in structure, substituents, and spatial conformation, each possesses the common biologic capacity to stimulate typical changes in the genital organs and maintain secondary sex characteristics. The presence, deficiency, or absence of these compounds also has potent effects on other organs and metabolic systems which will be discussed in other chapters. Some of the effects of estrogen deficiency, which for this discussion will be confined to loss of ovarian function from surgical or natural causes, can be ameliorated, postponed, or even reversed by replacement therapy. Although clinical applications of replacement therapy will be discussed in a subsequent chapter, it is important to understand the pharmacology of these various estrogenic compounds.

Natural and synthetic estrogens as well as compounds with estrogenic properties are numerous, but relatively few are used clinically. The three main naturally occurring compounds (17β-estradiol, estrone, and estriol), their conjugated metabolites, and the synthetic products, ethinyl estradiol and mestranol, are the chief exogenous estrogens used in replacement therapy (Table 5–1). Each drug, in spite of its unique chemical structure, expresses its desired effects through properties common to

TABLE 5–1. Oral Estrogen Preparations and Dosage Ranges.

GENERIC PREPARATION	DOSAGE RANGE	COMMERCIAL PREPARATION
Conjugated estrogens	0.3–1.25 mg/day	Premarin
Esterified estrogens	0.3–1.25 mg/day	Amnestrogen, Evex, Menest, Estratab
Piperazine estrone sulfate	0.625–2.5 mg/day	Ogen
Estradiol (micronized)	1.0–2.0 mg/day	Estrace
Combined estrogen preparations	1–2 tablets/day	Hormonin
Ethinyl estradiol	0.02–0.05 mg/day	Estinyl, Feminone
Quinestrol	100 µg/day for 1 week, then 100–200 µg/week	Estrovis
Diethylstilbestrol	0.2–0.5 mg/day	Diethylstilbestrol
Chlorotrianisene	12–25 mg/day	Tace

the entire class. Among these properties are the following:

1) Absorption, formulation, and administration.
2) Bioavailability: hormone binding and transport.
3) Metabolism, conjugation, and excretion.
4) Interaction with target organ: estrogen receptors.

ABSORPTION, FORMULATION, AND ADMINISTRATION. The naturally occurring estrogens would seem, at first glance, to be the most physiologic choice for replacement therapy in hormone-deficient states; but their use is plagued with problems. They are virtually insoluble in water, limiting parenteral administration to aqueous suspensions or solutions dissolved in oil which are rapidly absorbed and metabolized. For many years the oral administration of estrone, estradiol, estriol has been avoided due to a belief that they were inactive by that route. Vaginal application for local treatment of atrophic vaginitis is associated with significant systemic levels of estrogens.[40] Despite these drawbacks, the natural estrogens, especially estradiol and estrone sulfate preparations, have become the mainstay of hormonal replacement therapy.

Estradiol. Pharmacologic investigations of estrogen metabolism have improved our understanding of the limited effectiveness of oral administration and have guided means to improve it. The gastrointestinal tract is second only to placental tissue in its ability to convert estradiol to estrone.[41] After absorption, estrogens travel via the portal circulation to the liver where further metabolism and conjugation occur. This has been called the "first pass" metabolism. Thus, by the time 17β-estradiol has reached the systemic circulation a significant portion of it has been inactivated. Experimental efforts have been directed toward increasing the amount of estradiol presented for absorption and finding means to bypass the initial transport through the liver.

One method used in attempts to improve estradiol absorption after oral administration is micronization (Estrace). This process involves reduction in particle size to increase absorptive area and has been shown to be important for steroid administration.[42] Clinical studies have confirmed the efficacy of this mode of therapy.[43,44] Circulating levels of estrone and estradiol were also shown to increase with consequent suppression of gonadotropins. After oral administration of a 2-mg tablet of estradiol, levels of estrone were consistently three to six times greater than those of estradiol over a 24-hour period of examination (Fig. 5–4A).[45] Noteworthy was the change in the estrone/estradiol ratio (here 3–6:1). This ratio is usually less than one or unity in menstruating women, and reverses at menopause (usually 2–4:1) due to the increased level of estrone[46] from peripheral conversion of androgenic precursors.[47] Although the significance of the estrone-to-estradiol ratio remains unsettled, the problem of excessive estrone delivery in attaining sufficient levels of estradiol to relieve menopausal symptoms may prove to be important.

Efforts to bypass the initial local intestinal and liver metabolism of orally administered estrogens have centered around topical application via vaginal mucosa, nasal mucosa, oral mucosa, and skin. Micronized estradiol appears to be rapidly and efficiently absorbed through the vaginal mucosa. Higher levels of estradiol are achieved with small concomitant changes in estrone. Following vaginal administration of a 1-mg dose of micronized estradiol in saline, serum levels of estradiol were 100

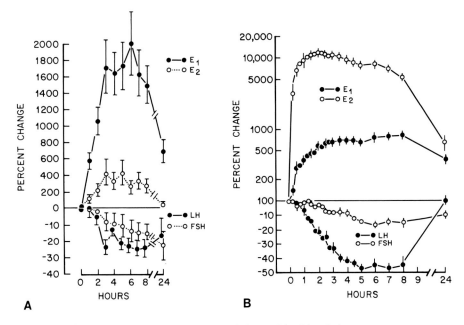

Fig. 5–4. Percentage change (mean ± SE) from basal levels in serum estrogen and gonadotropin concentrations following 2-mg oral (**A**) and 1-mg vaginal (**B**) administration of micronized estradiol. After oral administration estrone (E$_1$) is the principal estrogen recovered in blood, but with vaginal administration estradiol (E$_2$) is found in higher concentrations. Adapted from Henzel MR. Natural and synthetic female sex hormones. In: Yen SSC, Jaffe RB, eds. Reproductive endocrinology. Philadelphia: Saunders, 1978.

times greater than those following a 2-mg oral dose (Fig. 5–4B).[48] Although these serum concentrations of estradiol are clearly supraphysiologic, a smaller 0.2-mg dose of micronized estradiol in a cream base has been shown to produce levels of both estradiol and estrone similar to those in the follicular phase of the menstrual cycle.[40] With all dosages examined, incremental changes in estrone were dampened by vaginal administration. Presumably this is due to circumvention of changes in absorption across the intestinal mucosa and subsequent conjugation in the first pass through the liver via the portal circulation.[40,48–50] The persistence of a smaller but sustained increase in estrone levels is thought to be secondary to endogenous interconversion of estradiol to estrone after absorption.[51,52] A vaginal ring of polysiloxane containing estradiol has been utilized to deliver slow-release steroid for a 3-month period producing more physiologic estradiol levels; however, no description of estrone levels was given.[53] Serum levels of estrogens with intranasal[48] and sublingual[54] administration, although bypassing intestinal absorption, mimic those following oral administration with rapid, short-lived increases in estradiol levels followed by gradual, supraphysiologic increases in estrone. Local changes during absorption through these mucosal surfaces or contributions by the lymphatics of the head and neck may have produced conversion to estrone. Despite this drawback, a smaller 0.5-mg dose of estradiol administered sublingually was noted to produce serum levels of estradiol comparable to those seen with a 2.0-mg oral dose.[55] Percutaneous absorption of estradiol cream results in increased estrone levels, but individual variance in absorption is marked.[56] Other studies involving percutaneous administration, although complicated by the same variations in absorption, have suggested a greater increase in estradiol concentrations, maintaining a low estrone-to-estradiol ratio,[57] especially with prolonged therapy.[58]

Preparations for injection of estradiol have been developed through chemical alterations of the parent compound to prolong its availability. Organic esterification of estradiol with substituents of greater size makes it less polar and decreases the rate of absorption, enhancing the duration of action in solutions in oil.[29]

Long-acting preparations include estradiol benzoate (2–3 days), estradiol dipropionate (1–2 weeks), estradiol valerate (1–3 weeks), and estradiol cyclopentylpropionate (3–4 weeks).[30] The valerate and benzoate esters are also active when administered orally. Estradiol pellets for subcutaneous implantation have been used for many years when oral therapy was ineffective. When 25-mg pellets have been used, greater estrone than estradiol levels have been described.[59] Individual differences in absorption with pellets have caused vaginal bleeding from endometrial hyperplasia,[60] requiring cyclic progestogen therapy.

Estrone. Crystalline estrone is relatively inactive when administered orally, but it is used principally as estrone sulfate or as a part of a conjugated or esterified preparation for oral, vaginal, or parenteral administration. Although the parent compound is relatively insoluble in water, conjugation imparts solubility and stability to estrone for oral use. Conjugated estrogens are mixtures of naturally occurring compounds composed of 50–65% sodium estrone sulfate and 20–35% sodium equilenin sulfate, while the esterified preparations contain more estrone and less equilenin sulfate. The most popular formulation, Premarin, prepared from the urine of pregnant mares, contains 70% sodium estrone sulfate, 20% equilenin sulfate, and lesser amounts of other equine metabolites.[61] Orally administered estrone sulfate is absorbed and present in the circulation primarily in its natural form. It is then hydrolyzed to estrone or estradiol in the liver or at its target organ. Once again, there occurs a proportionately greater increase in serum levels of estrone than estradiol, compared to oral combination therapy[62,63] or vaginal creams.[40,49] Levels of equilenin following the ingestion of conjugated equine preparations exceeded peak levels of estradiol in the menstrual cycle. The significance of this remains to be elucidated.[64]

Estriol. Traditionally, estriol has been viewed as a metabolic product of estradiol and estrone with weak estrogenic properties.[32] Vaginal administration of estriol produces significant levels of unconjugated, but little conjugated, estriol, whereas oral use produces more of the latter, presumably due to intestinal metabolic changes.[65] In a comparison of equivalent dosages, only vaginal administration was associated with gonadotropin suppression, supporting the hypothesis that unconjugated estriol is the biologically active compound.[66] Although not widely used alone in hormone replacement therapy, estriol is available as a combined preparation, Hormonin (0.135 mg estriol, 0.7 mg estrone, 0.3 mg estradiol).

Synthetic Estrogens. Less is known about the absorption of the synthetic estrogens, for they are a more diverse group. Ethinyl estradiol is rapidly and fairly completely absorbed by the gastrointestinal tract,[67] reaching peak serum levels in the first hour after oral ingestion.[68,69] Mestranol has a more variable fate. Peak levels of both mestranol and its presumed active form, ethinyl estradiol, occur from 1 to 4 hours after ingestion.[69,70] Quinestrol is stored in body fat after oral ingestion, resulting in a prolonged duration of action.[71] Diethylstilbestrol is rapidly absorbed by the intestinal tract with a prolonged decline in serum levels over 2 to 3 days, but it is not used frequently in hormone replacement therapy.[72]

BIOAVAILABILITY: HORMONE BINDING AND TRANSPORT. Estrogens, like most of the other steroids, are present in the circulation in association with serum proteins, principally sex hormone binding globulin (SHBG) and albumin. SHBG, synthesized in the liver, is a glycoprotein with one binding site per molecule and a molecular weight of about 100,000 daltons. Estradiol, testosterone, and 5α-dihydrotestosterone bind to it competitively with affinities in ratios of approximately $0.4 : 1 : 3$.[73,74] Androstenedione, dehydroepiandrosterone, estrone, estrone sulfate, and estriol are poorly bound by SHBG. Albumin, although present in much greater concentration, has a lower affinity for estradiol but may act as an unsaturable source for estradiol binding;[73] it has higher affinities for estrone, estrone sulfate, and estriol.[75,76] Approximately 38% of estradiol is bound to SHBG, 60% is bound to albumin, and 2–3% is unbound or free in the circulation.[77] Recently another estrogen binding protein distant from SHBG and with high affinity, low capacity, and significant steroid specificity (high affinity for DES, but not testosterone or dihydrotestosterone) has been detected.[78] Further studies regarding its significance are awaited. Estrone sulfate is bound almost exclusively to albumin with a high affinity; over 90% of the circulating hormone is thought to be associated with its transport protein.[75]

SHBG, by influencing hormone availability, metabolism, and exposure to end-organ receptors, plays a central role in expression of estrogenic effects. As will be discussed later, it is felt that estradiol rather than estrone is the principal intracellular modulator of biologic effects. It is generally recognized that the unbound or absolutely free portion of a given hormone is the active form.[79] The concentration of unbound hormone then is a function of both the total hormone concentration and SHBG concentration, affinity, and capacity.[73] Changes in the extent of protein binding also dampen the effect of acute alterations in steroid secretion, thus maintaining a relatively stable free hormone level. The metabolic clearance rate and tissue extraction of a given steroid are inversely proportional to the extent of protein binding;[79] this may explain partially the lower potency and longer half-life of estrone sulfate.[80]

Different metabolic states and pathologic conditions influence both the levels of SHBG and free hormone, especially estradiol. It is known that conditions such as hyperthyroidism, cirrhosis, pregnancy, and estrogen therapy cause increased levels of SHBG,[79] whereas hypothyroidism, obesity, and androgen excess states are associated with decreased SHBG levels.[81] Obesity appears to be associated with target cell exposure to higher fractions of free estradiol due to efficient peripheral conversion of elevated androgenic precursors to estrogens and low SHBG levels. Siiteri has stressed that serum hormone levels, a function of production and metabolic clearance rates (MCR), do not always reflect true end-organ exposure. An obese woman with low SHBG levels, and therefore increased MCR and free estradiol levels, may be exposed to excessive amounts of active hormone despite normal serum levels.[81]

Several authors have suggested an active role for SHBG with regard to the association between estrogens and neoplasia, especially in uterine and breast cancer. Anderson first coined the term "estrogen amplifier" to describe the interaction between the transport protein and estradiol, noting increased free estradiol with low levels of SHBG.[82] De Moor noted an inverse correlation between weight and SHBG levels;[83] this was later confirmed by others.[84] Nisker showed higher percentages of free estradiol and lower levels of SHBG in women with endometrial cancer compared to postmenopausal controls, but this difference was not significant when women of similar weight were compared.[85] Davidson stressed that the obese postmenopausal woman has the dual risk of increased total estradiol levels and proportionately greater levels of free hormone when compared to a nonobese cohort.[86] He also noted a decreased binding capacity and an increased percentage of free estradiol in the face of normal SHBG concentrations in some women with breast cancer.[87] Although the etiology of this phenomenon is unknown, Siiteri has suggested that it may be due to a blood-borne, nonsteroidal lipid.[81] Thus, it would seem that in susceptible women, chronic exposure to elevated levels of free hormone mediated through SHBG may increase risks for breast[81,87,88] and endometrial cancer.[81,85,86]

METABOLISM, CONJUGATION, AND EXCRETION. The ultimate fate of estrogens, endogenous or exogenous, depends upon alterations occurring in their structure prior to elimination. Two terms are used frequently to describe these processes: metabolism and conjugation. Metabolism refers to biochemical transformations in the steroid moiety that are part of the activation or deactivation of a particular hormone. Conjugation refers to a specific metabolic transformation: the covalent linkage of a nonsteroidal substituent to the steroid moiety. This process usually involves addition of a more polar group, giving the steroid a greater solubility in water, thus facilitating excretion. Conjugation also can result in the formation of an intermediary steroid metabolite that may undergo further changes in the steroid nucleus to a more active form. Thus, while conjugation is included in the biotransformations during metabolism of steroid hormones, it has a second separate role for estrogens,[89] as will be emphasized in the discussion of the formation of the estrone sulfate pool.

Estrone Sulfate Pool. The natural estrogens undergo mainly oxidative metabolism. The initial step is a rapid and complete conversion of estradiol to estrone by 17β-dehydrogenase in the liver.[90] This process is reversible, but the equilibrium favors net formation of estrone. In humans, a distinct estrogenic intermediate exists in equilibrium with both estradiol and estrone, the conjugate estrone-3-sulfate.[80] It is formed in both liver and endometrium[91] by sulfurylation of estrone or estradiol and is found in higher concentrations in the peripheral circulation than either parent compound.[92,93]

Estrone sulfate is unique, for it is not secreted by any endocrine organ. Its production can be accounted for fully by conversion from estrone or estradiol.[80] Transfer constants reflect the extent to which this reversible equilibrium favors the formation of estrone sulfate: 54% of estrone and 65% of estradiol from both secretion and peripheral aromatization are converted to estrone sulfate, whereas only 1.4% of estradiol and 21% of estrone are formed from the sulfate intermediate (Fig. 5–5).[80] The reversible reactions that reform the parent compounds may occur in the liver by sulfatase and 17β-dehydrogenase catalyzed conversions.[94]

The metabolic fate of estrone sulfate in women has not been established, but it may be converted to estrone or estradiol in the liver[93] or in the target organ itself, e.g., the endometrium.[95] It has been shown that sulfurylation[95] and the activity of sulfatase[96] vary in the endometrium in a cyclic fashion and are inversely related, with the former yielding more of the inactive conjugate during the secretory phase.[97] One is tempted to postulate that this pool of estrone sulfate serves as a largely inactive reservoir for estradiol and estrone. Thus it is indirectly in equilibrium with free hormone and readily metabolized or formed in target tissues.

Steroid Nucleus Metabolism. After the initial conversion of estradiol to estrone, oxidative metabolism assumes a role of central importance. Within the endoplasmic reticulum of the liver, cytochrome P-450 dependent irreversible hydroxylation occurs with marked specificity. The major metabolic transformations involve reactions concerning either (1) the A ring, producing principally 2-hydroxyestrone or (2) the D ring producing estriol via 16α-hydroxyestrone. These pathways are competitive and mutually exclusive; they do not share interconversion of metabolic products.[98] Although es-

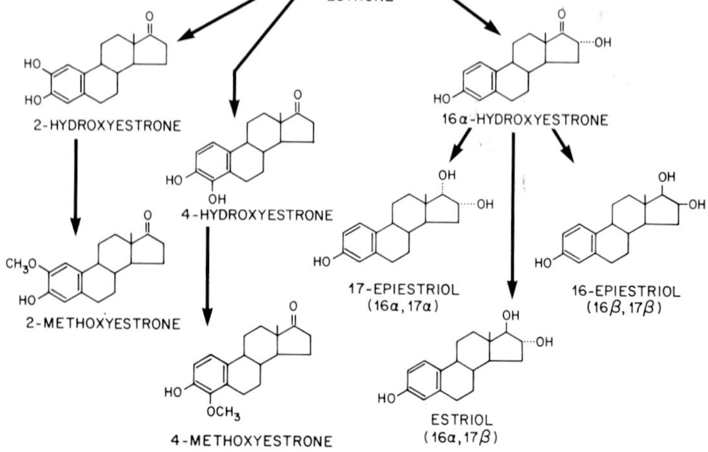

Fig. 5–5. Metabolism of the natural estrogens. Both estradiol and estrone exist in a reversible equilibrium with estrone sulfate, which may act as an inactive estrogen reservoir for both compounds. Once estrogen is metabolized to estrone by 17β-dehydrogenase, subsequent steps in degradation are principally oxidative. A-Ring hydroxylation produces catecholestrogens which then may undergo methylation prior to excretion. D-Ring metabolism produces mainly estriol with lesser amounts of the epiestriols.

triol previously was thought to be the main urinary excretory product of estradiol metabolism, 2-hydroxyestrone is quantitatively of equal importance.[99] Other metabolites of A-ring modulation, such as 4-hydroxyestrone, and D-ring metabolites such as the epiestriols, are formed but are of less significance (Fig. 5–5).

The competition and mutual exclusion of the two ring metabolic pathways are demonstrated in certain metabolic derangements. As will be described in the following section, the A-ring metabolites (catecholestrogens) have limited peripheral organ effects, but do bind to estrogen receptors; thus they may act as weak estrogens or antiestrogens. The D-ring metabolite estriol has been shown to bind to estrogen receptors[100] and with continuous infusion techniques has uterotrophic activity almost equal to estradiol.[101] Changes in metabolism of estradiol would tend to produce a hypoestrogenic state if D-ring metabolism were impeded, while decreased A-ring metabolism would enhance traditional end-organ response to estrogens. Body weight seems to influence estradiol metabolism. Women who have anorexia nervosa have impaired D-ring metabolism, whereas obese women tend to have fewer A-ring alterations.[102] Sensitivity to changes in thyroid hormone concentrations is demonstrated by impaired 16α-hydroxylation, favoring 2-hydroxylation in hyperthyroid patients; the reverse pattern is exhibited by hypothyroid persons.[103] Individuals with alcoholic cirrhosis have impaired formation of A-ring metabolites with increased formation of 16-hydroxyestrone, possibly potentiating the effects of endogenous estrogens.[104] Thus, amenorrhea, menstrual irregularities, gynecomastia, and other systemic metabolic derangements seen in the above disorders may be due in part to altered estrogen metabolism and may be reversed by correction of the underlying pathologic process.

Catecholestrogens. The catecholestrogens are a group of compounds whose existence has been known for many years, but whose importance has been realized, only recently. Due to their extreme instability, the catecholestrogens were difficult to obtain. As probable mediators of estrogenic activity, they have altered our concept of biologic activity with regard to the natural estrogens. Although their precise mechanism of action is yet to be determined, they may be important effectors of estrogen tissue specificity in target organs, especially in the central nervous system.

The catecholestrogens are so named because they possess adjacent hydroxyl groups on the phenolic A ring, either at C-2 and C-3 or C-3 and C-4 (Fig. 5–5). Although 2-hydroxyestrone is the most abundant catecholestrogen in the serum[105] and urine,[106] 2-hydroxyestradiol and 2-hydroxyestriol also are formed. 4-Hydroxylation also occurs; but the principal product, 4-hydroxyestrone, is present in only small amounts in urine.[107] The catecholestrogens have adjacent hydroxyl groups on an aromatic ring, as do the catecholamines dopa, dopamine, epinephrine, and norepinephrine; in addition they all are metabolized by methylation. Both 2- and 4-hydroxy estrogens are substrates for the enzyme catechol-*o*-methyl transferase (COMT) forming methoxy derivatives, and they are potent competitive inhibitors of COMT-mediated catecholamine degradation.[108]

Catecholestrogen formation occurs predominantly in liver tissue; but activity also has been documented in the pituitary, hypothalamus, and other peripheral organs.[109,110] Degradation occurs in the liver, brain, kidney, and erythrocytes via COMT and via conjugation mainly to glucuronides.[110] Due to the wide availability of inactivating enzymes, the half-life of 2-hydroxyestrone is very short, limiting its effectiveness as a circulating hormone.[111]

The biologic effects attributed to the catecholestrogens can be divided into two categories: (1) those traditional properties in peripheral organs and systems, usually reflected by uterotrophic assay; and (2) activities in the central nervous system, reflected by control of sexual behavior and neuroendocrine interrelationships. The 2- and 4-hydroxy compounds differ in observed effects on peripheral organs. 2-Hydroxyestrone and other catecholestrogen methoxy metabolites exhibit low affinity for uterine cytosolic receptors (affinity is a requirement for uterotrophic effect); estradiol, estrone, 4-hydroxyestrone, and estriol show higher affinity for the same receptors.[112] Curiously, in some studies 2-hydroxyestrone and its methoxy derivative have demonstrated negligible uterotrophic effect, whereas the 4-hydroxy catecholestrogens effected moderate changes in uterine weight.[113,114] These findings suggest that perhaps the 2-hydroxy compounds are peripheral antiestrogens,[115] a concept not confirmed by further studies, [114,116] which suggest that they are instead weak estrogens.[117] The influence on the central nervous system attributed to the catecholestrogens is less well understood, since peripheral administration of the compounds may not mimic central local formation and action. Since these compounds affect both catecholamine synthesis (by inhibiting tyrosine hydroxylase[118]) and metabolism (by inhibiting COMT[108]), it has been suggested that their central activity might be to alter the actions of biogenic amines that affect hypothalamic control of gonadotropin secretion,[119] thus explaining effects previously attributed to estradiol.[120] The effects of catecholestrogens on LH secretion and prolactin suppression are uncertain[110,121] and depend on dosage infused, the timing of measurements, the stage of the menstrual cycle, and other variables.[114–116,122] Recent evidence suggests that 2-hydroxyestrone is both a weak peripheral and central estrogen,[123] whereas 4-hydroxyestrone is a stronger peripheral estrogen with little central activity.[116]

In conclusion, it appears that both peripherally and locally synthesized catecholestrogens have important, albeit different, roles in the central nervous system and other target organs. The diversity of effects previously ascribed to estradiol may in part be explained by these compounds and their tissue-specific bioactivities.

Conjugation, Enterohepatic Circulation, and Excretion. Estrogens and their steroid nucleus metabolites are excreted predominantly as conjugates, mostly as glucuronides or sulfates, but also as double conjugates. As noted earlier, the process is thought to occur in the intestinal tract, during the first transit through the liver after absorption,[124] and in the kidney.[125] These now soluble compounds then undergo further metabolism or are excreted mainly in the urine; biliary and fecal excretion play a minor role in steroid excretion in humans owing to the enterohepatic circulation of steroid intermediates.

The prolonged effects of some orally admin-

istered estrogens have been attributed to the estrone sulfate pool, but some investigators have stressed the role of the estrogen "trap" formed by the enterohepatic circulation involving biliary excretion of estrogen metabolites.[89] It appears that the active estrogens enter this second pool readily in proportional amounts: 65% of estradiol, about 50% of estrone, and 23% of estriol are present in bile, predominantly as D-ring metabolites.[126] Using estradiol or estrone as examples, approximately one-half of an injected dose can be accounted for through urinary excretion, with the remainder found in the bile during the first 24 hours.[127] The biliary estrogens, which are mostly in a conjugated state, undergo hydrolysis and approximately 80% are reabsorbed. The reabsorbed estrogens are either (1) reconjugated locally and returned to the liver to repeat the biliary cycle or be excreted; (2) returned to the liver where they are again conjugated and then excreted in the urine or bile; or (3) returned to the liver, escaping conjugation, and then released into the systemic circulation as free hormone.[127] After oral administration of labeled estrogen, dual peaks of estrogen conjugates are recovered in the urine 4 to 5 hours apart, reflecting the reappearance of the enterohepatic metabolites in the circulation.[128] Over a 4- to 6-day period, 50–80% of the injected steroid will be excreted in urine, whereas only about 10% ultimately will be lost in feces.

Although further discussion of conjugation and the enterohepatic circulation is beyond the scope of this section, several interesting points merit mention. Two unique conjugates are associated with the biliary excretion and reabsorption process. The double conjugate estriol-3-sulfate-16-glucuronide is the principal estrogenic metabolite in bile,[129] with other glucuronides present in lesser amounts. Estriol-3-glucuronide is formed uniquely during reabsorption and intestinal mucosal conjugation; subsequently it is excreted rapidly without further metabolism, making it a good marker for evaluation of the functional state of the enterohepatic circulation.[130] Various gastrointestinal disorders that alter or disrupt the enterohepatic circulation may diminish estrogen effects.[126] Antibiotic administration may decrease estrogen reabsorption and alter expression of bioactivity by decreasing hydrolysis by intestinal bacteria prior to reabsorption of the estrogen conjugates.[131]

Synthetic Estrogens. The synthetic steroidal estrogens mestranol and ethinyl estradiol are of particular interest, for they long have been known to be more potent oral agents than the naturally occurring estrogens. It was thought previously that the intestinal and initial-pass liver metabolism noted with oral administration of the natural estrogens was avoided, owing to steric hindrance of 16α-hydroxylation by the 17α-ethinyl group present on both compounds. Thus, theoretically more active hormone was presented to the systemic circulation, explaining the greater bioactivity seen with oral synthetic agents. Bolt believes that the lack of D-ring metabolism of ethinyl estradiol is due to preferential 16α-hydroxylation of estrone rather than the synthetic compound in the liver.[132] It is known that ethinyl estradiol is the biologically active form of both synthetic compounds.[133] In the liver, mestranol undergoes C-3 demethylation, which converts it to ethinyl estradiol. This is reflected by a delayed rise in serum levels of the latter compound after oral administration of mestranol.[69] The demethylation appears to be about 54% effective,[134] which agrees with the relative potency of the two drugs.

The degradation and excretion of mestranol and ethinyl estradiol proceed in a manner analogous to that of estradiol, with several exceptions. With D-ring metabolism impeded, biologic alteration occurs predominantly in the A ring, characteristically at C-2.[135] Conjugation occurs to an appreciable extent, reflected by the presence of glucuronides in urinary excretion.[136] An ethinyl estradiol sulfate pool exists which is similar to that of estrone, possibly explaining its delayed clearance from the circulation.[137] Unlike the natural estrogens, lesser amounts of the metabolites of mestranol and ethinyl estradiol are excreted in urine with greater biliary and fecal excretion[132] despite an active enterohepatic circulation.[138]

Several other synthetic nonsteroidal and steroidal estrogens are used in therapy in the menopause; for information on the metabolism of all but diethylstilbestrol, the reader is directed to several excellent recent reviews.[132,139] The stilbene derivative, DES, undergoes conjugation to glucuronides prior to excretion in urine and feces,[72] but also undergoes several oxidative steps, the products of which are epoxides, semiquinones, and quinones that may bind covalently with nucleic acids and proteins of DNA.[140] The oncogenic potential of DES in susceptible tissues has been investigated extensively.[141]

INTERACTION WITH TARGET ORGAN: ESTROGEN RECEPTORS. The interaction of the estrogens with specific receptors in hormone-sensitive tissues is the final common pathway in expression of the biologic effects of these compounds. Estrogen receptors are found in the cytoplasm of estrogen-sensitive tissues and function by selective high-affinity binding of steroid hormones to begin the process of transforming molecular events into physiologic responses.[142] The relative binding affinities of the estrogenic hormones are reflective of the hormones' potency as peripheral estrogens. Ethinyl estradiol, estradiol, estrone, DES, 4-hydroxyestrone, and estriol are bound with significant affinity, whereas 2-hydroestrone and estrogen sulfates demonstrate low binding affinity.[112,143–145]

The mechanism of estrogen interaction with the individual cell in estrogen-sensitive tissue is common to all steroid-sensitive tissues. It involves diffusion of free hormone into the cytoplasm, followed by translocation of a receptor-hormone complex to the nucleus.[146] The free hormone circulating in the plasma is generally agreed to be the biologically active form. Both the concentration of unbound hormone and its receptor affinity determine the degree of receptor binding.[79] Target organs also may contribute to the expression of bioactivity by metabolizing active forms to less active metabolites or to conjugates which do not bind to receptors. This is seen in secretory phase endometrium, which demonstrates increased 17β-estradiol dehydrogenase[147] and sulfotransferase[91] activities. Conversely, synthetic compounds (such as mestranol[134] and quinestrol,[71] which have low estrogen receptor affinity) must be metabolized to their active form, ethinyl estradiol, which has a high receptor affinity. This last observation supports the hypothesis that the phenolic C-3 hydroxyl group is essential for estrogenic effect.[143]

Unbound estrogen diffuses freely into the cytoplasm of sensitive tissue cells, binding initially to the estrogen receptor. The estrogen has a higher affinity for the receptor than for its circulating transport protein. The interaction is a specific, reversible, noncovalent binding. The cell has a limited number of receptors; thus estrogen binding is a saturable process. The receptor is a macromolecular protein that seems to exist in one of several forms, defined by patterns of migration in sucrose density gradient ultracentrifugation analysis. Under hypotonic conditions the receptor sedimentation pattern is 8S (molecular weight, about 236,000 daltons), whereas more hypertonic conditions show a 4S (molecular weight, 61,000 daltons) migration. It may be that the 8S form is an aggregation of molecules that dissociates in the more hypertonic state.[148] Although not demonstrated conclusively, the 4S form is thought to be the native form of the receptor in the cytoplasm. An intermediate 5S form (molecular weight, 110,000–130,000 daltons) also has been detected and is thought to be the active form of the receptor molecule in the nucleus of the hormone-sensitive cell.

Once estrogen is bound by the native receptor protein in the cytoplasm, it is translocated to the nucleus.[142] During this step the receptor-hormone complex undergoes a conformational change or transformation[149] to a form with higher affinity for acceptor sites on nuclear chromatin.[150] It is not known if this processing occurs before, during, or after translocation to the nucleus, but this activated form appears to be the 5S complex.[144] After binding with nuclear chromatin, transcription is initiated with a subsequent increase in RNA polymerase activity.[151] As a result, synthesis of messenger and total RNA is enhanced. This is followed by an increase in directed protein synthesis in the ribosomes. The newly synthesized protein may then have a local effect, altering intrinsic cellular mechanisms (e.g., cellular proliferation); or it may be released into the circulation to affect other organs and systems.

Cytosolic estrogen receptors are replenished following translocation of the estrogen-receptor complex to the nucleus. This process is essential to the continued responsiveness of the cell to further exposure to free estrogen. It appears that both recycling of receptors after dissociation from estrogen[152] as well as an estrogen-stimulated de novo synthesis of new receptor proteins are involved.[153] The latter process is inhibited by progesterone, which has been shown to block full replenishment after treatment with estradiol and progesterone in rats.[154]

A group of compounds called "antiestrogens" has been used for the induction of ovulation in infertility, in treatment of hormone-sensitive tumors, and as a cyclic adjunct to hormone replacement therapy.[155] The term "antiestrogen" is a misnomer, for these compounds bind estrogen receptors and in short-term use act as weak estrogens.[156] They may act as competitive inhibitors of actual estrogen binding with receptors; or, more importantly, they may block replenishment of cytoplasmic receptor levels. This is accomplished by prolonged nuclear retention of the antiestrogen-receptor complex.[157] This impairs the recycling process, lowers the cytosolic receptor level, and renders the cell less capable of responding to further estrogen availability.[158] Examples of these compounds, which are nonsteroidal synthetic analogs, include tamoxifene, nafoxidine, and hydrochlorine clomiphene citrate (Fig. 5–6). The chemistry and use of antiestrogens have been reviewed recently by Devi.[156]

Clinical Implications. Both estrogen and progesterone receptors have been shown to play an important role in treatment planning and in the prognosis for tumors involving estrogen-dependent tissues, e.g., endometrial carcinoma (see Chapter 8) and breast carcinoma. Approximately 75% of breast carcinomas contain significant levels of estrogen receptors.[158] Prior to the advent of estrogen receptor assays, approximately 30% of patients responded to endocrine therapy (ablative surgery, estrogens, corticosteroids, or antiestrogens). With the ability to detect and then treat receptor-positive tumors, regression after endocrine therapy can be expected in 56%, whereas only 10% of receptor-negative tumors will respond to this therapy.[158] Progesterone receptors are present in most estrogen-sensitive tissues. The synthesis of these proteins is estrogen-induced, and their levels reflect the responsiveness of the tissue to estrogen. Indeed, using the presence of both hormonal receptors as a guide to therapy, almost 80% of patients can be shown to respond to endocrine therapy,[159] giving the clinician an excellent

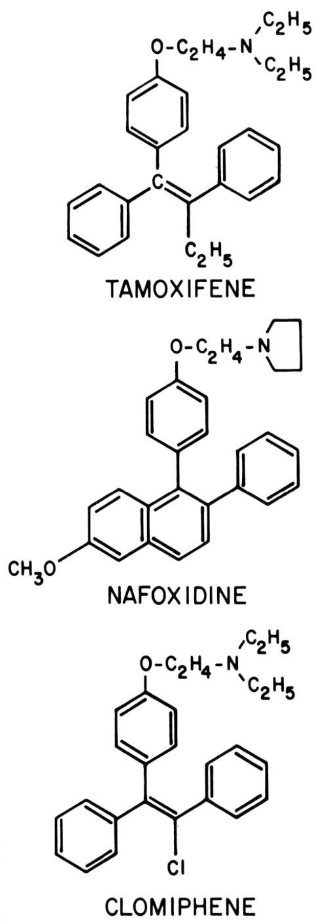

Fig. 5–6. The antiestrogens.

means to select the most hormone-sensitive tumors prior to treatment. Other recent investigations have shown higher rates of DNA synthesis[160] and more frequent recurrences in patients with tumors that lack estrogen receptors.[161] It was hoped that the lack of estrogen receptors in a tumor might reflect a more aggressive tumor that would respond to cytotoxic chemotherapy. Available studies have not supported the concept of using receptor status as a criterion for instituting systemic chemotherapy.[162–164]

Summary

Although much is known about the paradoxical physiologic hormone-deficient state in the menopause, the ideal method of estrogen replacement is still uncertain. Both structure and formulation are important in selecting a route of administration, which then determines ab-

sorption and early metabolism. Although conclusive evidence is lacking, the unphysiologic levels and proportions of estrone and estradiol after certain forms of administration may play a role in increasing risks for untoward side-effects. Different pathologic states may alter estrogen metabolism, producing compounds with more potent effects in hormone-sensitive tissues, probably causing increased risks for neoplasia in these organs. The best method of estrogen replacement therapy is one with the lowest risk/benefit ratio for the particular patient: it must relieve undesired menopausal symptoms while avoiding systemic effects of estrogen replacement. With an understanding of the chemistry, metabolism, and mechanism of action of the various estrogenic preparations, the clinician should be better equipped to formulate a treatment plan and individualize therapy for the menopausal patient.

REFERENCES

1. Murray JA, Bradley H, Craigie WA, Onions CT. The Oxford English dictionary, Vol 7. Oxford: Clarendon Press, 1933: (letter O)66.
2. Speert H. Iconographia gyniatrica: a pictorial history of gynecology and obstetrics. Philadelphia: Davis, 1973:1–42.
3. van Horne, JC. Opuscula Anatomico-chirurgica. Leipzig: Thomas Fritschius, 1707.
4. Baer KE. De Ovi Mammalium et Hominis Benesi. Leipzig: L Voss, 1827.
5. Kurzrok R. The endocrines in obstetrics and gynecology. Baltimore: Williams & Wilkins, 1937:1–8.
6. Hegar A. Die Castration Der Frauen. Leipzig: Breitkopf Hartel, 1878.
7. Brown-Séquard CE. Demontrant la poissance dynamogenique chez l'homme d'un liquide extrait de testicules d'animaux. Arch Physiol. 1889; 21:651–658.
8. Greenblatt RB. Some historic and biblical aspects of endocrinology. In: Givens JR, ed. Gynecologic endocrinology. Chicago: Yearbook Medical, 1976:313–324.
9. Mainzer F. Vorshlag zur Behandlung der Ausfallserscheinungen nach Castration. Dtsche Med Wochenschr. 1896; 22:188.
10. Morris RT. The ovarian graft. NY Med J. 1895; 62:436–437.
11. Fraenkel L. Die Funktion des corpus luteum. Arch Gynaekol. 1903; 68:438–545.
12. Burnam CF. Corpus luteum extract. JAMA. 1912; 59:698–703.
13. Knauer E. Einige Verusche uber Ovarien-

transplantation bei Kaninchen. Zentralbl Gynekol. 1896; 20:524–528.

14. Knauer E. Die Ovarientransplantation. Experimentelle Studie. Arch Gynaekol. 1900; 60:322–376.

15. Halban J. Ueber den Einfluss der Ovarien auf die Entwicklung des Genitales. Monatschr Geb Gynakol. 1900; 12:496–506.

16. Adler L. Zur Physiologie und Pathologie der Ovarialfunktion. Arch Gynaekol. 1912; 95:349–424.

17. Iscovesco H. Le lipoipe utero-stimulant de l'ovarie proprietes physiologiques. CR Soc Biol. 1912; 73:104–106.

18. Fellner 00. Untersuchungen über die Wirkung von Gewebsextrakten aus der Placenta und den weiblichen Sexualorganen auf das Genitale. Arch Gynaekol. 1913; 100:641-719.

19. Frank RT. The ovary and the endocrinologist. JAMA. 1922; 78:181–185.

20. Allen E, Doisy EA. An ovarian hormone: A preliminary report on its localization, extraction, and partial purification and action in test animals. JAMA. 1923; 81:819–821.

21. Stockard CR, Papanicolaou GN. The existence of a typical oestrus cycle in the guinea pig—with a study of its histological and physiological changes. Am J Anat. 1917; 22:225–283.

22. Aschheim S, Zondek B. Hypophysenvorderlappenhormon und Ovarialhormon im Harn von Schwangeren. Klin Wochenschr. 1927; 6:1322.

23. Zondek B. Die Hormone des Ovariums und des Hypophysenvorderlappens. Berlin: Springer, 1931.

24. Doisy EA, Veler CD, Thayer SA. Folliculin from the urine of pregnant women. Am J Physiol. 1929; 90:329–330.

25. Butenandt A. Uber Progynon ein kristallisiertes weibliches Sexualhormon. Naturwissenschaften. 1929; 17:879.

26. Marrian GF. Chemistry of oestrin; improved method of preparation and isolation of active crystalline material. Biochem J. 1930; 24:435–445.

27. Butenandt A. Uber physikalische und chemische Eigenschaften des krystallisierten Follikelhormons. Hoppe-Seyler's Physiol Chem. 1930; 191:140–156.

28. MacCorquodale DW, Thayer SA, Doisy EA. The isolation of the principle estrogenic substance of liquor folliculi. J Biol Chem. 1936; 115:435–448.

29. Dodds EC, Goldberg L, Lawson W, Robinson R. Oestrogenic activity of certain synthetic compounds. Nature. 1938; 141:247–248.

30. Inhoffen HH, Hohlweg W. Neue per oswirksame weibliche Keimdrusenhormon Derivate: 17-Aethinyl-oestradiol und Pregnen-inon-3-ol-17. Naturwissenschaften. 1938; 26:96.

31. Murad F, Haynes RC. Estrogens and progestins. In: Gilman AG, Goodman LS, Gilman A, eds. The pharmacological basis of therapeutics. New York: MacMillan, 1980:1420–1447.

32. Edgren R. The biology and chemistry of progestogens and estrogens used in therapy. In: Gold JJ, Josimovich JB, eds. Gynecologic endocrinology. Philadelphia: Lippincott, 1980:369–384.

33. Ryan KJ. Steroid hormones and prostaglandins. In: Reid DE, Ryan KJ, Benirschke K, eds. Principles and management of human reproduction. Philadelphia: Saunders, 1972:4-27.

34. Short RV. Steroids in the follicular fluid and the corpus luteum of the mare. A "two cell type" theory of ovarian steroid synthesis. J Endocrinol. 1962; 24:59–63.

35. Yen SSC. The human menstrual cycle. In: Yen SSC, Jaffe RB, eds. Reproductive endocrinology. Philadelphia: Saunders, 1978:126-151.

36. Ryan KJ, Petro Z, Kaiser J. Steroid formation by isolated and recombined ovarian granulosa and thecal cells. J Clin Endocrinol. 1968; 20:355–358.

37. Erickson GF. Follicular growth and development. In: Sciarra JJ, Speroff L, Simpson JL, eds. Gynecology and obstetrics, Vol. 5. Hagerstown: Harper & Row, 1982:(12)1–16.

38. Erickson GF. Normal ovarian function. Clin Obstet Gynecol. 1978; 21:31–52.

39. Ryan KJ. Endocrine organs of reproduction—ovary. In: Reid DE, Ryan KJ, Benirschke K, eds. Principles and management of human reproduction. Philadelphia: Saunders, 1972: 72–81.

40. Rigg LA, Hermann H, Yen SSC. Absorption of estrogen from vaginal creams. N Engl J Med. 1978; 298:195–197.

41. Ryan KJ, Engel LL. The interconversion of estrone and estradiol by human tissue slices. Endocrinology. 1953; 52:287–291.

42. Fincher JH. Particle size of drugs and its relation to absorption and activity. J Pharmacol Sci. 1968; 57:1825–1835.

43. Martin PL, Burnier AM, Greaney MO. Oral menopausal therapy using 17β micronized estradiol. Obstet Gynecol. 1972; 39:771–774.

44. Callantine MR, Martin PL, Bolding OT, Warner PO, Greaney MO. Micronized 17β estradiol for oral estrogen therapy in menopausal women. Obstet Gynecol. 1975; 46:37–41.

45. Yen SSC, Martin PL, Burnier AM, et al. Circulating estradiol, estrone, and gonadotropin levels following the administration of orally active 17β estradiol in postmenopausal

women. J Clin Endocrinol Metab. 1975; 40:518–521.

46. Judd HL, Judd GE, Lucas WE, Yen SC. Endocrine function of the postmenopausal ovary: Concentration of androgens and estrogens in ovarian and peripheral vein blood. J Clin Endocrinol Metab. 1974; 39:1020–1024.

47. Grodin JM, Siiteri PK, MacDonald PC. Source of estrogen production in postmenopausal women. J Clin Endocrinol Metab. 1973; 36:207–214.

48. Rigg LA, Milanes B, Villanueva B, Yen SSC. Efficacy of intravaginal and intranasal administration of micronized estradiol 17-β. J Clin Endocrinol Metab. 1977; 45:1261–1264.

49. Schiff I, Tulchinsky D, Ryan KJ. Vaginal absorption of estrone and 17β-estradiol. Fertil Steril. 1977; 28:1063–1066.

50. Martin P, Yen SSC, Burnier AM, Hermann H. Systemic absorption and sustained effects of vaginal estrogen creams. JAMA 1979; 242:2699–2700.

51. Longcope C, Tait JF. Validity of metabolic clearance and interconversion rates of estrone and 17β-estradiol in normal adults. J Clin Endocrinol Metab. 1971; 32:481–489.

52. Longcope C, Williams KIH. The metabolism of estrogens in normal women after pulse injections of ³H-estradiol and ³H-estrone. J Clin Endocrinol Metab. 1974; 38:602–607.

53. Stumpf PG, Maruca J, Santen RJ, Demers LM. Development of a vaginal ring for achieving physiologic levels of 17β-estradiol in hypoestrogenic women. J Clin Endocrinol Metab. 1982; 54:208–210.

54. Casper RF, Yen SSC. Rapid absorption of micronized estradiol-17β following sublingual administration. Obstet Gynecol. 1980; 57:62–64.

55. Burnier AM, Martin PL, Yen SSC, Brooks P. Sublingual absorption of micronized 17β-estradiol. Am J Obstet Gynecol. 1981; 140:146–150.

56. Lyrenas S, Carlstrom K, Backstrom T, Von Scoultz B. A comparison of serum oestrogen levels after percutaneous and oral administration of oestradiol-17β. Br J Obstet Gynecol. 1981; 88:181–187.

57. Whitehead MI, Townsend PT, Kitchin Y, et al. Plasma steroid and protein hormone profiles in postmenopausal women following topical administration of oestradiol 17β. In: Mauvais-Jarvis P, Vickers CF, Wepierre J, eds. Percutaneous absorption of steroids. London: Academic Press, 1980:231–248.

58. Basdevant A, de Lignieres B. Treatment of menopause by topical administration of oestradiol. In: Mauvais-Jarvis P, Vickers CF, We-

pierre J, eds. Percutaneous absorption of steroids. London: Academic Press, 1980: 249–258.

59. Greenblatt RB, Bryner JR. Estradiol pellet implantation in the management of menopause. J Reprod Med. 1977; 18:307–316.

60. Jarolim C, Bernard LI, Strauss H. Estrogenic substitution therapy with estradiol pellet implantation. Am J Obstet Gynecol. 1966; 94:170–177.

61. Carol J, Kunze FM, Banes D. Analysis of conjugated estrogen preparations. J Pharmacol Sci. 1961; 50:550–555.

62. Englund DE, Johansson EDB. Plasma levels of oestrone, oestradiol, and gonadotropins in postmenopausal women after oral and vaginal administration of conjugated equine oestrogens (Premarin). Br J Obstet Gynecol. 1978; 85:957–964.

63. Townsend PT, Dyer GI, Young O, Whitehead MI, Collins WP. The absorption and metabolism of oral oestradiol, oestrone and oestriol. Br J Obstet Gynecol. 1981; 88:846–852.

64. Morgan MRA, Whittaker PG, Dean PD, et al. Plasma equilin concentrations in an oophorectomized woman following ingestion of conjugated equine oestrogens (Premarin). Eur J Clin Invest. 1979; 9:473–474.

65. Dickfalusy E, Levitz, M. Formation, metabolism and transport of estrogen conjugates. In: Bernstein S, Solomon S, eds. Chemical and biological aspects of steroid conjugation. New York: Springer-Verlag, 1970:291–320.

66. Schiff I, Tulchinsky D, Ryan K, et al. Plasma estriol and its conjugates following oral and vaginal administration of estriol to postmenopausal women: Correlations with gonadotropin levels. Am J Obstet Gynecol. 1980; 138:1137–1141.

67. Cargill DI, Steinetz BG, Gosnill E, et al. Fate of ingested radiolabeled ethynylestradiol and its 3-cyclopentyl ether in patients with bile fistulas. J Clin Endocrinol Metab. 1969; 29:1051–1061.

68. Warren RJ, Fotherby K. Plasma levels of ethynyloestradiol after administration of ethynyloestradiol or mestranol to human subjects. J Endocrinol. 1973; 59:369–370.

69. de la Pena A, Chenault CB, Goldzieher JW. Radioimmunoassay of unconjugated plasma ethynylestradiol in women given a single oral dose of ethynylestradiol or mestranol. Steroids. 1975; 25:773–780.

70. Goldzieher JW, Tazewell SD, de la Pena A. Plasma levels and pharmacokinetics of ethynyl estrogens in various populations. II. Mestranol. Contraception. 1980; 21:17–27.

71. Williams KI, Layne DS, Hobkirk R, Nilsen M. Metabolism of doubly-labelled ehtynylestra-

diol-3-cyclopentyl ether in women. Steroids. 1967; 9:275–287.

72. Metzler M. Metabolic activation of carcinogenic diethylstilbestrol in rodents and humans. J Toxicol Environ Health. 1976; 1(S):21–35.

73. Anderson DC. The role of sex hormone binding globulin in health and disease. In: James VHT, Serio M, Guisti G, eds. The endocrine function of the human ovary. London: Academic Press, 1976:141–158.

74. Moll GW, Rosenfield RL, Helke JH. Estradiol-testosterone binding interactions and free plasma estradiol under physiologic conditions. J Clin Endocrinol Metab. 1981; 52:868–874.

75. Rosenthal HE, Pietrzak E, Slaunwhite WR, Sanberg AA. Binding of estrone sulfate in human plasma. J Clin Endocrinol Metab. 1972; 34:805–813.

76. Murphy BE. Protein binding and radioassays of estrogens and progestins. In: Greep RO, Astwood EB, eds. Handbook of physiology, Vol. 2. Washington, DC: American Physiologic Society, 1973:631–642.

77. Chung-Hsiu W, Motohashi T, Abdel-Rahman HA, Flickinger GL, Mikhail G. Free and protein bound plasma estradiol 17β during the menstrual cycle. J Clin Endocrinol Metab. 1976; 43:436–445.

78. O'Brien TJ, Higashi M, Kanasugi A, et al. A plasma/serum estrogen-binding protein distinct from testosterone-estradiol-binding globulin. J Clin Endocrinol Metab. 1982; 54:793–797.

79. Anderson DC. Sex-hormone binding globulin. Clin Endocrinol. 1974; 3:69–96.

80. Ruder HJ, Loriaux L, Lipsett MB. Estrone sulfate production rate and metabolism in man. J Clin Invest. 1972; 51:1020–1033.

81. Siiteri PI. Extraglandular oestrogen formation and serum binding of oestradiol: Relationship to cancer. J Endocrinol. 1981; 89:119–129.

82. Burke CW, Anderson DC. Sex-hormone binding globulin is an oestrogen amplifier. Nature. 1972; 240:38–40.

83. De Moor P, Joossens JV. An inverse correlation between body weight and the activity of the steroid binding globulin in human plasma. Steroidologia. 1970; 1:129–136.

84. Nisker JA, Hammond GL, Siiteri PK. More on fatness and reproduction. N Engl J Med. 1980; 303:1124.

85. Nisker JA, Hammond GL, Davidson BJ, et al. Serum sex hormone-binding globulin capacity and the percentage of free estradiol in postmenopausal women with and without endometrial carcinoma. Am J Obstet Gynecol. 1980; 138:637–642.

86. Davidson BJ, Gambone JC, Lagasse LD, et al. Free estradiol in postmenopausal women with and without endometrial cancer. J Clin Endocrinol Metab. 1981; 52:404–408.

87. Hammond GL, Nisker JA, Siiteri PK. Elevated percent free estradiol in breast cancer patients. Proc Soc Gynecol Invest. Denver 1980; 90, Abstract.

88. Nisker JA, Siiteri PK. Estrogen and breast cancer. Clin Obstet Gynecol. 1981; 24:301–322.

89. Slaunwhite WR, Kirdani RY, Sandberg AA. Metabolic aspects of estrogens in man. In: Greep RO, Astwood EB, eds. Handbook of physiology, Vol. 2. Washington, DC: American Physiologic Society, 1973:485–523.

90. Fishman J, Bradlow HL, Gallagher TF. Oxidative metabolism of estradiol. J Biol Chem. 1960; 235:3104–3107.

91. Pack BA, Tovar R, Booth E, Brooks SC. The cyclic relationship of estrogen sulfurylation to the nuclear receptor level in human endometrial curettings. J Clin Endocrinol Metab. 1979; 48:420–424.

92. Loriaux DL, Ruder HJ, Lipsett MB. The measurement of estrone sulfate in plasma. Steroids. 1971; 18:463–472.

93. Roberts KD, Rochefort JG, Bleau G, Chapdelaine A. Plasma estrone sulfate levels in postmenopausal women. Steroids. 1980; 35:179–187.

94. Roy AB. Enzymological aspects of steroid conjugation. In: Bernstein S, Solomon S, eds. Chemical and Biological Aspects of Steroid Conjugation. New York: Springer-Verlag, 1970:74–130.

95. Hahnel R, Twaddle E, Ratajczak T. The specificity of the estrogen receptor of human uterus. J Steroid Biochem. 1973; 4:21–31.

96. Gurpide E, Stoles A, Tseng L. Quantitative studies of tissue uptake and disposition of hormones. Acta Endocrinol (Suppl). 1971; 153:247–278.

97. Hawkins RA, Oakey RE. Estimation of oestrone sulfate, oestradiol-17β and oestrone in peripheral plasma: Concentrations during the menstrual cycle and in men. J Endocrinol. 1974; 60:3–17.

98. Fishman J, Cox RI, Gallagher TF. 2-Hydroxyestrone: a new metabolite of estradiol in man. Arch Biochem Biophys. 1960; 90:318–319.

99. Fishman J. Role of 2-hydroxyestrone in estrogen metabolism. J Clin Endocrinol Metab. 1963; 23:207–210.

100. Anderson JN, Peck JN, Clark JH. Estrogen-induced uterine responses and growth: Relationship to receptor estrogen binding by uterine nuclei. Endocrinology. 1975; 96:160–167.

101. Fishman J, Martucci CP. New concepts of es-

trogenic activity: The role of metabolites in the expression of hormone action. In: Pasetto N, Paoletti R, Ambrus JL, eds. The menopause and postmenopause. Lancaster: MTP Press, 1980:43–52.

102. Fishman J, Boyar RM, Hellman L. Influence of body weight on estradiol metabolism in young women. J Clin Endocrinol Metab. 1975; 41:989–991.

103. Fishman J, Hellman L, Zumoff B, Gallagher TF. Effect of thyroid on hydroxylation of estrogen in man. J Clin Endocrinol Metab. 1965; 25:365–368.

104. Zumoff B, Fishman J, Gallagher TF, Hellman L. Estradiol metabolism in cirrhosis. J Clin Invest. 1968; 47:20–25.

105. Yoshizawa I, Fishman J. Radioimmunoassay of 2-hydroxyestrone and 2-methoxyestrone in human placenta. J Clin Endocrinol Metab. 1971; 32:3–6.

106. Ball P, Gelbke HP, Knuppen R. The excretion of 2-hydroxyestrone during the menstrual cycle. J Clin Endocrinol Metab. 1975; 40:406–408.

107. Williams JG, Longcope C, Williams KJH. 4-Hydroxyestrone: A new metabolite of estradiol-17β from humans. Steroids. 1974; 24:687–701.

108. Ball P, Knuppen R, Haupt M, Breuer H. Interactions between estrogens and catecholamines. III. Studies on the methylation of catechol estrogens, catecholamines and other catechols by the catechol-o-methyltransferase of human liver. J Clin Endocrinol Metab. 1972; 34:736–746.

109. Ball D, Haupt M, Knuppen R. Comparative studies on the metabolism of oestradiol in the brain, the pituitary and liver of the rat. Acta Endocrinol. 1978; 87:1–11.

110. MacLusky NJ, Naftolin F, Krey LC, Franks S. The catecholestrogens. J Steroid Biochem. 1981; 15:111–124.

111. Merriam GR, Brandon DO, Kono S, et al. Rapid metabolic clearance of the catecholestrogen 2-hydroxyestrone. J Clin Endocrinol Metab. 1980; 51:1211–1213.

112. Martucci C, Fishman J. Uterine estrogen receptor binding of catechol estrogens and estetrol. Steroids. 1976; 27:325–333.

113. Martucci C, Fishman J. Direction of estradiol metabolism as a control of its hormonal action—uterotrophic activity of estradiol metabolites. Endocrinology. 1977; 101:1709–1715.

114. Martucci C, Fishman J. Impact of continuously administered catecholestrogens on uterine growth and LH secretion. Endocrinology. 1979; 105:1288–1292.

115. Naftolin F, Morishita H, Davies J, et al. 2-Hydroxyestrone induced rise in serum luteinizing hormone in the immature male rat. Biochem Biophys Res Commun. 1975; 64:905–910.

116. Ball P, Emons G, Gethmann U. Effect of low doses of continuously administered catecholestrogens on peripheral and central target organs. Acta Endocrinol. 1981; 96:470–474.

117. Jellinck PH, Krey L, Davis PG, et al. Central and peripheral action of estradiol and catecholestrogens administered at low concentration by constant infusion. Endocrinology. 1981; 108:1848–1854.

118. Lloyd T, Weisz J. Direct inhibition of tyrosine hydroxylase activity by catecholestrogens. J Biol Chem. 1978; 253:4841–4843.

119. Frohman LA. Neurotransmitters as regulators of endocrine function. Hosp Pract. 1975; 10(4):54–67.

120. Cramer OM, Parker CR, Porter JC. Estrogen inhibition of dopamine release into hypophysial portal blood. Endocrinology. 1979. 104:419–422.

121. Fishman J. Biological action of catecholestrogens. J Endocrinol. 1981; 89:59–65.

122. Schinfield JS, Tulchinsky D, Schiff I, Fishman J. Suppression of prolactin and gonadotropin secretion in postmenopausal women by 2-hydroxyestrone. J Clin Endocrinol Metab. 1980; 50:408–410.

123. Merriam GR, Kono S, Loriaux DL, Lipsett MB. Does 2-hydroxyestrone suppress prolactin in women? J Clin Endocrinol Metab. 1982; 54:753–756.

124. Fishman J, Goldberg S, Rosenfeld RS, et al. Intermediates in the transformation of oral estradiol. J Clin Endocrinol. 1969; 29:41–46.

125. Kirdani RY, Sampson D, Murphy GP, Sandberg AA. Studies on phenolic steroids in human subjects. XVI. Role of the kidney in the disposition of estriol. J Clin Endocrinol Metab. 1972; 34:546–557.

126. Aldercreutz H, Martin F. Biliary excretion and intestinal metabolism of progesterone and estrogens in man. J Steroid Biochem. 1980; 13:231–244.

127. Sandberg A, Slaunwhite WR. Studies on phenolic steroids in human subjects. II. The metabolic fate and hepato-biliary-enteric circulation of C^{14}-estrone and C^{14}-estradiol in women. J Clin Invest. 1957; 36:1266–1278.

128. Howard CM, Robinson H, Schmidt FH, et al. Evidence for a two-pool system governing the excretion of radioactive urinary estrogen conjugates during the first 8 hours following the administration of estrone-6,7-^{3}H to male subjects. Probable role of the enterohepatic circu-

lation. J Clin Endocrinol Metab. 1969; 29:1618–1629.

129. Støa KF, Skulstad PA. Biliary and urinary metabolites of intravenously and intraduodenally administered 17β-oestradiol and oestriol. Steroid Lipid Res. 1972; 3:299–314.

130. Aldercreutz H. Hepatic metabolism of estrogens in health and disease. N Engl J Med. 1974; 290:1081–1083.

131. Aldercreutz N, Martin F, Pulkkinen M, et al. Intestinal metabolism of estrogens. J Clin Endocrinol Metab. 1976; 43:497–505.

132. Bolt HM, Metabolism of estrogens—natural and synthetic. Pharmacol Ther. 1979; 4:155–181.

133. Kappus H, Bolt HM, Remmer H. Affinity of ethynyl-estradiol and mestranol for the uterine estrogen receptor and for microsomal mixed function oxidase of the liver. J Steroid Biochem. 1973; 41:121–128.

134. Bolt HM, Bolt WH. Pharmacokinetics of mestranol in man in relation to its estrogenic activity. Eur J Clin Pharmacol. 1974; 7:295–305.

135. Bolt WH, Kappus H, Bolt HM. Ring A oxidation of 17α-ethinylestradiol in man. Horm Metab Res. 1974; 6:432.

136. Stimmel BF, May JA, Randolph JA, Conn WM. The metabolism of ethinyl estradiol in man. J Clin Endocrinol Metab. 1951; 11:408–415.

137. Bird CE, Clark AF. Metabolic clearance rates and metabolism of mestranol and ethynylestradiol in normal young women. J Clin Endocrinol Metab. 1973; 36:296–302.

138. Hanasono GK, Fischer LJ. The excretion of tritium-labeled chlormanidone acetate, mestranol norethindrone and norethynodrel in rats and the enterohepatic circulation of metabolites. Drug Metab Disp. 1974; 2:159–168.

139. Fotherby K, James F. Metabolism of synthetic steroids. In: Briggs MH, Christie GA, eds. Advances in steroid biochemistry and pharmacology, Vol. 3. London: Academic Press, 1972:57–165.

140. Metzler M. Diethylstilbestrol metabolism in humans and experimental animals. In: Herbst Al, Bern HA, eds. Developmental effects of diethylstilbestrol (DES) in pregnancy. New York: Taieme-Stratton, 1981:158–166.

141. Krishna G, Corsini GU, Gillette J, Brodie BB. Biochemical mechanisms for hepatotoxicity produced by diethylstilbestrol. Toxicol Appl Pharmacol. 1972; 23:794.

142. Jensen EU, De Sombre E. Mechanism of action of the female sex hormones. Ann Rev Biochem. 1972; 41:203–230.

143. Korenman SG. Comparative binding affinity of estrogens and its relation to estrogenic activity. Steroids. 1969; 13:163–177.

144. Segal SJ, Koide SS. Molecular pharmacology of estrogens. Pharmacol Ther. 1979; 4:183–220.

145. Fanchenko ND, Sturchark JV, Shchedrina RN, et al. The specificity of the human uterine receptor. Acta Endocrinol. 1979; 90:167–175.

146. Jensen EV, Suzuki T, Kawashina T, et al. A two-step mechanism for the interactions of estradiol with the rat uterus. Proc Natl Acad Sci. 1968; 59:632–638.

147. Tseng L, Gurpide E. Induction of human estradiol dehydrogenase by progestins. Endocrinol. 1975; 97:825–833.

148. Keenan EJ. The physiological and pathophysiological significance of steroid hormone receptors. In: Sciarra JJ, Speroff L, Simpson JL, eds. Gynecology and obstetrics, Vol. 5. Philadelphia: Harper & Row, 1982:(4)1–19.

149. Notides AC, Nielsen S. The molecular mechanism of the in vitro 4S to 5S transformation of the uterine estrogen receptor. J Biol Chem. 1974; 249:1866–1873.

150. McGuire WL, Huff K, Chamness G. Temperature-dependent binding of estrogen receptor to chromatin. Biochem. 1973; 11:4562–4565.

151. Chan L, O'Malley BW. Steroid hormone action: recent advances. Ann Intern Med. 1978; 89:694–701.

152. Kassis JA, Gorski J. Estrogen receptor replenishment. J Biol Chem. 1981; 256:7378–7382.

153. Gorski J, Sarff M, Clark J. Regulation of uterine concentration of estrogen binding protein. Adv Biosci. 1971; 7:5–20.

154. Hsueh AJ, Peck EJ, Clark JH. Control of uterine estrogen receptor levels by progesterone. Endocrinology. 1976; 98:438–444.

155. Kauppila A, Janne O, Kivinen S, et al. Postmenopausal hormone replacement therapy with estrogen periodically supplemented with antiestrogen. Am J Obstet Gynecol. 1981; 140:787–792.

156. Devi PK. Antiestrogens. Pharmacol Ther. 1981; 12:439–447.

157. Clark JH, Anderson JN, Peck EJ. Estrogen receptor antiestrogen complex: Atypical binding by uterine nuclei and effects on uterine growth. Steroids. 1973; 22:707–718.

158. McGuire WL, Carbone PP, Sears ME, Escher GC. Estrogen receptors in human breast cancer. An overview. In: McGuire WL, Carbone PP, Volmer EP, eds. Estrogen receptors in human breast cancer. New York: Raven Press, 1974:1–8.

159. Knight WA, Osborne CK, Yochmowitz MG, McGuire WL. Steroid hormone receptors in

the management of human breast cancer. Ann Clin Res. 1980; 12:202–207.

160. Meyer JS, Rao BR, Stevens SC, White WL. Low incidence of estrogen receptors in breast carcinomas with rapid rates of cellular replication. Cancer. 1977; 40:2290–2298.

161. Knight WA, Livingston RB, Gregory EJ, McGuire WL. Estrogen receptor as an independent prognostic factor for early recurrence in breast cancer. Cancer Res. 1977; 37:4669–4671.

162. De Sombre ER, Carbone PP, Jensen EV, et al. Steroid receptors in breast cancer. N Engl J Med. 1979; 301:1011–1012.

163. Lippman ME, Allegra JC, Thompson EB, et al. The relation between estrogen receptors and response rate to cytotoxic chemotherapy in metastatic breast cancer. N Engl J Med. 1978; 298:1223–1228.

164. Kiang DT, Frenning DH, Goldman AI, et al. Estrogen receptors and responses to chemotherapy and hormonal therapy in advanced breast cancer. N Engl J Med. 1978; 299:1330–1334.

Estrogen Replacement Therapy 6

Clare D. Edman

Estrogen replacement therapy has been scrutinized closely and the biologic effects of various estrogens have been examined extensively during the past 5 years.[1-14] During the early 1960s, estrogens were used liberally in an attempt to perpetuate youth for menopausal women. It was common practice at that time to prescribe estrogens routinely to nearly every postmenopausal woman on the premise that estrogens protected women against the ravages of aging. This "feminine forever" concept was challenged in the mid-1970s when several investigators noted an increased incidence of endometrial cancer in the United States.[15,16] They suggested that the prolonged exposure of women with uteri to unopposed estrogen was responsible for these findings. These suggestions provoked widespread concern among laypersons and physicians about the potential risks of estrogen replacement therapy.

Currently, specific benefits of low-dose estrogen therapy in menopausal women include relief of vasomotor symptoms, urogenital atrophy, and the prevention of osteoporosis (Table 6–1). Some investigators have suggested that estrogens improve mental status and prevent cardiovascular disease and aging changes of the skin in menopausal women, although these conditions are not recognized as specific indications for estrogen treatment.

Potential risks of estrogen therapy include endometrial cancer, hypertension, gallbladder disease, abnormal uterine bleeding, and possibly breast cancer. Presently, there is no concensus about the last risk. There is no evidence that estrogen therapy increases or decreases the risk of developing a primary psychiatric disorder, myocardial infarction, cerebral vascular accident, pulmonary embolus, or abnormal glucose metabolism.

Estrogens circulate primarily in three forms: free, conjugated, and protein-bound. The free estrogens are lipophilic, cross cell membranes readily and exert biologic activity by binding to a specific high-affinity, low-capacity receptor in the cytoplasm of the target cell. Once the steroid-receptor complex has formed, it is transported into the nucleus of the cell where it stimulates the production of messenger ribonucleic acid (mRNA) and protein synthesis. The potency of a specific estrogen depends upon the length of time that the specific estrogen-receptor complex resides in the nucleus of the cell.[5,9,11] Estrogens are conjugated in the liver as sulfates or glucuronides; as such, they are biologically inactive, water soluble, and excreted into bile and urine. These conjugated estrogens are activated to a free form in the tissue site of action by specific enzymes. The protein-bound estrogens, especially those bound to sex hormone binding globulin (SHBG), are thought to be biologically inactive.

Recommendations for Management of Estrogen Replacement Therapy

Considering the potential risks of estrogen therapy, every woman should be evaluated thoroughly before therapy is initiated. The evaluation should include a detailed history of medical problems with particular attention di-

TABLE 6–1. Potential Benefits and Risks of Low-dose Estrogen Therapy in Menopausal Women.

Potential Benefits
  Relief of vasomotor symptoms
  Relief of atrophic urogenital symptoms
  Prevention of severe osteoporosis
  Improvement of emotional status
Potential Risks
  Development of endometrial cancer
  Exacerbation of hypertension
  Increased incidence of cholelithiasis
  Abnormal uterine bleeding
  Development of breast cancer
No Apparent Benefit or Risk
  Prevention of psychiatric disorders
  Alterations in the incidence of arteriosclerotic cardio-
    vascular disease, stroke, or thromboembolic disease
  Alterations in glucose metabolism

rected to the contraindications of estrogen therapy (Table 6–2). The physical examination should include a blood pressure check and breast and pelvic examination. The latter should include cervical cytology (Pap smear) and a sampling of the endometrium for histologic evaluation. The patient should be advised of the specific indications for estrogen therapy, as well as the general benefits and risks.

THERAPY BY AGE GROUP. Guidelines for estrogen replacement therapy in specific age groups are given below.

TABLE 6–2. Contraindications to Estrogen Replacement Therapy.

Absolute Contraindications
  Undiagnosed vaginal bleeding
  Acute liver disease
  Chronic impaired liver function
  Acute vascular thrombosis (with or without emboli)
  Neuroophthalmologic vascular disease
  Breast carcinoma
  Chronic thrombophlebitis
Relative Contraindications
  Preexisting hypertension
  Fibrocystic disease of breast
  Uterine leiomyomata
  Familial hyperlipidemia
  Severe varicose veins
  Gallbladder disease
  Severe obesity
  Heavy cigarette smoking
  Porphyria

Hypogonadal Individuals. All sexually immature, adolescent girls with hypogonadism should start estrogen therapy as soon as the diagnosis has been established. In order to achieve maximal breast development, the dosage of unopposed estrogen should be low initially (0.3 mg/day) and increased gradually over 6- to 12-months before a progestin is added to the therapy. Unless complications occur, therapy should be continued until age 50 when menopause would occur naturally.

Premenopausal Women. All nonobese women who develop *premature menopause* by natural or surgical causes prior to age 40 should receive estrogen replacement until age 50 if there are no contradindications to estrogen therapy. Unless obese women are symptomatic, they should not be treated with estrogens since they will produce sufficient quantities of estrone by peripheral aromatization to protect them against osteoporosis (see Chapter 1). Obesity is defined as body weight that exceeds 15% of ideal body weight (determined by height and estimated size of body frame).

Postmenopausal Women. All postmenopausal women do *not* require long-term estrogen therapy. The exception is the thin, small-framed, Caucasian woman who smokes, weighs less than 120 pounds, and is at risk of developing osteoporotic fractures. Short-term estrogen therapy should be reserved for symptomatic, menopausal women with vasomotor or atrophic urogenital symptoms.

DOSAGE AND METHOD OF ADMINISTRATION. Therapy should be administered cyclically (during the first 25 days of each month) using the lowest dosage that controls symptoms effectively (Table 6–3).

ROUTES OF ADMINISTRATION. Currently, the oral route is the preferred method of administration. Injectable therapy is effective, but not recommended on the basis of cost, high dosage requirement, and the hazards of prolonged action. Subcutaneous estrogen implants are not recommended for similar reasons. Vaginal creams containing estrogen may be used effectively for urogenital atrophy. The risks of estrogens administered by this route are similar to those for the oral route. Many

TABLE 6–3. Commonly Used Oral Estrogen Preparations in Postmenopausal Women.

GENERIC NAME	LOWEST EFFECTIVE DAILY DOSE (mg)
Conjugated estrogens	0.3–0.6
Ethinyl estradiol	0.01–0.02
Micronized estradiol	1.0
Diethylstilbestrol	0.2
Quinestrol	0.1

Adapted and reproduced with permission from Carr BR, Mac-Donald PC (1983) Estrogen treatment of postmenopausal women. In Stollerman GH, et al., eds. Advances in internal medicine, Vol. 28. Chicago: Year Book Medical.

women reject vaginal creams as being messy and requiring too much effort to maintain continuous therapy.

Recently, it has been shown that the topical application of an ointment containing 17β-estradiol (E2) to the abdominal skin, may provide an effective alternative to the oral administration of estrogens. The percutaneous administration of E2, in contrast to the conjugated estrogens, produces plasma levels of estradiol and estrone similar to those observed during the early follicular phase of the menstrual cycle with less toxicity (i.e., little or no alterations in renin substrate, SHBG, triglycerides, and antithrombin III) than with oral estrogens.[14]

ENDOMETRIAL BIOPSY. Histologic evaluation of the endometrium is mandatory in all women with uteri before estrogen therapy is initiated. Whether tissue for evaluation of endometrial status is obtained by dilatation and curettage, office biopsy, jet washing, aspiration of the endometrium, or by a progestogen challenge test[10] will depend upon the preference of the physician and the facilities available. Estrogen replacement therapy should not be started if the tissue sampling reveals endometrial hyperplasia or carcinoma.

SURVEILLANCE OF PATIENTS. All women receiving estrogen therapy should be evaluated regularly at 6- to 12-month intervals; a blood pressure check, breast examination, pelvic examination, and review of the indications for therapy are conducted at each visit. If vaginal bleeding has occurred, histologic evaluation of the endometrium is mandatory.

DURATION OF USE. The duration of therapy must be individualized for each woman. Lifelong therapy may be indicated for some postmenopausal women at high risk of developing osteoporosis; but therapy should be discontinued within 2 to 5 years for other indications. It is important to keep in mind that estrogen replacement therapy is a substitution for but does *not* recapitulate, the physiologic, cyclic production of 17β-estradiol and progesterone during reproductive life.

COMBINED THERAPY. Combinations of estrogen-progestins may be advantageous over unopposed estrogen therapy in reducing the risk of developing endometrial disease and osteoporosis.[17] The effectiveness of long-term progestin therapy for the prevention of urogenital atrophy and cardiovascular complications has not been clearly defined at this time. Moreover, combined therapy may result in withdrawal bleeding in many menopausal women. (For a detailed discussion see Chapter 7.)

PATIENT COUNSELING. The risks and complications of estrogen therapy must be explained to each woman with empathy for her dilemma, especially if long-term therapy is contemplated. Some women are unaware of the risks (e.g., they know a friend who was helped by estrogen and now they want it). They may be hesitant to take estrogens because they were afraid to ask about such therapy, or they were frightened by stories in the media, a misinformed friend, or a family member. When information regarding estrogen therapy is presented to women in an understandable form, they often make the correct decision about long-term estrogen therapy.

Specific Benefits of Estrogen Replacement Therapy

RELIEF OF VASOMOTOR SYMPTOMS. Although vasomotor symptoms subside spontaneously within 1 to 5 years after the menopause for nearly all women, only one-third of menopausal women will suffer from severe symptoms that cause them to seek medical help. Estrogens provide prompt relief from vasomotor symptoms by reducing the frequency and severity of hot flushes and relieving insomnia in most postmenopausal women.[8] However, they do not abolish symptoms in all menopausal women.

Hot flushes can generally be controlled by the use of 0.62–1.25 mg of conjugated estrogen (CE) or 0.02–0.05 mg of ethinyl estradiol (EE) daily.[5,11] The dosage may be titrated to control symptoms and then reduced periodically until the medication is discontinued, usually within 6 to 24 months. The rapidity with which therapy can be withdrawn may be assessed by the occurrence of symptoms during the estrogen-free interval when the medication is administered cyclically. If symptoms do not occur during that interval, therapy may be discontinued abruptly. If symptoms recur or intensify during that interval, the individual will experience hot flushes when therapy is discontinued. Women should be forewarned about this possibility before therapy is begun and before it is discontinued.

Although estrogen is *the* therapy for vasomotor instability, other drugs may be used effectively for this problem in women who are unable or unwilling to take estrogens. Medroxyprogesterone acetate, a progestin, provides prompt relief of vasomotor symptoms, is well tolerated, and is effective when given orally, 30 mg/day, or intramuscularly, 150 mg every other week, to menopausal women.[18] Approximately 10% of women taking this drug will experience side-effects, i.e., irregular uterine bleeding, fluid retention, and mild depression. Other drugs, such as tranquilizers and sedatives, may be used; they probably act through a placebo effect. Drugs which suppress gonadotropins (i.e. danazol) are ineffective. Propranolol offers little benefit over the placebo effect. Although clonidine may reduce the severity and frequency of hot flushes in some women, it is generally ineffective in most cases.

RELIEF OF ATROPHIC UROGENITAL SYMPTOMS. Estrogen is effective for the relief of urogenital atrophy.[9] Symptoms such as atrophic vaginitis and urethritis (urethral syndrome) respond readily to low-dose estrogen replacement. Less estrogen is required for the relief of these symptoms than is required for vasomotor symptoms. Vaginal creams may be used effectively for these disorders. It should be remembered that estrogens (both estrone and estradiol) are absorbed readily from the vagina and may yield supraphysiologic blood levels systemically for 5–6 hours (Fig. 6–1). Estrogens administered vaginally have a pronounced effect on vaginal cornification and may produce endometrial stimulation and uterine bleeding if therapy is continued for several months. Thus, estrogen administration by this route should be subject to the same contraindications and safeguards as that by the oral route (see also Chapter 9).

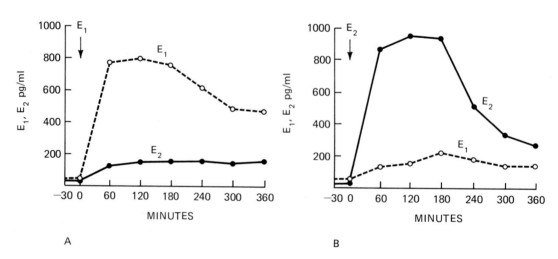

Fig. 6–1. Plasma concentrations of estrone (E1) and 17β-estradiol (E2) following vaginal administration of 0.05 mg estrone (*left*) and 0.5 mg micronized estradiol (*right*). Redrawn from Vaughn TC, Hammond CB. Estrogen replacement therapy. Clin Obstet Gynecol. 1981, 24:278–279.

PREVENTION OF SEVERE OSTEOPOROSIS.

Low-dose estrogen therapy does arrest and retard bone resorption up to 8 years if therapy is begun shortly after the loss of ovarian estrogens[8,12]; however, more longevity studies are needed before these observations may be used as the premise for long-term therapy. Such therapy does prevent the development of bone fragility and reduces the incidence of fractures.[4,9,10,12,19] Discontinuation of the early initiated estrogen therapy often results in a rapid loss of bone density similar to that observed in nonuser individuals.[9]

The protective effect of estrogen administration on the bony skeleton appears to be dose-dependent. Several studies have shown that 0.625 mg of CE or 0.025 mg of EE or mestranol will maintain constant levels of bone density in young and menopausal women. Mandel and coworkers[11] have shown that as little as 0.01 mg of EE significantly lowers the calcium/creatinine baseline below that observed in ovulatory premenopausal women. However, they point out that the protective effect of that dosage of EE may not hold during long-term studies.

Despite the effect of long-term estrogen therapy on bone, there is still the question of whether all postmenopausal women need estrogen therapy routinely, especially now that progestins have been found to enhance new bone formation in postmenopausal women.[17] Most clinicians do not place all menopausal women on replacement therapy to protect 25–30% of the population. They would recommend that Caucasian women with small body frames who smoke or were castrated prior to age 40 be started on prophylactic replacement therapy.

Nearly all clinicians recommend calcium supplementation and daily exercise for postmenopausal women. Riggs et al.[19] found that treatment with calcium carbonate alone (1500 mg/day) reduced the rate of vertebral fractures by 36% of that observed in untreated women (Table 6–4). Moreover, the fracture rate was reduced by 50% and 65% when vitamin D and sodium fluoride were added, respectively. When calcium and estrogen (1.3 mg/day) were combined, the fracture rate decreased by 78%. If calcium, estrogen, sodium fluoride, and vitamin D were given simultaneously, the fracture rate decreased by 94% to

TABLE 6–4. Effect of Various Combinations of Calcium (Ca), Estrogens (E), Sodium Fluoride (NaF), and Vitamin D (D) on Vertebral Fractures in Postmenopausal Osteoporosis.

THERAPY	FRACTURE RATE/ 1000 PATIENT YEARS	
Untreated	834	
Ca alone	532	$p < 0.001$
Ca + D	419	$p < 0.001$
Ca + NaF	344	
Ca + NaF + D	304	NS
Ca + E	191	
Ca + E + D	181	NS
Ca + NaF + E	125	
Ca + NaF + E + D	53	NS

Adapted from Riggs BL, et al.[17]

levels of 53 fractures/1000 patient years. Thus, these investigators found that the fracture rate could be reduced significantly in all treatment groups. The combined use of calcium, estrogen, fluoride, and vitamin D seemed to provide the best protection. Fluoride and estrogen seemed to act independently of each other.

Sixty percent of women treated with sodium fluoride had an apparent increase in vertebral bone mass radiographically. Fluoride appears to be a potent stimulator of bone formation whereas estrogen appears to be a potent inhibitor of bone resorption. However, the addition of vitamin D to these therapeutic regimens did not reduce the incidence of fractures significantly, except when added with calcium. Vitamin D is known to cause hypercalcemia, hypercalciuria, and potential renal stone formation. Calcium supplementation maintains a positive calcium balance in menopausal women by slowing bone resorption and increasing renal tubular and intestinal reabsorption of calcium. Tums, an antacid, provides a ready source of calcium carbonate for this purpose (see also Chapter 4).

MENTAL STATUS. As discussed in Chapter 3, irritability, fatigue, depression, anxiety, decreased psychic efficiency, impaired recent memory, and insomnia occur frequently during the climacteric and postmenopausal years. Although estrogen does appear to improve the sense of well-being, relieve depression, and slow the natural deterioration in perception and memory in some menopausal women, they do so indirectly by a *domino effect.* That is, irritability and fatigue improve as insomnia abates at hot flushes and night sweats are controlled by estrogen therapy. Estrogens do alter sleep patterns by shortening the latency period required to fall asleep and by increasing the length of REM sleep. (See Chapter 12.)

Specific Risks of Estrogen Replacement Therapy

DEVELOPMENT OF ENDOMETRIAL CANCER. The use of estrogens in postmenopausal women increases the risk of developing endometrial cancer.[1-3,6-9] This risk appears to be dose and duration dependent, and appears greater when the estrogen is administered continuously. The development of endometrial cancer during estrogen exposure frequently occurs as a localized process. The 5-year survival rate of women with a well-differentiated endometrial cancer is 95%.[9] If these lesions are recognized and treated early in the course of the disease process, they are curable in most cases. This may explain, in part, why there has not been a demonstrable increase in mortality from endometrial carcinoma recently despite the surge of estrogen use during the early 1970s.

According to the Third National Cancer Survey, the annual incidence of endometrial cancer is 0.7/1000 women. Estrogens increase that incidence rate by three to four fold to 2.3–3.0/1000 women.[8] It was suggested recently that the addition of a progestin during the last 7 to 10 days of estrogen therapy may prevent the development of endometrial hyperplasia and carcinoma. However, the effectiveness and safety (especially with regard to cardiovascular and thromboembolic risks) of such therapy must be evaluated thoroughly before this recommendation is practiced routinely.

EXACERBATION OF HYPERTENSION. At present, the relationship between estrogen replacement therapy and the risk of hypertension is unresolved. Theoretically, estrogens should induce the renin-angiotensin system and cause or exacerbate hypertension. Serum concentrations of renin substrate rose 180% or threefold following the oral administration of 1.25 mg of CE or 0.05 mg of EE and were much higher than levels found in nonuser premenopausal or postmenopausal women.[11,14] Interestingly, the percutaneous application of E2 ointment to the abdominal wall skin does not alter plasma levels of renin or antithrombin III as is found after administration of conjugated estrogens. This observation may alter the preferred route of estrogen administration in menopausal women.

Despite the potential risk of hypertension during oral estrogen therapy, there was no apparent increased incidence of hypertension during short-term, low-dose estrogen use in several large, well-controlled studies.[8,9] If hypertension does occur during therapy, it usually abates after the medication is discontinued. Hypertensive changes are seen less frequently during estrogen replacement therapy than during oral contraceptive therapy.

CHOLELITHIASIS. Bile may become saturated with cholesterol during estrogen therapy and combine with other metabolic salts to form stones. The incidence of surgically proven cholelithiasis is 2.5 times higher in healthy postmenopausal women using estrogens than in nonusers. The risk of gallstone formation is higher in obese women on estrogen. It is not feasible to screen all postmenopausal women for occult gallbladder disease before estrogen therapy is begun, but it is prudent to instruct all women about the early signs of cholelithiasis when therapy is started.

UTERINE BLEEDING. Uterine bleeding is a worrisome side-effect of estrogen therapy in postmenopausal women. One-third of postmenopausal women on estrogen will have bleeding at some time during therapy.[10] High dosage and prolonged use of estrogen enhances the risk of developing endometrial cancer in menopausal women with uteri. Thus, uterine bleeding in postmenopausal women on estrogen therapy (breakthrough, withdrawal, or otherwise) requires a histologic evaluation of the endometrium.

Combinations of estrogen-progestin therapy would seem to have distinct advantages over the administration of estrogen alone in menopausal women with a uterus. It has been shown that combined therapy results in periodic uterine bleeding and does reduce the incidence of hyperplasia and endometrial cancer. With cyclic combined therapy (0.62 mg of CE + 10 mg progestogen), 97% of women in one study experienced withdrawal bleeding for 3–4 days each month.[10] The frequency of uterine bleeding can be reduced if the dosage of both hormones is reduced. Progestogens apparently have to be given at least 10 days each month to obtain its protective effect on the endometrium.

DEVELOPMENT OF BREAST CANCER. Recently, concern has been expressed regarding the relationship of estrogen replacement therapy and benign and malignant breast disease. Several studies have addressed this issue.[3,20] In two of these studies, it was found that the risk of breast cancer was increased after 10 to 15 years of estrogen use; whereas, a third study found no relationship between risk of cancer and length of exposure. In that study (a case-control epidemiologic investigation), it was found that the risk of developing breast cancer was increased only in those women with ovaries who were exposed to at least 1500 mg of estrogen accumulatively. These dosages are equivalent to the daily consumption of 1.25 mg CE for 3 years.[20] Patients receiving 0.62 mg CE did not develop breast tumors unless they had preexisting benign breast disease. Other investigators, using equally well-designed case-controlled studies, found no relationship between chronic estrogen use and breast cancer.[1–3,6–10] If these epidemiologic data for breast cancer are age-adjusted, the incidence and death rates of this disease have not changed in the United States for several decades despite the surge in estrogen usage recently.

Although the evidence suggests that estrogen replacement therapy neither contributes to nor prevents breast cancer, the possibility cannot be ignored since breast tissue is a target organ for estrogen action. Estrogen therapy should not be given if breast disease exists and should be discontinued if benign or malignant breast disease develops during therapy.

THROMBOEMBOLIC DISEASE. Synthetic estrogens in oral contraceptives are associated with a high incidence of deep vein thrombosis and myocardial infarction after age 40.[9] Despite these well-documented observations in premenopausal women, long-term estrogen therapy in postmenopausal women has not been associated with an increased incidence of occlusive arterial or venous thromboembolic disease.[2,9,10] This is somewhat surprising since risk factors such as hypertension, hyperlipidemia, and obesity are common in menopausal women. Many investigators attribute these observations to the predominant use of *natural estrogens* during estrogen replacement therapy.

ALTERATIONS IN GLUCOSE METABOLISM. Presently, data regarding the effect of estrogen on glucose metabolism in menopausal women are conflicting.[9] Some investigators find that glucose metabolism is altered and that a tolerance test is often abnormal, but more have found frank diabetes mellitus in menopausal women treated with estrogens. Others could not confirm these observations even when high dosages of estrogens were used. Therefore, we do not consider estrogen therapy to be contraindicated in symptomatic diabetic menopausal women. It would, however, be prudent to monitor blood glucose levels closely during the first 3 months of therapy.

REFERENCES

1. Shoemaker ES, Forney JP, MacDonald PC. Estrogen treatment of postmenopausal women: benefits and risks. JAMA. 1977; 238:1524–1530.
2. Greenblatt RB, Causa H, Studd J (eds). The menopause. Clin Obstet Gynecol. 1977; 4(1):1–258.
3. Hulka BS. Effect of exogenous estrogen on postmenopausal women: the epidemiologic evidence. Obstet Gynecol Survey 1980; 35:389–399.
4. Schiff I, Ryan KJ. Benefits of estrogen replacement. Obstet Gynecol Survey 1980; 35:400–411.
5. Geola FL, Frumar AM, Tataryn IV, et al. Biological effects of various doses of conjugated equine estrogens in postmenopausal women. J Clin Endocrinol Metab. 1980; 51:620–625.
6. Worley FJ (ed). The menopause. Clin Obstet Gynecol. 1981; 24(1):163–324.
7. Mosher BA, Whelan EM. Postmenopausal estrogen therapy: a review. Obstet Gynecol Survey 1981; 36:467–475.
8. Judd HL, Cleary RE, Creasman WT, et al. Estrogen replacement therapy. Obstet Gynecol. 1981; 58:267–275.
9. Hammond CB, Maxson WS. Current status of

estrogen therapy for the menopause. Fertil Steril. 1982; 37:5–25.

10. Gambrell RD. The menopause; benefits and risks of estrogen-progestogen replacement therapy. Fertil Steril. 1982; 37:457–473.

11. Mandel FP, Geola FL, Lu JK, et al. Biologic effects of various doses of ethinyl estradiol in postmenopausal women. Obstet Gynecol. 1982; 59:673–679.

12. Upton GV. The perimenopause: physiologic correlates and clinical management. J Reprod Med. 1982; 27:1–28.

13. Carr BR, MacDonald PC (1983) Estrogen treatment of postmenopausal women. In: Siperstein MD, Advances in internal medicine, 28:491. Chicago: Year Book Medical.

14. Elkik F, Gompel A, Mercier-Bodard C, et al. Effects of percutaneous estradiol and conjugated estrogens on the level of plasma proteins and triglycerides in postmenopausal women. Am J Obstet Gynecol. 1982; 143:888–892.

15. Smith DC, Prentice R, Thompson DJ, Hen-mann WL. Association of exogenous estrogen and endometrial carcinoma. N Engl J Med 293: 1164–1167, 1975.

16. Mack TM, Pike MC, Henderson BE, et al. Estrogens and endometrial carcinoma in a retirement community. N Engl J Med 294:1262–1267, 1976.

17. Mandel FP, Davidson BJ, Erlik Y, et al. Effects of progestins on bone metabolism in postmenopausal women. J Reprod Med. 1982; 27:511–514.

18. Schiff I. The effects of progestins on vasomotor flushes. J Reprod Med. 1982; 27:498–502.

19. Riggs BL, Seeman E, Hodgson SF, et al. Effect of the fluoride/calcium regimen on vertebral fracture occurrence in postmenopausal osteoporosis. N Engl J Med. 1982; 306:446–450.

20. Ross RK, Paganini-Hill A, Gerkins VR, et al. A case-control study of menopausal estrogen therapy and breast cancer. JAMA 1980; 243:1635–1639.

The Role of Progestational Agents in Hormone Replacement Therapy

7

Marc A. Fritz and Leon Speroff

Women seeking medical attention for complaints of vasomotor phenomena and symptoms related to the deterioration of estrogen-dependent tissues comprise an ever-increasing proportion of gynecologic care as the population ages and life expectancy beyond reproductive age continues to rise. There can be no question that estrogen replacement therapy can effectively relieve many of the disturbing and sometimes disabling symptoms of the perimenopausal and postmenopausal periods. The value of estrogen replacement in the arrest and prevention of osteoporosis and in reducing the general incidence of malignant disease and overall mortality has also become apparent. Enthusiasm over the benefits of postmenopausal estrogen has been tempered, however, by an appreciation for its causative link to the rise in incidence of endometrial cancer. Legitimate concerns have also been raised over estrogen-induced alteration of carbohydrate and lipid metabolism, its influence on clotting mechanisms, and impact on both benign and malignant breast disease.

Progestins have important clinical applications in the care of the menopausal patient. The effects of estrogen on target tissues may be significantly altered by progestational therapy. A detailed discussion of the benefits of estrogen replacement as well as its inherent and potential risks is provided in Chapter 6. Accordingly, the discussion to follow will focus on the role of progestational agents in hormone replacement and the influence that progestins, alone and in combination with estrogen, exert on common target tissues and pertinent metabolic pathways. The action and effects of estrogen are included where necessary to illustrate the modulation or contrasting action of progestational agents.

The Mechanism of Progestin Action

The many clinical applications of progestational agents in the management of the menopausal patient require a knowledge of their mechanism of action. Estrogens serve principally to stimulate growth whereas the actions of progesterone are directed more toward cellular differentiation. As steroid hormones, both exert their effects through binding to specific, high affinity protein receptors present in the cytoplasm of target tissues.

Binding of the hormone to its receptor results in "transformation," a conformational change in the hormone-receptor complex which allows "translocation," the migration and binding of the complex to specific acceptor sites on nuclear chromatin. This latter interaction regulates the levels of specific messenger ribonucleic acids (mRNA) which direct the synthesis of proteins mediating the steroid hormone response. The proteins synthesized include enzymes and other receptors. Once the hormone-receptor complex is released from the nucleus it dissociates and is metabolized. Alternatively, the receptor may be recycled to the cytoplasm for reuse.

Acting through this mechanism, estrogen both stimulates an increase in the synthesis of its own cytoplasmic receptor and induces the synthesis of cytoplasmic progesterone receptors (PgR), actions resulting in enhanced tissue sensitivity to progesterone.[1–3] In turn, acting through its estrogen-induced cytoplasmic receptor, progesterone reduces the concentration of estrogen receptors (ER) by interfering with their replenishment.[3–6]

The replenishment of cytoplasmic ER involves both recycling and the synthesis of new receptors. Progesterone does not interfere with the recycling of existing receptors nor does it alter receptor binding specificity or affinity.[4] Progesterone does not inhibit translocation of the estrogen-receptor complex.[7] It is the synthesis of new ER that appears to be blocked by progestational agents.[4] The ultimate result is a reduction in the number of cytoplasmic ER which can be subsequently bound by estrogens and translocated to the nucleus to affect growth of the cell.[4–6] The action of progesterone is dose dependent, specific, and correlates with a reduced tissue sensitivity to the subsequent administration of estrogen. Since PgR synthesis is an ER-mediated process, progesterone indirectly antagonizes the synthesis of its own receptor and exerts a self-limiting action. Thus, under normal conditions in estrogen-dependent tissues, the proliferative action of estrogen is modified and limited by progesterone in a delicately balanced system in which each hormone regulates the other through modulation of its specific cytoplasmic receptor concentration.

Endometrial cytoplasmic ER and PgR concentrations throughout the menstrual cycle correlate well with the mechanism observed in vitro. During the proliferative phase, ER concentrations progressively rise. Cytoplasmic PgR levels are initially low but gradually increase to reach a peak coincident with the preovulatory rise of estradiol and a marked shift of ER to the nuclear fraction.[8,9] With luteinization, cytoplasmic PgR levels steadily fall. ER concentrations in the cytoplasm remain low while levels of both in the nucleus rise. Both receptors then gradually fall to their lowest levels, in the cytosol and nuclear fraction, late in the secretory phase.[8]

Synthetic progestins also exhibit a characteristic progestational effect on ER concentrations. Oral medroxyprogesterone acetate (MPA), administered during the proliferative phase, reduces endometrial cytoplasmic ER to levels below that normally observed in untreated patients.[10] Although the PgR binds both natural and synthetic progestins, receptor affinity and relative potency vary.[11] MPA exhibits the greatest relative potency of six commonly employed progestins, judged on ability to induce glycogen accumulation in human endometrium in vitro.[12] Relative receptor affinity, determined by ability to displace labeled progesterone from its receptor, correlates well with relative potency, although MPA demonstrates a greater receptor affinity than progesterone itself.[12] The synthetic progestins may differ in other regards. MPA has been reported to influence glandular transformation more than decidualization of stroma and may be contrasted with the 19-nortestosterone derivatives which appear to have the opposite effect.[11]

In addition to the modulation of steroid receptor concentrations, progesterone is important in the induction of enzymes involved in estrogen metabolism. It is well established that progesterone induces 17β-estradiol dehydrogenase activity in the human endometrium.[10,13–15] The enzyme mediates the conversion of estradiol to estrone. Its activity in secretory endometrium is increased more than tenfold over levels found in the proliferative phase.[13,14] Progesterone stimulates activity of the dehydrogenase in a dose-dependent manner when added to proliferative human endometrium cultured in vitro.[15] The effect can also be demonstrated in vivo and occurs in response to a variety of synthetic progestins as well as the natural hormone.[10,15] The ultimate result of progesterone-induced estradiol dehydrogenase activity is a reduction in the tissue concentration of estradiol and a rise in the intracellular estrone/estradiol ratio.

Recent evidence suggests that progesterone plays a similar role in the induction of estrogen sulfotransferase, the enzymatic catalyst for the production of estrogen sulfate conjugates.[16,17] Enzyme activity is detectable only in the secretory phase where it serves to sulfurylate estrone produced through prior action of estradiol dehydrogenase. Having no affinity for the ER, estrone sulfate is rapidly excreted from the cell. The actions of estradiol dehydrogenase and the sulfotransferase are closely coupled and may combine to effect a rapid decline in the intracellular concentration of estrogen.

Thus, in reducing the cytoplasmic ER population and inducing metabolic enzymatic activity, progestational agents act both to decrease binding and to stimulate the metabolism of estrogens. In so doing, progestins effectively limit estrogenic influence on cellular growth.

Progestins and the Endometrium

The evidence supporting a causal relationship between long-term exposure to an unopposed estrogen stimulus and the development of endometrial hyperplasia, progressive atypia, and potential malignant degeneration is compelling. Several risk factors have long been identified in association with the development of endometrial cancer. Obesity confers a relative risk of three times normal incidence in patients 20–25 pounds overweight.[18] Nulliparity carries a relative risk twice that of women having delivered a single child. Diabetes and late menopause (after age 52) increase the risk of developing endometrial cancer 2.8 and 2.4 times, respectively.[18] In addition, infertility, functioning ovarian tumors, polycystic ovaries, anovulation, and dysfunctional uterine bleeding have all been implicated as predisposing conditions. The common denominator that would appear to link the majority, if not all, of such risk factors is their association with continuous, long-term exposure to the unopposed proliferative stimulus of estrogen.

A dramatic rise in the incidence of endometrial cancer occurred coincident with the growth in popularity of estrogen replacement therapy.[19] Subsequent studies of the association appear to have provided sufficient evidence to establish causality. Several retrospective studies of women exposed to postmenopausal estrogen have demonstrated a relative risk of endometrial cancer four to eight times the normal incidence.[20–24] Estrogen replacement therapy is most highly correlated with the development of early stage, low grade, superficially invasive endometrial malignancy. Risk is both dose and duration related and is higher with continuous treatment regimens than with "cyclic" administration.[22]

The endometrial hyperplasias may be considered a spectrum of epithelial alterations associated with the anovulatory state. They are now recognized as lesions reflecting a chronic estrogenic environment which, if uninterrupted, promotes gradual progression. In later stages, endometrial hyperplasia must be considered a premalignant lesion. Indeed, foci of varying degrees of hyperplasia have been shown to coexist with adenocarcinoma.[25]

The risk of developing endometrial hyperplasia in response to the administration of estrogens has been reported to be from 12 to 33% and is directly related to both dose and duration of exposure.[26–29] Hyperplastic change can often develop rapidly and has been observed within 6 to 7 months after initiation of therapy.[26,30] Once present, the risk of progression to frank carcinoma appears dependent on the degree of hyperplasia and accompanying atypia as well as the subsequent duration of unopposed estrogen stimulation. Endometrial carcinoma will develop in approximately 1% of patients with proven cystic hyperplasia.[26] Persistent adenomatous hyperplasia has been observed to antedate invasive adenocarcinoma in 25–30% of patients.[25,31] Over eight to 10 years, 80% of patients with persistent atypical hyperplasia will develop endometrial cancer, whereas malignant degeneration has been observed without exception in patients diagnosed as having adenocarcinoma in situ and left untreated.[25]

Fortunately, estrogen replacement therapy need not subject patients to a greater risk of endometrial hyperplasia and adenocarcinoma. It is now well established that the addition of cyclic progestational therapy to both cyclic and continuous estrogen replacement regimens is protective. The addition of a progestin to hormone replacement therapy not only eliminates the increase in relative risk but reduces the incidence of endometrial cancer in treated patients to below that of the untreated population.

Several large series comparing the incidence of endometrial cancer in untreated patients with that observed in groups treated with estrogen, alone and in combination with cyclic progestins, have been reported.[23,24,32–34] In all cases, when compared to untreated patients, a higher incidence of endometrial cancer was confirmed in those treated with estrogen alone. More significantly, patients treated with a combination of estrogen and cyclic progestins developed endometrial cancer with a frequency lower than in untreated controls. Although the addition of cyclic progestins did not entirely prevent the development of adenocarcinoma, nearly all patients in whom endometrial cancer has been diagnosed while receiving combination therapy have received only 5–7 days of progestational relief.[24,32,33,35] When administered for 10 or more days per month, in a manner more closely resembling the pattern characteristic of the normal cycle, progestins have been almost universally effective in preventing malignant endometrial disease.[23] A rare patient will develop endometrial cancer despite even 10 days of cyclic progestin. Although disappointing, we would be naive to think that unopposed estrogenic stimulation is the *only* etiologic influence on endometrial cancer.

Predictably, the incidence of endometrial hyperplasia is also markedly reduced in patients receiving combination replacement therapy. The addition of norethindrone or MPA to estrogen replacement regimens employing a variety of agents can reduce the incidence of associated hyperplasia to 5% or less.[26] Here again, the need to administer progestational agents for a minimum of 10 days has become apparent. Hyperplasias developing in the face of combined therapy have all been observed when only a 5- to 7-day course of progestin has been employed. When progestin was administered for 13 days in a cyclic fashion combined with daily estrogen, not a single case of endometrial hyperplasia was observed to develop in more than 200 patients over 4 years of observation.[28] The fact should not, perhaps, be surprising but only serve to emphasize that, to be optimally effective while not imposing added risk, hormone replacement therapy should be structured so as to simulate the normal ovulatory cycle. Unfortunately, the consequences of a failure to do so were graphically illustrated by past experience with sequential oral contraceptives.

Adenocarcinoma of the endometrium developed in a significant number of women on sequential contraceptive pills.[36,37] The cycles employed a relatively large dose of a potent estrogen, administered alone for a period of 14–16 days, followed by a relatively weak progestin for 5–7 days. Sequential pill users were subject to a relative risk seven times the normal incidence of endometrial cancer. In contrast, women taking combination contraceptive preparations had only half the risk of nonusers.[37,38]

Unopposed estrogen replacement increases the concentration of both ER and PgR to three to four times that found in the proliferative phase in normal women.[39] Conjugated equine estrogens (CEE) are known to induce cytoplasmic ER levels in a dose-dependent fashion when administered to postmenopausal women.[40] Elevated receptor concentrations have been demonstrated in association with endometrial hyperplasia and well-differentiated adenocarcinomas.[9,39,41] In contrast, the levels of cytoplasmic ER and PgR observed in patients receiving estrogen replacement combined with cyclic progestins are similar to those of normally cycling preovulatory women.[39] As little as 2.5 mg MPA daily, provided as 10 days of cyclic progestational relief, can effectively return levels of cytoplasmic ER induced with 0.3 or 0.625 mg CEE to baseline concentrations. A 5.0- or 10.0-mg dose of MPA appears necessary if 1.25 mg CEE is used.[40] Progestins can also reduce ER levels in the hyperplastic endometrium and even in some cases of frank adenocarcinoma.[10,39]

Poor patient acceptance has been a criticism often raised when cyclic progestins are recommended as a component of hormone replacement. Speculation has been that postmenopausal women seeking estrogen replacement for relief of menopausal symptoms would be reluctant to accept a return of cyclic menses. Support for this contention has, however, not been forthcoming. In fact, 90% of women managed with combination hormone replacement therapy may be expected to elect to continue treatment 16 months after initiated.[42] When the rationale for combined hormone replacement is adequately explained, patient acceptance has been excellent. Although cyclic menses may be expected to return in a number of patients, the incidence of more worrisome breakthrough bleeding is significantly reduced from that observed in patients receiving cyclic estrogens alone.[42] In addition, titration of the administered dose of estrogen to the lowest level compatible with symptomatic relief will minimize the number of patients experiencing a return of menses.

Progestational agents may be used not only

to reduce the risk of endometrial cancer in patients receiving hormone replacement therapy but also as a means to lower the risk for patients not requiring treatment. In fact, the individual at highest risk among the untreated peri-/postmenopausal population may be the asymptomatic woman producing sufficient endogenous estrogen. Estrone has been established as the principal estrogen of the postmenopausal state, derived almost entirely from the extraglandular conversion of androstenedione in adipose tissue.[43] The peripheral aromatization of androgen is increased with aging, obesity, liver disease, and other factors. Moreover, there is evidence that a greater rate and efficiency of extraglandular conversion may exist in women who develop endometrial hyperplasia or adenocarcinoma.[43,44]

The "progesterone challenge test" has been proposed as a method of identifying the patient at high risk.[32] The progestin "challenge," administered to asymptomatic postmenopausal women, seeks to identify those patients with sufficient endogeneous estrogen to promote endometrial proliferation. Should the progestin induce subsequent withdrawal bleeding, it has been recommended that such patients be managed with continued cyclic administration of progestins until they no longer generate a withdrawal response. In this fashion, the patient may be spared the consequences of an apparent unopposed estrogen stimulus until she no longer produces sufficient endogenous estrogen to support endometrial growth.

In addition to their use as effective prophylactic agents, serving to interrupt otherwise unopposed estrogen, progestins have been repeatedly shown capable of normalizing the already hyperplastic endometrium.[24–26,28,32,33,45] Reversal of endometrial hyperplasia has been observed over the entire spectrum, from simple and cystic varieties to adenomatous, and even atypical adenomatous, hyperplasia. A variety of progestational agents have been employed. Norethindrone acetate,[24,32,33] norethindrone,[28] MPA,[26,32,33] dimethisterone or megestrol,[25] 17-hydroxyprogesterone caproate,[45] and various combination oral contraceptives[24,33,45] have all proven similarly effective. In all series, various degrees of hyperplasia were converted to normal with not less than 95% effectiveness. The induction of cyclic withdrawal bleeding for 3–6 months appears to be as effective as shorter-term, continuous treatment regimens. Indeed, cyclic progestins have proven effective in normalizing hyperplastic states even when employed in the continuing presence of estrogen replacement.[26,45]

Treatment failures tend to occur when cyclic progestins have been administered for intervals less than 10 days in duration or when the lesion under treatment is of advanced degree or demonstrates significant atypia. In no case has the degree of hyperplasia been observed to progress while under treatment. Such results would seem to warrant a trial of progestational agents in the management of virtually all patients found to harbor endometrial hyperplasia. Care must be taken, however, to confirm normalization of the lesion and continuing management in the form of cyclic progestational withdrawal must be provided lest the conditions which predisposed to the hyperplastic state be allowed to persist and prompt recurrence, or worse, progression. Surgical management may be safely reserved for the occasional treatment failure. Advanced lesions, particularly those with significant atypia, are perhaps those most likely to demonstrate a loss of ability to respond appropriately to a progestational stimulus.

Progestins and Bone Mineral

The incidence of postmenopausal osteoporosis and its consequences in the affected patient have been well documented.[29] Its impact on the delivery of health care is substantial and may be expected to assume still greater significance as the size of the population at risk continues to grow. Recognition of the potential magnitude of the problem has prompted a great deal of investigation and the evaluation of various approaches to prevention and treatment.

Several factors have been identified as predisposing to the development of osteoporosis. A low calcium intake or its malabsorption and dietary deficiencies of vitamin D and fluoride may be involved. Smoking, physical inactivity, alcohol consumption, and race (Oriental and Caucasian) also appear to be related.[46] A hypoestrogenic state has long been recognized as a major risk factor. Indeed, the onset of clinically significant osteoporosis is closely related in time to the climacteric. With the onset of menopause, bone mineral content declines, rapidly at first, then stabilizing in a gradual downward trend. Bone mineral is depleted at a rate of 2–3% per year in the first 3 years after menopause, falling an additional 1% per year thereafter.[47–49] It is estimated that approximately 15% of skeletal calcium is lost every 10 years beyond the cessation of menses.[49]

The management of postmenopausal osteoporosis has met with variable success but no single measure has proven as effective as estrogen.[29,50] The mechanism through which estrogen influences the dynamic equilibrium between bone resorption and deposition remains unclear. Estrogen appears to operate through enhancement of both intestinal and renal tubular absorption of calcium as well as inhibition of bone resorption.[51] Numerous investigators have demonstrated the effectiveness of estrogen replacement therapy in the prevention of postmenopausal osteoporosis.[23,48,49,52–55] Estrogen reduces urinary calcium and hydroxyproline excretion and effectively prevents the progressive loss of bone mineral observed in untreated controls. Both "natural" and synthetic estrogens have proven efficacy.

The role of progestational agents in the prevention and management of postmenopausal osteoporosis is not yet well defined. Certainly, it is clear that the addition of a cyclic progestin to estrogen replacement therapy in no way detracts from its effectiveness.[56] On the contrary, there is evidence to suggest that progestins may enhance the effects of estrogen in preventing loss of bone mineral. The incidence of fractures in postmenopausal patients on estrogen replacement may be significantly reduced when cyclic progestational therapy is also provided.[23]

Combined therapy may actually increase bone mineral content.[48,49,54] In a 10-year double-blind prospective study comparing matched pairs of randomly chosen postmenopausal patients, the group receiving CEE and cyclic MPA experienced a significant gain in bone mineral if therapy was begun within 3 years after menopause.[48] Another study involving combination therapy demonstrated a 2.5% gain in bone mineral over 2 years,

whereas placebo-treated controls experienced a 3.3% decline.[54] In yet another recent clinical investigation, combined hormone replacement therapy was observed to result in a significant increase in bone mineral content, whereas placebo-treated controls suffered a 4% loss over a 2-year period. Importantly, when treatment was initiated in a subgroup of those previously receiving placebo, photon absorptiometry revealed an increase in bone mineral over the subsequent year, whereas those remaining on placebo experienced continuing loss.[49]

It is not yet clear whether an increase in bone mineral is unique to replacement regimens including cyclic progestational therapy. If these data are confirmed, combination hormone replacement may offer effective treatment to the patient with *established* osteoporosis. Although both single and combined hormone replacement have proven to be effective prophylaxis, the postmenopausal loss of bone mineral has generally been regarded as irreversible. The most recent prospective study suggests that may not be so.[49]

There is evidence that progestational agents may spare bone mineral through actions of their own, in a manner distinct from that of estrogen. Ethynodiol diacetate was found to be effective in preventing significant loss of bone mineral in postmenopausal women.[57] An earlier investigation documented the ability of norethindrone to produce a fall in plasma and urinary calcium.[58] Recently, MPA reduced urinary calcium excretion in postmenopausal women to levels similar to those observed in premenopausal patients.[59] Megestrol acetate, in high dose, had similar effects. Parenteral gestranol hexanoate also effectively prevented bone mineral depletion when administered to postmenopausal patients. After 1 year, when bone density was compared with baseline determinations, the progestin was found equally as effective as the daily administration of mestranol.[60] Interestingly, unlike mestranol, progestin therapy was not associated with a reduction in urinary hydroxyproline excretion, an indicator of bone resorption. The finding suggested a separate and distinct mechanism of action.

High affinity glucocorticoid receptors have been identified in rat bone.[61,62] Glucocorticoids are known to promote osteopenia, both enhancing bone resorption and inhibiting new bone deposition. Consistent with its known affinity for corticosteroid binding globulin, progesterone can effectively compete for cortisol receptors at physiologic concentrations.[61] In high dosage, MPA exhibits some intrinsic cortisollike activity and is even capable of suppressing adrenal function.[11] In the rodent model, progestin administration has been associated with an increase in periosteal new bone formation.[57] Such action might explain the apparent intrinsic bone-sparing properties of progestational agents and their tendency to promote an actual increase in bone mineral when used in combination with estrogens.

Further research is needed to better document and define the role of progestins in the prevention and management of osteoporosis. Certainly, they hold promise as effective adjuncts to existing therapy.

Progestins and Lipid Metabolism

The menopause has been associated with a change in cholesterol transport mechanisms. The decline of ovarian function is related to an increase in low density lipoprotein (LDL) concentrations, accompanied by a fall in high density lipoprotein (HDL) levels.[63] The climacteric redistribution of cholesterol to the LDL fraction appears to result from the gradual fall in circulating levels of estrogen. Administration of exogenous estrogen can reverse the postmenopausal trend of plasma lipoprotein concentrations. Although data are conflicting, a majority of investigators have observed lower LDL concentrations and a 20–30% rise in HDL in women receiving estrogen replacement therapy.[63–67]

A striking inverse correlation exists between circulating levels of HDL and the incidence of coronary heart disease.[68] A fall in HDL appears to be involved in the pathogenesis of coronary atherosclerosis. HDL serves to accelerate lecithin/cholesterol acyltransferase activity, promoting the transfer to cholesterol from tissue to plasma and facilitating its subsequent transport to the liver for metabolism and excretion.[69] The plasma concentration of HDL may be rate limiting in the process, with reduced levels slowing the clearance of cholesterol from vessel walls. The overall decrease in cholesterol and "beneficial" direction of the

shift in relative lipoprotein levels have led some to consider estrogen a therapeutic approach to the management of hypercholestrolemic states.[67,70]

Although both synthetic and "natural" forms of estrogen produce similar effects on lipoproteins, the two may differ in their effect on triglyceride (TG) concentrations. Ethinyl estradiol and mestranol tend to increase TG levels.[64,65,71] In contrast, estradiol valerate, estrone sulfate, and CEE have no effect.[64,65,71,72] Although increased serum cholesterol levels are regarded as an important etiologic factor in atheroma formation, the effect of elevated TG concentrations is less well established. However, many consider the lack of effect on TG levels an advantage of "natural" estrogens over synthetic preparations since both appear to be of otherwise equal efficacy.

With growing recognition of a need for cyclic progestational relief during estrogen replacement therapy, concern has arisen regarding the influence progestins might exert on serum lipid profiles. Several investigations have sought to address the question. When administered in depot form and provided as contraceptive agents to women of reproductive age, progestins had no effect on cholesterol, TG, and phospholipid concentrations.[73] A change to combined hormone replacement therapy was without effect on altered lipid levels previously induced by the administration of estrogen alone.[71] Some investigators have suggested that the addition of cyclic progestins may actually enhance the action of estrogen in reducing total serum cholesterol concentrations.[65]

There is evidence to suggest that the ultimate effect of hormone replacement therapy on circulating lipid levels may depend on the choice of progestational agent. A comparison of lipoprotein profiles among women receiving one of three progestins, in addition to replacement with a "natural" estrogen, demonstrated that progestins may differ in their impact on lipid metabolism.[63] Replacement with estradiol valerate raised HDL concentrations. The subsequent addition of cyclic norgestrel or norethindrone acetate reduced HDL to a level 20% below that observed *prior* to treatment with estrogen alone. In contrast, while also preventing the estrogen-induced rise in HDL, the addition of cyclic MPA had no such effect.[63] The two 19-nortestosterone (19-nor) derivatives not only blocked, but effectively reversed the beneficial effect of postmenopausal estrogen on HDL-cholesterol, whereas the hydroxyprogesterone derivative, MPA, did not. A similar observation had been made earlier when norethindrone was added to ethinyl estradiol replacement therapy.[66]

The effect of the 19-nor progestins on lipoproteins may reflect their androgenic derivation. In general, androgens reduce the concentration of HDL in both man and experimental animals.[74] Androgens may act to selectively inhibit synthesis of apolipoprotein A, characteristically the principal component of HDL.[74] Their administration may also induce a rise in LDL levels.

Patients in need of hormonal support may be treated without adverse effect on lipid profiles and raising the risk of atherosclerotic disease. Consideration of potential impact on lipid metabolism should be kept in mind when selecting each component of hormone replacement therapy.

Progestins and Carbohydrate Metabolism

The diabetogenicity of pregnancy with its well-established insulin resistance and progressive hyperinsulinemia has implicated the sex steroids as causative agents. Similar observations of elevated blood glucose and insulin have been made in association with oral contraceptives (OCP). As a result, the effects of hormone replacement therapy on carbohydrate metabolism have also been examined.

Estrogens are known to exert a tropic effect on the pancreatic z-cell and thereby increase insulin secretion.[75] Despite such insulinotropic action, postmenopausal estrogen replacement has been associated with impaired glucose tolerance in a significant number of women.[76–78] As with observed effects on serum lipids, many have suggested that synthetic estrogens are more diabetogenic than the "natural" preparations.[78–81] It is not yet clear whether the distinction is only a reflection of dose and relative potency or an inherent property of the estrogen employed. Further confusion stems from the finding that intravenous glucose tolerance tests (GTT) were invariably normal in a group of women in which 70% had an abnormal oral GTT.[82] Estrogen appears to induce a delay in glucose absorption and postpone the peak of plasma insulin following a glucose load.[76,81,83] Whether real or apparent, there is evidence that any estrogen-induced alteration in carbohydrate metabolism may, in fact, be only a transient phenomenon, resolving within 3 to 6 months.[79,84,85]

Although most have focused on estrogen as the component responsible for the observed diabetogenic influence of OCP, recent investigations have implicated the progestational component. The type of progestin and relative ratio to estrogen have been emphasized.[86] Any negative influence of progestational agents on carbohydrate metabolism appears more marked with the 19-nor progestins than with hydroxyprogesterone derivatives and may be dose related.[86] Nevertheless, progestins of both varieties have been associated with significant elevations of both blood glucose and plasma insulin.[87–89]

Progesterone itself has been implicated as etiologic in impaired glucose tolerance. Diabetic control may be more difficult during the luteal phase. In high dosage, exogenous progesterone may induce a rise in plasma insulin levels similar to that seen in late pregnancy.[90] Progesterone can bind to pancreatic β-cells at physiologic concentrations and may act to "down-regulate" insulin receptor concentrations in association with hyperinsulinemia.[91]

Several studies have failed to demonstrate impaired carbohydrate metabolism in association with progestin administration. The addition of norethindrone acetate, megestrol, or norgestrel to treatment with ethinyl estradiol or mestranol had no effect on glucose tolerance in premenopausal women.[92] The administration of neither norethindrone nor MPA for contraception had any effect on glucose or insulin levels in women of reproductive age.[73] Similarly, ethynodiol diacetate did not impair glucose tolerance when evaluated 3 months after therapy was initiated.[78] Although estrogen has induced abnormal glucose tolerance when administered to baboons, the subsequent addition of a progestin reversed the abnormality.[92] In addition, at least one investigator has reported *improved* carbohydrate metabolism in women with endometrial cancer treated with 17-hydroxyprogesterone caproate.[93]

It is important to note that short-term progestin therapy is generally not associated with altered carbohydrate metabolism. If at all, the effect of progestational agents may take months to become manifest, in contrast to that exerted by estrogens.[91] Many of the discrepancies between individual studies can be resolved if duration of therapy and time of evaluation are considered. Furthermore, it is perhaps both unrealistic and misleading to attempt to examine the impact of progestins alone on carbohydrate metabolism. Since progestational agents have little or no effect on target tissues in the absence of estrogen, it is quite possible that the end result of the administration of either will reflect the action of both.

The role of hormonal changes during menopause in glucose tolerance has not been clearly separated from the known impairment associated with advancing age.[91] The menopause itself does not appear to be diabetogenic in the absence of underlying disease. Likewise, the use of hormone replacement therapy rarely will result in precipitation of frank diabetes. In general, the use of an appropriate dose of estrogen does not result in significant or prolonged alteration in glucose tolerance and diabetes is not an absolute contraindication to replacement therapy. The use of cyclic progestational therapy is also unlikely to have significant impact on carbohydrate metabolism. Assessment of any associated risk must await further studies in women receiving hormone replacement therapy in the low doses currently recommended.

Progestins and Coagulation

Studies of clotting function in women receiving hormone replacement therapy inevitably followed the recognition of an increased relative risk of thromboembolic disease in association with use of OCP. An increase in factors II, VII, X, and fibrinogen has been attributed to use of the birth control pill.[94] A decrease in prothrombin time and antithrombin III activity has also been described.[94] Synthetic estrogens are considered to cause a hypercoagulable state, an effect which appears to be dose related.[95]

Evidence regarding an association of estrogen replacement with thromboembolism has

been conflicting. Replacement with CEE is reported to induce an increase in factors VII and X and in thrombin-induced platelet aggregation.[96,97] The analysis of clotting profiles suggested hypercoagulability in a majority of women receiving postmenopausal estrogens when compared to untreated controls.[98] Others have failed to demonstrate any significant impact of estrogen replacement on clotting function.[99,100] As a result, it has been recommended that the use of postmenopausal estrogen be approached with caution in patients with conditions otherwise predisposing to thromboembolism.[29]

In contrast, progestational agents do not appear to have adverse effects on the clotting mechanism. Conclusions drawn from studies of progestational impact on coagulation have been consistent. Neither clotting nor platelet aggregation appears to be altered by progestins in the absence of estrogen.[101] The addition of either cyclic norethindrone or norgestrel to replacement with any of three "natural" estrogens had no observed effect on coagulation factors or platelet function.[102] No change has been observed in plasma antithrombin III activity after treatment with progestins alone.[103] Not only did chlormadinone acetate not alter clotting function but its administration was observed to reverse elevated levels of factors VII and X previously induced by estrogen.[104] Similar results were obtained in studies involving the use of norethindrone and norgestrel.[104,105]

Concern remains over the risk of thromboembolism that may accompany the use of postmenopausal estrogen replacement. Just as "natural" and synthetic estrogens appear to differ in their effects on lipid and carbohydrate metabolism, some maintain that synthetics are relatively more thrombogenic.[102] Available data suggest that if estrogen replacement is to be used, cyclic progestational therapy may be added without fear of inducing or potentiating the risk of thromboembolic disease.

Progestins and the Breast

The breast, like the endometrium, is well recognized as a target tissue for sex hormones. Discovery of a dose- and duration-related rise in the risk of endometrial hyperplasia and adenocarcinoma in association with unopposed endogenous and exogenous estrogen suggested a similar etiology for malignant breast disease. Although studies of the epidemiology of breast cancer have provided considerable evidence to support the contention, proof of such a causative role for estrogens has been rather elusive.

Patients who develop breast malignancy exhibit several characteristics commonly observed in women with endometrial cancer. In fact, carcinoma of the breast and endometrium not infrequently occur in the same individual.[106] Early menarche, nulliparity, late menopause, and obesity are all conditions predisposing to the development of breast cancer.[107] As the age of menarche has gradually fallen, the incidence of carcinoma of the breast has steadily risen.[108] Women choosing to postpone pregnancy, or who are otherwise unable to conceive until after the age of 35, have twice the incidence of breast cancer observed in those delivered before the age of 20.[108] Women continuing to menstruate after age 55 are twice as likely to develop breast cancer. Obesity has been correlated with both an increased urinary excretion of estrogen and malignant breast disease.[109,110] Oligomenorrhea, infertility, and luteal phase defects have also been associated with higher relative risk.[43,111] Thus, it is not surprising that many have regarded long-term unopposed estrogenic stimulation as etiologic in both carcinoma of the breast and endometrium.

Estrogen replacement therapy has inevitably been indicted for inducing malignant degeneration in the breast. A case-control study of patients in retirement communities concluded that women treated for 7 or more years were almost twice as likely to develop breast cancer.[112] Curiously, risk appeared still greater in treated women with intact ovaries. A higher-than-expected incidence of breast cancer was observed in women receiving CEE for relief of menopausal symptoms.[113] Risk appeared to be both dose- and duration-related, reaching a plateau after 15 years of use. After 10 years, the relative "protection" offered by multiparity and oophorectomy was no longer in evidence.[113] Recently, the use of injectable estrogens was associated with a fourfold increase in breast cancer risk among naturally postmenopausal women.[114] In defense, several studies

have contested the link between estrogen replacement and carcinoma of the breast.[115–117] Some have even suggested that postmenopausal estrogen reduces the risk of developing breast cancer.[118] Needless to say, a verdict must await the presentation of more conclusive evidence.

Several theories have been offered on a possible mechanism through which estrogen may be related to breast cancer. The "estrone hypothesis" suggested unopposed estrone as carcinogenic, drawing support from epidemiologic evidence cited earlier.[43] The "estrogen window hypothesis" views unopposed estrogenic stimulation as the most favorable environment in which carcinogens may induce malignancy in a susceptible mammary gland.[119] Two main induction intervals are postulated, the perimenarchial period, from onset of pubertal development to establishment of regular ovulatory cycles, and the perimenopausal period. Both are characterized by relatively unopposed estrogenic influence. The "intensive differentiation" which accompanies pregnancy is seen as limiting "inducibility" and ultimately closing the first "window." Similarly, a second "estrogen window" may open as oligoovulation and luteal inadequacy usher in the perimenopause.[119] The use of unopposed estrogen replacement may serve to keep the second "window" open.

Estrogen replacement has been associated with a higher incidence of benign breast disease, a recognized predisposition to breast cancer.[120] The use of postmenopausal estrogen may impose a distinctly higher risk in women observed to develop benign breast disease after the onset of therapy.[113] Radiologic studies have called attention to apparent estrogen-induced mammographic changes. A higher incidence of epithelial hyperplasia has been noted in women receiving postmenopausal estrogens.[121] Cystic and dysplastic elements have been observed to regress after cessation of estrogen replacement therapy.[122] Studies of the opposite breast in women with breast cancer treated with estrogen have described epithelial changes, extension of smaller ducts, development of ductal alveoli, and formation of new breast lobules. Such proliferation was considered atypical and not resembling a normal premenopausal configuration.[123] Any association of postmenopausal estrogen to a higher risk of breast cancer might operate, at least in part, through induction of benign breast disease. Some investigators, however, have reported that the risks associated with fibrocystic disease and estrogen replacement are not only independent, but synergistic.[112]

Combination OCP are related to a lower incidence of benign breast disease and, in fact, are often therapeutic. The longer the duration of use, the lower is the incidence of fibrocystic disease. The effect has been offered as a mechanism through which OCP may reduce the risk of breast cancer. Women using oral contraception were observed to develop breast cancer with a frequency significantly lower than that predicted by the Third National Cancer Survey.[124] By inducing a "pseudopregnancy," through prolonged progestational influence, OCP may also simulate parity, a characteristic considered protective.

There is some evidence to suggest that cyclic progestational therapy may reduce the risk of breast cancer. Four of 84 untreated controls developed breast carcinoma in one double-blind, prospective study of combined hormone replacement therapy.[125] None of the age-matched patients in a treated group of the same size developed breast cancer over the 10 years of observation. The incidence of malignant breast disease in postmenopausal women treated with a combination of estrogen and cyclic progestational therapy appears to be lower than in those treated with estrogen alone. Figures from the largest ongoing prospective study comparing the two forms of management are approaching statistical significance.[126]

Available data would seem to suggest that estrogen and progesterone interact in a similar fashion in all target tissues. Although best characterized in the endometrium, progesterone has been demonstrated to reduce estrogen binding capacity in the monkey oviduct as well.[127] The PgR content of the breast is increased severalfold following estrogen treatment. The effect is rapid in onset and antagonized by the simultaneous administration of progesterone.[5]

The metabolic enzyme activities of normal and pathologic breast tissue have been examined.[128] The levels of 5α-reductase activity found in carcinomas were second only to those in fibrocystic disease. The production of 5α-reduced metabolites was correlated with increasing epithelial cellularity. Such compounds may compete for the PgR.[129] The receptor content of breast cancers is now well established as predictive of response to palliative endocrine therapy.[5,130,131] Response is correlated both qualitatively and quantitatively with tumor ER content.[5] If both receptors are present, remissions are observed in a larger proportion of patients than would be predicted on the basis of ER alone.[130]

Whereas estrogen acts to promote proliferation of ductal elements of the breast, progesterone induces differentiation and mitotic rest. During the latter half of pregnancy, progesterone induces mammary alveolar cell differentiation in conjunction with diminished mammary DNA synthesis.[132] The increase in 17β-estradiol dehydrogenase activity in pregnancy may serve to decrease the proliferative effect of estrogen on mammary epithelium.[133] Progesterone has been suggested to be protective by opposing the proliferative action of estrogens.[134]

If estrogen and progesterone exert actions on the breast like those observed in the endometrium and unopposed estrogenic stimulation is indeed etiologic in the development of breast cancer, why has such a relationship been so difficult to demonstrate conclusively in investigations conducted to date? Development and normal differentiation of the breast requires the collective actions of insulin, cortisol, thyroxine, prolactin, and growth hormone, in addition to the influence of estrogen and progesterone. By comparison, our current understanding of the hormonal requirements of the endometrium is relatively more simplistic. It may be that carcinoma of the breast is considerably more multifactorial in etiology than its endometrial counterpart. Our inability to adequately and appropriately control for other variables may underlie the failure of attempts to define the role, if any, of unopposed estrogen in the pathogenesis of breast cancer. Until such time as the pathophysiology of carcinoma of the breast is better characterized, it may be prudent to consider the addition of cyclic progestins to estrogen replacement therapy even for patients previously subjected to hysterectomy.

Progestins and Menopausal Symptoms

Estrogen has long been the mainstay of effective therapy for relief of menopausal symptoms. Treatment may be difficult in patients who do not tolerate estrogen-related side-effects or who have an underlying condition contraindicating estrogen therapy. The results of recent trials of progestational therapy in such patients have been promising.

Both parenteral and oral progestins may be employed with reasonable expectation of success. Parenteral depot-MPA (150 mg every 3 months) provided effective relief from disturbing menopausal symptoms in 89% of treated patients compared to reports of subjective response in only 25% of saline-treated controls.[135] These encouraging results have been recently confirmed. Forty-eight postmenopausal women were studied in a randomized, double-blind fashion with change in the number of hot flushes serving as the basis of comparison between MPA-treated patients and placebo-treated controls.[136] Treated patients received 50, 100, or 150 mg of depot-MPA. No patient receiving 100 or 150 mg MPA discontinued the study because of treatment failure, whereas 75% of the placebo group discontinued after 6–10 weeks for lacks of response. Seventy-five to 100% of treated patients reported relief of symptoms between 2 and 4 weeks after onset of therapy. In general, response was noted within the first week after injection and was maximal at 4 weeks.[136] A double-blind crossover study comparing the effects of oral MPA (20 mg daily) and placebo on vasomotor flushes has provided additional evidence that progestational agents are effective in the management of menopausal symptoms.[137] Women receiving MPA initially observed subjective relief by the second week of therapy with an overall 74% reduction in the frequency of hot flushes by 9–12 weeks. When subsequently treated with placebo, patients experienced a marked exacerbation of symptoms with frequency ultimately greater than that reported prior to entering the study. Placebo was effective if offered initially but even this group experienced a further 35% reduction in symptoms when switched to the active drug regimen.[137]

The loss of ovarian function is associated with an increase in catecholamine synthesis and metabolism in the central nervous system.[138] Progesterone appears to reduce tyrosine hydroxylase activity, the rate-limiting step in catecholamine synthesis, in an action facilitated by the presence of small amounts of estrogen.[138] Progestins may thus modulate the turnover of biogenic amines and alter sympathetic outflow.[46] MPA has been found to reduce both skin conductance and heart rate variability.[139] Besides their influence on the autonomic nervous system, progestational agents have been shown to affect cortical function and behavior.[140]

In addition to providing relief from vasomotor symptoms, progestins may have other actions of benefit to the postmenopausal woman. Both cyproterone acetate, an antiandrogen with potent progestational action, and norgestrel have been found to alter electroencephalograms in a manner similar to that seen after administration of antidepressants or anxiolytics.[140] Progestins have been employed successfully in the management of aggressive psychiatric patients and were found to promote an earlier sleep.[141] In high dosage, progestational agents may even act as hypnotic sedatives.[142]

When estrogen replacement therapy is poorly tolerated or contraindicated, progestational agents may be of significant benefit in the relief of disturbing vasomotor symptoms. If combined with estrogen replacement in a cyclic fashion, progestins may further enhance the effectiveness of postmenopausal estrogen. Their action on cortical centers may offer additionally therapeutic benefits to the symptomatic postmenopausal woman.

Summary

Estrogens and progestins exert mutually dependent actions on target tissues. Through modulation of its concentration of specific cytoplasmic receptor protein, each hormone limits the action of the other. Progestational agents also induce the activity of enzymes involved in estrogen metabolism. By both decreasing the binding and stimulating the metabolism of estrogens, progestins effectively limit the influence of estrogen on cellular growth in hormone-dependent tissues.

Unopposed estrogenic stimulation promotes progressive hyperplastic growth of the endometrium and may ultimately induce malignant degeneration. Cyclic progestational agents, administered for at least 10 days per month, can virtually eliminate the risk of endometrial hyperplasia and adenocarcinoma associated with estrogen replacement therapy. Cyclic MPA, 10 mg daily, has consistently proven effective. Although recent data suggest that as little as 2.5 mg MPA may be sufficient, recommendation of such low dosages must await appropriate clinical trials. Should progestin therapy with MPA be poorly tolerated a trial with a reduced dosage regimen may be offered with reasonable expectation of equal effectiveness, although it would be prudent to obtain a confirmatory biopsy. Although withdrawal bleeding may be induced in some postmenopausal patients, its frequency can be minimized with titration to the lowest effective dose of estrogen and its occurrence is unlikely to affect compliance in the informed patient.

A progestational "challenge," administered annually to asymptomatic postmenopausal women, will identify those patients at highest risk for development of endometrial disease. A positive withdrawal response is indicative of sufficient endogenous estrogen production to support continued endometrial proliferation, and signals the need for continued cyclic progestational therapy until the response is no longer elicited. Progestins may also be employed as effective therapy for endometrial hyperplasia, once present. Reversal of even advanced lesions is commonly observed. Although care must be taken to document success, progestational therapy may be expected to normalize the endometrium with 95% effectiveness and obviate the need for surgical management in all but a few cases.

Estrogen replacement is the single most effective form of treatment in the prevention of postmenopausal osteoporosis. Estrogen enhances calcium absorption in both the intestine and renal tubule and inhibits bone resorption. The addition of a cyclic progestin to estrogen replacement in no way detracts from its effectiveness. In fact, progestational agents may enhance the bone-sparing effect of estrogen through actions of their own. Combined hormone replacement therapy may actually induce an increase in bone mineral content. Competition by progestins for glucocorticoid receptors in bone may mediate their action, promoting bone deposition and inhibiting osteoporotic change.

The menopause is associated with a significant fall in HDL concentrations which has been linked to increased risk of atherosclerotic disease. Estrogen replacement elevates HDL concentrations and lowers LDL levels. "Natural" estrogens tend not to alter TG levels, whereas their synthetic counterparts often raise TG concentrations. The addition of cyclic progestational therapy to estrogen replacement will prevent the estrogen-induced rise in HDL levels, although hydroxyprogesterone derivatives such as MPA have less effect than do the 19-nortestosterone derivatives.

Estrogens may induce an elevation in blood glucose and plasma insulin although the effect is usually transient. Progestational agents, too, may impair glucose tolerance, an effect more marked with 19-nor progestins. However, an appropriate dose of estrogen, alone or combined with cyclic progestins, is unlikely to result in significant or prolonged alteration in glucose tolerance.

While estrogens frequently alter coagulation profiles, progestational agents do not appear to have an adverse effect on the clotting mechanism. Progestins may be administered in either a cyclic or continuous fashion without fear of increased risk of thromboembolic disease.

An etiologic role for unopposed estrogen has not been established in the development of breast cancer, although considerable epidemiologic evidence supports an association. There is no reason to believe that the nature of the interaction between estrogen and progesterone differs among their target tissues. There is evidence that progestational agents may reduce the risk of developing carcinoma of the breast. It is prudent to consider the addition of cyclic progestational therapy to estrogen replacement until the multifactorial pathogenesis of breast cancer is better understood.

When estrogen replacement is poorly tolerated or contraindicated progestational therapy can be most effective in alleviating disturbing vasomotor symptoms. Combined hormone replacement therapy may take advantage of the additional mild anxiolytic and sedative actions of progestational agents.

It should be clear that the progestins have an important role in the successful management of the peri- and postmenopausal patient. They may be used to counter successfully many of the less desirable effects of estrogen replacement while imposing few, if any, of their own. In fact, progestational agents often enhance the effectiveness of postmenopausal estrogen. Progestins should be considered an integral component of hormone replacement therapy. Administered alone, progestins have several therapeutic actions and offer an effective alternative when estrogen has failed or cannot be given.

REFERENCES

1. Sarff M, Gorski J. Control of estrogen binding protein concentration under basal conditions and after estrogen administration. Biochemistry. 1971; 10:2557–63.
2. Milgrom E, et al. Mechanisms regulating the concentration and the conformation of progesterone receptor(s) in the uterus. J Biol Chem. 1973; 248:6366–74.
3. Leavitt WW, et al. A specific progesterone receptor in the hamster uterus: physiologic properties and regulation during the estrous cycle. Endocrinology. 1974; 94:1041–53.
4. Hsueh AJW, et al. Control of uterine estrogen receptor levels by progesterone. Endocrinology. 1976; 98:438–44.
5. Keenan EJ. The physiological and pathophysiological significance of steroid hormone receptors. In: Sciarra JW, ed. Gynecology and obstetrics, Vol. 5, Chap. 4. Philadelphia: Harper & Row, 1982:1–19.
6. Hsueh AJW, et al. Progesterone antagonism of the oestrogen receptor and oestrogen-induced uterine growth. Nature. 1975; 254:337–39.
7. Anderson J, et al. Oestrogen and nuclear binding sites. Biochem J. 1972; 126:561–67.
8. Bayard F, et al. Cytoplasmic and nuclear estradiol and progesterone receptors in human endometrium. J Clin Endocrinol Metab. 1978; 46:635–48.
9. Gurpide E, et al. Estrogen metabolism in normal and neoplastic endometrium. Am J Obstet Gynecol. 1977; 129:809–16.
10. Tseng L, et al. Estradiol receptor and 17β-dehydrogenase in normal and abnormal human endometrium. Ann NY Acad Sci. 1977; 286:190–98.
11. Wentz AC. Assessment of estrogen and progestin therapy in gynecology and obstetrics. Clin Obstet Gynecol. 1977; 20:461–82.
12. Shapiro SS, et al. Synthetic progestins: in vitro potency on human endometrium and specific binding to cytosol receptor. Am J Obstet Gynecol. 1978; 132:549–54.
13. Tseng L, Gurpide E. Estradiol and 20α-dihydroprogesterone dehydrogenase activities in human endometrium during the menstrual cycle. Endocrinology. 1974; 94:419–23.
14. Gurpide E, Tseng L. Factors controlling intracellular levels of estrogens in human endometrium. Gynecol Oncol. 1974; 2:221–27.
15. Tseng L, Gurpide E. Induction of human endometrial estradiol dehydrogenase by progestins. Endocrinology. 1975; 97:825–32.
16. Tseng L, Ching Liu H. Stimulation of arylsulfotransferase activity by progestins in human endometrium in vitro. J Clin Endocrinol Metab. 1981; 53:418–21.
17. Clarke CL, et al. Induction of estrogen sulfotransferase in the human endometrium by progesterone in organ culture. J Clin Endocrinol Metab. 1982; 55:70–75.
18. Gusberg SB. The individual at high risk for endometrial carcinoma. Am J Obstet Gynecol. 1976; 126:535–42.
19. Weiss NS, et al. Increasing incidence of endometrial cancer in the United States. N Engl J Med. 1976; 294:1259–62.
20. Smith DC, et al. Association of exogenous estrogen and endometrial carcinoma. N Engl J Med. 1975; 293:1164–67.
21. Ziel HK, Finkle WD. Increased risk of endometrial carcinoma among users of conjugated estrogens. N Engl J Med. 1975; 293:1167–70.
22. McDonald TW, et al. Exogenous estrogen and endometrial carcinoma: case-control and incidence study. Am J Obstet Gynecol. 1977; 127:572–80.
23. Hammond CB, et al. Effects of long-term estrogen replacement therapy. II. Neoplasia. Am J Obstet Gynecol. 1979; 133:537–47.
24. Gambrell RD. Estrogens, progestogens, and endometrial cancer. J Reprod Med. 1977; 18:301–6.
25. Wentz WB. Progestin therapy in endometrial hyperplasia. Gynecol Oncol. 1974; 2:362–67.
26. Campbell S, et al. The modifying effect of progestogen on the response of the postmenopausal endometrium to exogenous oestrogens. Postgrad Med J. 1978; 54(Suppl. 2):59–64.
27. Campbell S, Whitehead M. Oestrogen therapy and the menopausal syndrome. Clin Obstet Gynaecol. 1977; 4:31–47.
28. Thom MH, et al. Prevention and treatment of

endometrial disease in climacteric women receiving oestrogen therapy. Lancet. 1979; 1:455–57.

29. Hammond CB, Maxson WS. Current status of estrogen therapy for the menopause. Fertil Steril. 1982; 37:5–25.

30. Aylward M, et al. Endometrial factors under treatment with oestrogen and oestrogen/progestogen combinations. Postgrad Med J. 1978; 54(Suppl. 2):74–81.

31. Gusberg S. The individual at high risk for endometrial carcinoma. Am J Obstet Gynecol. 1976; 126:535–42.

32. Gambrell RD, et al. Use of the progestogen challenge test to reduce the risk of endometrial cancer. Obstet Gynecol. 1980; 55:732–38.

33. Gambrell RD, et al. Reduced incidence of endometrial cancer among postmenopausal women treated with progestogens. J Am Geriatr Soc. 1979; 27:389–94.

34. Greenblatt RB, et al. Update on the male and female climacteric. J Am Geriatr Soc. 1979; 27:481–90.

35. Budoff PW, Sommers SC. Estrogen-progesterone therapy in perimenopausal women. J Reprod Med. 1979; 22:241–47.

36. Silverberg SG, Makowski EL. Endometrial carcinoma in young women taking oral contraceptive agents. Obstet Gynecol. 1975; 46:503–6.

37. Weiss NS, Sayvetz TA. Incidence of endometrial cancer in relation to the use of oral contraceptives. N Engl J Med. 1980; 302:551–54.

38. Kaufman DW, et al. Decreased risk of endometrial cancer among oral contraceptive users. N Engl J Med. 1980; 303:1045–47.

39. Natrajan PK, et al. The effect of progestins on estrogen and progesterone receptors in the human endometrium. J Reprod Med. 1982; 27:227–30.

40. Gibbons WE, et al. Evaluation of estrogen receptor status in the endometria of postmenopausal women on sequential estrogen-progestin therapy. The Endocrine Society, 64th Annual Meeting, San Francisco, 1982; Abstract #1079.

41. McCarty KS, et al. Correlation of estrogen and progesterone receptors with histologic differentiation in endometrial adenocarcinoma. Am J Pathol. 1979; 96:171–82.

42. Whitehead MI, et al. Clinical considerations in the management of the menopause: the endometrium. Postgrad Med J. 1978; 54(Suppl. 2):69–73.

43. Siiteri PK, et al. Estrogen receptors and the estrone hypothesis in relation to endometrial and breast cancer. Gynecol Oncol. 1974; 2:228–38.

44. Schindler AE, et al. Conversion of androstenedione to estrone by human fat tissue. J Clin Endocrinol Metab. 1972; 35:627–30.

45. Kistner RW. Histological effects of progestins on hyperplasia and carcinoma in situ of the endometrium. Cancer. 1959; 12:1106–11.

46. Upton GV. The perimenopause: physiologic correlates and clinical management. J Reprod Med. 1982; 27:1–27.

47. Lindsay R, et al. Bone response to termination of oestrogen treatment. Lancet. 1978; 2:1325–27.

48. Nachtigall LE, et al. Estrogen replacement therapy. I. A 10-year prospective study in the relationship to osteoporosis. Obstet Gynecol. 1979; 53:277–81.

49. Christiansen C, et al. Bone mass in postmenopausal women after withdrawal of oestrogen/gestagen replacement therapy. Lancet. 1981; 1:459–61.

50. Riggs BL, et al. Effect of the fluoride/calcium regimen on vertebral fracture occurrence in postmenopausal osteoporosis. N Engl J Med. 1982; 306:446–50.

51. Gallagher JC, et al. Effect of estrogen on calcium absorption and serum vitamin D metabolites in postmenopausal osteoporosis. J Clin Endocrinol Metab. 1980; 51:1359–64.

52. Lindsay R, et al. Long-term prevention of postmenopausal osteoporosis by oestrogen. Lancet. 1976; 2:1038–40.

53. Marshall DH, et al. The prevention and management of postmenopausal osteoporosis. Acta Obstet Gynecol Scand. 1977; 65(Suppl.):49–56.

54. Christiansen C, et al. Prevention of early postmenopausal bone loss: controlled 2-year study in 315 normal females. Eur J Clin Invest. 1980; 10:273–79.

55. Horsman A, et al. Prospective trial of oestrogen and calcium in postmenopausal women. Br Med J. 1977; 2:789–92.

56. Crilly RG, et al. The effect of oestradiol valerate and cyclic oestradiol valerate/DL-norgestrel on calcium metabolism. Postgrad Med J. 1978; 54(Suppl. 2):47–49.

57. Lindsay R, et al. The effect of ovarian sex steroids on bone mineral status in the oophorectomized rat and in the human. Postgrad Med J. 1978; 54(Suppl. 2):50–58.

58. Gallagher JC, Nordin BEC. Effects of oestrogen and progestogen therapy on calcium metabolism in postmenopausal women. In: van Keep PA, Lauritzen C, eds. Estrogens in the postmenopause. Frontiers of hormone research. Basel: Karger, 1975: 150–76.

59. Mandel FP, et al. Effects of progestins on bone

metabolism in postmenopausal women. J Reprod Med. 1982; 27:511–14.

60. Lindsay R, et al. Comparative effects of oestrogen and a progestogen on bone loss in postmenopausal women. Clin Sci Mol Med. 1978; 54:193–95.

61. Manolagas SC, Anderson DC. Detection of high-affinity glucocorticoid binding in rat bone. J Endocrinol. 1978; 76:379–80.

62. Chen TL, Feldman D. Glucocorticoid receptors and actions in subpopulations of cultured rat bone cells. Mechanism of dexamethasone potentiation of parathyroid hormone-stimulated cyclic AMP production. J Clin Invest. 1979; 63:750–58.

63. Hirvonen E, et al. Effects of different progestogens on lipoproteins during postmenopausal replacement therapy. N Engl J Med. 1981; 304:560–63.

64. Wallentin L, Larsson-Cohn U. Metabolic and hormonal effects of postmenopausal oestrogen replacement treatment. Acta Endocrinol. 1977; 86:597–607.

65. Paterson MEL, et al. The effect of various regimens of hormone therapy on serum cholesterol and triglyceride concentrations in postmenopausal women. Br J Obstet Gynaecol. 1980; 87:552–60.

66. Gustafson A, Svanborg A. Gonadal steroid effects on plasma lipoproteins and individual phospholipids. J Clin Endocrinol Metab. 1972; 35:203–7.

67. Tikkanen MJ, Nikkila EA. Natural oestrogen as an effective treatment for type-II hyperlipoproteinaemia in postmenopausal women. Lancet. 1978; 2:490–91.

68. Gordon T, et al. High density lipoprotein as a protective factor against coronary heart disease. The Framingham study. Am J Med. 1977; 62:707–14.

69. Miller GJ, Miller NE. Plasma high-density-lipoprotein concentration and development of ischaemic heart disease. Lancet. 1975; 1:16–19.

70. Tikkanen MJ, et al. Treatment of postmenopausal hypercholesterolaemia with estradiol. Acta Obstet Gynecol Scand. 1979; 88(Suppl.):83–8.

71. Maddock J. Effects of progestogens on serum lipids in the postmenopause. Postgrad Med J. 1978; 54(Suppl. 2):38–41.

72. Bolton CH, et al. Comparison of the effects of ethinyl oestradiol and conjugated equine oestrogens in oophorectomized women. Clin Endocrinol. 1975; 4:131–38.

73. Dhall K, et al. Short-term effects of norethisterone oenanthate and medroxyprogesterone acetate on glucose, insulin, growth hormone, and lipids. Fertil Steril. 1977; 28:156–58.

74. Solyom A. Effect of androgens on serum lipids and lipoproteins. Lipids. 1972; 7:100–105.

75. Costrini NV, Kalkhoff RK. Relative effects of pregnancy, estradiol, and progesterone on plasma insulin and pancreatic islet insulin secretion. J Clin Invest. 1971; 50:992–99.

76. Ajabor LN, et al. Effect of exogenous estrogen on carbohydrate metabolism in postmenopausal women. Am J Obstet Gynecol. 1972; 113:383–87.

77. Notelovitz M. Metabolic effect of conjugated oestrogens (USP) on glucose tolerance. S Afr Med J. 1974; 48:2599–2603.

78. Thom M, et al. Effect of hormone replacement therapy on glucose tolerance in postmenopausal women. Br J Obstet Gynaecol. 1977; 84:776–83.

79. di Paola G, et al. Estrogen therapy and glucose tolerance test. Am J Obstet Gynecol. 1970; 107:124–32.

80. Gow S, Mac Gillivray I. Metabolic, hormonal, and vascular changes after synthetic oestrogen therapy in oophorectomized women. Br Med J. 1971; 2:73–77.

81. Larsson-Cohn U, Wallentin L. Metabolic and hormonal effects of postmenopausal oestrogen replacement treatment. Acta Endocrinol. 1977; 86:583–96.

82. Buchler D, Warren JC. Effects of estrogen on glucose tolerance. Am J Obstet Gynecol. 1966; 95:479–83.

83. Spellacy WN, et al. The effect of estrogens on carbohydrate metabolism: glucose, insulin, and growth hormone studies on 171 women ingesting Premarin, mestranol, and ethinyl estradiol for 6 months. Am J Obstet Gynecol. 1972; 114:378–92.

84. Notelovitz M. The effect of long-term oestrogen replacement therapy on glucose and lipid metabolism in postmenopausal women. S Afr Med J. 1976; 50:2001–3.

85. Spellacy WN, et al. Effect of estrogen treatment for one year on carbohydrate and lipid metabolism in women with normal and abnormal glucose tolerance test results. Am J Obstet Gynecol. 1978; 131:87–90.

86. Wynn V, et al. Comparison of effects of different combined oral contraceptive formulations on carbohydrate and lipid metabolism. Lancet. 1979; 1:1045–49.

87. Spellacy WN, et al. The effects of norgestrel on carbohydrate and lipid metabolism over one year. Am J Obstet Gynecol. 1976; 125:984–86.

88. Spellacy WN, et al. The effects of medroxy-progesterone acetate on carbohydrate metabolism: measurements of glucose, insulin, and growth hormone after 12 months use. Fertil Steril. 1972; 23:234–44.

89. Spellacy WN, et al. Lipid and carbohydrate metabolic studies after on year of megestrol acetate treatment. Fertil Steril. 1976; 27:157–61.

90. Kalkhoff RK, et al. Progesterone, pregnancy, and the augmented plasma insulin response. J Clin Endocrinol Metab. 1970; 31:24–28.

91. Notelovitz M. Carbohydrate metabolism in relation to hormonal replacement therapy. Acta Obstet Gynecol Scand. 1982; 106(Suppl.):51–56.

92. Goldzieher JW, et al. Comparative studies of the ethinyl estrogens used in oral contraceptives. VI. Effects with and without progestational agents on carbohydrate metabolism in humans, baboons, and beagles. Fertil Steril. 1978; 30:146–53.

93. Benjamin F, Casper DJ. Alterations in carbohydrate metabolism induced by progesterone in cases of endometrial carcinoma and hyperplasia. Am J Obstet Gynecol. 1966; 94:991–96.

94. Zador G. Estrogens and thromboembolic diseases. Present concept of a controversial issue. Acta Obstet Gynecol Scand. 1976; 54(Suppl.):13–28.

95. Conard J, et al. Antithrombin II and the oestrogen content of combined oestrogen-progestogen contraceptives. Lancet. 1972; 2:1148–49.

96. Coope J, et al. Effects of "natural oestrogen" replacement therapy on menopausal symptoms and blood clotting. Br Med J. 1975; 4:139–43.

97. Poller L, et al. Conjugated equine oestrogens and blood clotting: a follow-up report. Br Med J. 1977; 1:935–36.

98. Stangel JJ, et al. The effect of conjugated estrogens on coagulability in menopausal women. Obstet Gynecol. 1977; 49:314–16.

99. Toy JL, et al. The comparative effects of a synthetic and a "natural" oestrogen on the haemostatic mechanism in patients with primary amenorrhoea. Br J Obstet Gynaecol. 1978; 85:359–62.

100. Notelovitz M, Greig HBW. Natural estrogen and antithrombin III activity in postmenopausal women. J Reprod Med. 1976; 16:87–90.

101. Poller L, et al. Progesterone oral contraception and blood coagulation. Br Med J. 1969; 1:554–56.

102. Aylward M. Coagulation factors in opposed and unopposed oestrogen treatment at the climacteric. Postgrad Med J. 1978; 54(Suppl. 2):31–37.

103. Conard J, et al. AT III content and antithrombin activity in oestrogen-progestogen and progestogen-only treated women. Thromb Res. 1980; 18:675–81.

104. Poller L. Oral contraceptives, blood clotting, and thrombosis. Br Med Bull. 1978; 34:151–56.

105. Lorrain J, Harel P. Effects of certain contraceptive hormones on blood coagulation. Fertil Steril. 1972; 23:422–27.

106. Sall S, Calanog A. Steroid excretion patterns in postmenopausal women with benign and neoplastic endometrium. Am J Obstet Gynecol. 1972; 114:153–61.

107. Vorherr H, Messer RH. Breast cancer: potentially predisposing and protecting factors. Am J Obstet Gynecol. 1978; 130:335–58.

108. Sherman BM, Korenman SG. Inadequate corpus luteum function: a pathophysiological interpretation of human breast cancer epidemiology. Cancer. 1974; 33:1306–12.

109. de Waard F, et al. The bimodal age distribution of patients with mammary carcinoma. Cancer. 1964; 17:141–51.

110. Thijssen JHH, et al. Postmenopausal estrogen production, with special reference to patients with mammary carcinoma. In: van Keep PA, Lauritzen C, eds. Estrogens in the postmenopause. Frontiers of Hormone Research. Basel: Karger, 1975:45–56.

111. Swain MC, et al. Ovulatory failure in a normal population and in patients with breast cancer. J Obstet Gynaecol Br Commonw. 1974; 81:640–43.

112. Ross RK, et al. A case-control study of menopausal estrogen therapy and breast cancer. JAMA. 1980; 243:1635–39.

113. Hoover R, et al. Menopausal estrogens and breast cancer. N Engl J Med. 1976; 295: 401–05.

114. Hulka BS, et al. Breast cancer and estrogen replacement therapy. Am J Obstet Gynecol. 1982; 143:638–44.

115. Sartwell PE, et al. Exogenous hormones, reproductive history, and breast cancer. J Natl. Cancer Inst. 1977; 59:1589–92.

116. Brinton LA, et al. Breast cancer risk factors among screening program participants. J Natl Cancer Inst. 1979; 62:37–43.

117. Kelsey JL, et al. Exogenous estrogens and other factors in the epidemiology of breast cancer. J Natl Cancer Inst. 1981; 67:327–33.

118. Gambrell RD, et al. Estrogen therapy and

breast cancer in postmenopausal women. J Am Geriatr Soc. 1980; 28:251–57.

119. Korenman SG. The endocrinology of breast cancer. Cancer. 1980; 46:874–78.

120. Nomura A, Comstock GW. Benign breast tumor and estrogenic hormones: a population-based retrospective study. Am J Epidemiol. 1976; 103:439–44.

121. Fechner RE. Benign breast disease in women on estrogen therapy. Cancer. 1972; 29:273–79.

122. Peck DR, Lowman RM. Estrogen and the postmenopausal breast. JAMA. 1978; 240:1733–35.

123. Huseby RA, Thomas LB. Histological and histochemical alterations in the normal breast tissues of patients with advanced breast cancer being treated with estrogenic hormones. Cancer. 1954; 7:54–74.

124. Gambrell RD, et al. Breast cancer and oral contraceptive therapy in premenopausal women. J Reprod Med. 1979; 23:265–71.

125. Nachtigall LE, et al. Estrogen replacement therapy. II. A prospective study in the relationship to carcinoma and cardiovascular and metabolic problems. Obstet Gynecol. 1979; 54:74–79.

126. Gambrell RD. The menopause: benefits and risks of estrogen-progestogen replacement therapy. Fertil Steril. 1982; 37:457–74.

127. Brenner RM, et al. Cyclic changes in oviductal morphology and residual cytoplasmic estradiol binding capacity induced by sequential estradiol-progesterone treatment of spayed rhesus monkeys. Endocrinology. 1974; 95:1094–1104.

128. Lloyd RV. Studies on the progesterone receptor content and steroid metabolism in normal and pathological human breast tissues. J Clin Endocrinol Metab. 1979; 48:585–93.

129. Pinchon MF, Milgrom E. Characterization and assay of progesterone receptor in human mammary carcinoma. Cancer Res. 1977; 37:464–71.

130. McGuire WL, Horwitz KB. A role for progesterone in breast cancer. Ann NY Acad Sci. 1977; 286:90–99.

131. Allegra JC, et al. Relationship between the progesterone, androgen, and glucocorticoid receptor and response rate to endocrine therapy in metastatic breast cancer. Cancer Res. 1979; 39:1973–79.

132. Nagasawa H, Vorherr H. Rat mammary deoxyribonucleic acid synthesis during the estrous cycle, pregnancy, and lactation in relation to mammary tumorigenesis. Am J Obstet Gynecol. 1977; 127:590–93.

133. Gurpide E. Hormones and gynecologic cancer. Cancer. 1976; 38:503–508.

134. Hertz R. The estrogen-cancer hypothesis. Cancer. 1976; 38:534–40.

135. Bullock JL, et al. Use of medroxyprogesterone acetate to prevent menopausal symptoms. Obstet Gynecol. 1975; 46:165–68.

136. Morrison JC, et al. The use of medroxyprogesterone acetate for relief of climacteric symptoms. Am J Obstet Gynecol. 1980; 138:99–104.

137. Schiff I, et al. Oral medroxyprogesterone in treatment of postmenopausal symptoms. JAMA. 1980; 244:1443–45.

138. Beattie CW, et al. Influence of ovariectomy and ovarian steroids on hypothalamic tyrosine hydroxylase activity in the rat. Endocrinology. 1972; 91:276–79.

139. Carter Little B, et al. Physiological and psychological effects of progesterone in men. J Nerv Ment Dis. 1974; 159:256–62.

140. Herrmann WM, Beach RC. Experimental and clinical data indicating the psychotropic properties of progestogens. Postgrad Med J. 1978; 54(Suppl. 2):82–87.

141. Blumer D, Migeon C. Hormone and hormonal agents in the treatment of aggression. J Nerv Ment Dis. 1975; 160:127–37.

142. Merrymann W. Progesterone "anaesthesia" in human subjects. J Clin Endocrinol Metab. 1954; 14:1567–69.

Adenocarcinoma of the Endometrium

8

Samuel Lifshitz and Steven G. Bernstein

Endometrial carcinoma is the most common malignancy of the female genital tract, with an estimated 39,000 new cases of invasive carcinoma of the endometrium and 3000 deaths in 1982.[1] During the three decades before 1970 the incidence of cancer of the uterine corpus in the United States had been stable. Weiss et al.[2] examined the incidence rates of endometrial cancer from eight areas in the United States served by population-based cancer reporting systems and concluded that the incidence of endometrial cancer had risen sharply in the 1970s. The use of estrogen preparations by postmenopausal women is presumed to be responsible for this increasing incidence of endometrial cancer. More recently, a trend in decreasing incidence of endometrial carcinoma has been noted. This is speculated to be due to an increased number of hysterectomies being performed and a decreasing use of estrogen preparations by postmenopausal women.[3]

Epidemiology

Endometrial carcinoma is a disease of the postmenopause; the average age at diagnosis is 58 years. Only 5% of cases are diagnosed in women less than 40 years of age.

A number of risk factors have been identified for endometrial cancer. Many of these factors suggest an underlying endocrine-metabolic disorder. The increased risks for endometrial carcinoma for these factors are listed in Table 8–1. Wynder et al.[5] in an epidemiologic study identified obesity as the most important factor relating to cancer of the endometrium and speculated that the most practical preventive measure that could be taken to decrease the possibility of developing endometrial cancer was reduction of body weight. Armstrong and Doll[6] have correlated cancer incidence data from 23 countries with several environmental factors including diet. They found that the incidence of endometrial cancer was closely related to fat consumption and that caloric intake is a significant factor in determining the risk of endometrial cancer.

Estrogens and Endometrial Cancer

Data reported in the last decade indicate that estrogens may act as a carcinogen when unopposed by an adequate amount of progesterone. Interest in estrogen as an etiologic factor in the development of endometrial carcinoma stems from the observation that unopposed estrogen stimulation leads to the development of endometrial hyperplasia. Endometrial hyperplasia in turn is frequently associated with endometrial carcinoma.[7] Three groups of women are at increased risk of developing endometrial carcinoma: (1) postmenopausal women on estrogen replacement therapy; (2) women who took sequential oral contraceptives; and (3) women with ovarian dysgenesis who received unopposed estrogen therapy at puberty. Similarly, four groups of women appear to be at risk of developing cancer from endogenous estrogen sources: (1) women with granulosa-theca cell tumors of the ovary; (2) anovulatory

Table 8–1. Risk Factors in Endometrial Carcinoma.

FACTOR	RISK RATIO
Overweight (age 50–59)	
20–50 lbs.	3
> 50 lbs.	10
Nulliparity vs. one child	2
vs. five children	5
Late menopause	
(age 52 or later vs. < age 49)	2.4
Diabetes by history	2.8
Radiation to pelvis	8
Exogenous estrogen	6

From Morrow CP.[4]

women with polycystic ovarian syndrome; (3) obese postmenopausal women; and (4) women with chronic liver disease.[3]

Premenopausal patients rarely develop endometrial carcinoma. Young women with polycystic ovarian syndrome are at higher risk of developing endometrial carcinoma as are girls with ovarian dysgenesis on long-term estrogen replacement therapy. Granulosa-theca cell tumors characterized by abnormally high and unopposed estrogen stimulation are associated with endometrial hyperplasia in 50%, and with endometrial carcinoma in 6–8%, of cases. The extensive use of oral contraceptives has provided the opportunity to study the effects of exogenous estrogen in young women. Silverberg and Makowski[8] collected 21 cases of endometrial carcinoma in oral contraceptive users. Eleven of these patients had used sequential medication; all were young and without the usual predisposing factors for endometrial cancer.

Case-control studies published since 1975 have demonstrated an increased risk of endometrial cancer following exogenous estrogen administration in postmenopausal women (Table 8–2). These studies have been questioned with respect to statistical evaluation, choice of controls, and histologic diagnosis.[14] A prospective study would be the only way of circumventing the retrospective methodology and its inherent problems. It has been suggested that some studies may have exaggerated the hazard of estrogen therapy by including patients with atypical hyperplasia. Gordon and coworkers[15] independently reviewed the histology slides from the Ziel and Finkle study, finding that 74% (66/89) were correctly diagnosed. In the 66 patients with correct diagnosis, 61% (40/66) had used conjugated estrogens, vs. 57% (54/94) in the original study. On the basis of 66 patients and 132 matched controls the revised risk-ratio estimate was 8.1, validating the original estimate. Smith and coworkers,[16] at the University of Washington, reviewed the pathology material on 182 endometrial cancer patients from their previous study reported in 1975. The purpose of this study was to compare histopathologic characteristics with the

TABLE 8–2. Case-control Studies of Endometrial Carcinoma Following Exogenous Estrogen Administration.

	SEATTLE (SMITH[9])	LOS ANGELES (ZIEL[10])	LOS ANGELES (MACK[11])	ROCHESTER (MCDONALD[12])	BALTIMORE (ANTUNES[13])
Excluded "in situ" cancer	No	No	No	Yes	No
Further slide review	No	Later	No	Yes	10% sample
Controls	Gynecologic cancers	Community	Community	Clinic admissions	Hospital admissions; gynecologic admissions not analyzed
Definition of estrogen use	Any estrogen ≥ 6 months	Conjugated	Any estrogen ≥ 6 months	Conjugated	Any estrogen
Data sources	Hospital and clinic records	Clinic records	Clinic and pharmacy records and some interviews	Clinic records	Hospital records and some interviews
Relative risk	4.5	7.6	8.0	4.9	6.0

clinical behavior of endometrial adenocarcinoma in estrogen users and nonusers. They found that estrogen users were more likely to develop stage IA grade 1 disease than nonestrogen users. The relative risk ratio calculated was 9.4. The duration of use has been identified as the single most important factor in determining the risk of developing this neoplasm. Increasing dosage of estrogen administration also seems to increase risk. This increase in risk seems to be incurred by the nonobese woman and falls quickly after the discontinuation of estrogen.[17]

Screening of Endometrial Cancer

Screening is an effort to detect a disease in asymptomatic individuals. To date, no satisfactory technique is available for the routine screening of large populations for endometrial carcinoma. Koss and coworkers[18] reported the results of a study of detection of endometrial carcinoma in asymptomatic women. Only eight of 1280 women, evaluated by endometrial cytologic smear techniques and by two endometrial biopsy sampling methods, had histologically documented endometrial carcinoma diagnosed. Many devices have been used to obtain cytologic and histologic specimens in the outpatient setting (Table 8–3). Anderson et al.[19] found that cytologic specimens were not satisfactory for interpretation in 17–32% of samples obtained. The reasons for unsatisfactory preparations included insufficient number of cells, blood only, fractured cell membranes, loss of nuclear detail, and degeneration of cells. Endometrial biopsy is the only method that has been proven reliable in detecting both endometrial hyperplasia and carcinomas.[20] Hofmeister[21] reported that 17% of endometrial carcinomas diagnosed by office biopsy occurred in asymptomatic perimenopausal women. At present, annual endometrial biopsies cannot be recommended for all women. Periodic endometrial biopsy is indicated for postmenopausal women taking estrogen or having the clinical stigmata associated with endometrial cancer. Although the cervical Pap smear occasionally detects endometrial cancer, it is too unreliable to be utilized as a screening test.

Symptomatology

The most important single symptom in endometrial carcinoma is postmenopausal bleeding. The great majority of patients who develop endometrial cancer are in the postmenopausal years and in over 90% of them vaginal bleeding is the initial and only complaint. There are many causes of postmenopausal bleeding, but nearly 20% of patients with postmenopausal vaginal bleeding have a gynecologic malignancy, usually endometrial carcinoma.

Patients who present with a purulent, blood-tinged vaginal discharge and cramping lower abdominal pain may have pyometra. Pain in the lower abdomen or back is generally associated with metastatic disease.

A high index of suspicion must be maintained if the diagnosis of endometrial carcinoma is to be made in the young and in the perimenopausal patient. These patients present with abnormal vaginal bleeding often characterized as menometorrhagia. Endometrial cancer should be considered in the young woman with abnormal vaginal bleeding that is persistent or recurrent, especially if obesity or anovulation is present.

TABLE 8–3. Comparison of Outpatient Techniques for the Detection of Endometrial Cancer.

TECHNIQUE	NO. OF PATIENTS	CANCERS DETECTED	CANCERS AT D & C	FALSE-NEGATIVE RESULTS
Saline irrigation	1251	45	64	29%
Brush cytology	191	7	11	36%
Vacuum aspiration	122	5	10	50%
Jet washer	181	6	10	40%
Endometrial biopsy	811	60	62	3%

Modified from Anderson DG, et al.[19]

Diagnosis

The diagnosis of endometrial carcinoma requires examination of tissue obtained from the endometrium. Traditionally a dilatation and fractional curettage (D & C) has been the definitive diagnostic procedure in endometrial carcinoma. This procedure consists of (1) scraping the endocervical canal; (2) sounding of the uterus; (3) a thorough endometrial curettage; and (4) exploration of the uterine cavity with a Randall-Stone polyp forceps. The specimens are submitted to the laboratory in separate containers. The fractional D & C will demonstrate extension of disease into the endocervix or may detect an occult primary endocervical cancer. If any lesion is detected in the cervix or vagina, this should be biopsied.

Many patients suspected of having endometrial carcinoma can be evaluated in the physician's office with a Pap smear, endocervical sampling, uterine sounding, and endometrial biopsy. Negative findings necessitate fractional D & C under anesthesia. Patients with stenosis of the endocervical canal or with unsatisfactory pelvic examination in the office also require examination under anesthesia and fractional D & C. It is not appropriate to attribute post-menopausal bleeding to atrophic vaginitis or other benign conditions unless the results of a fractional D & C are negative.

Pathology

Endometrial carcinoma may occur simultaneously with or may be preceded by endometrial hyperplasia. Hyperplasia results from prolonged and unopposed estrogen stimulation of the endometrium. Endometrial hyperplasia is characterized by a morphologically abnormal proliferative-type endometrium and an abnormally increased endometrial volume.

Endometrial hyperplasia has been classified by the World Health Organization into cystic and adenomatous types. In cystic hyperplasia most of the endometrial glands are large and cystically dilated; in adenomatous hyperplasia, there is glandular crowding, budding, and branching. The presence of dysplasia in conjunction with glandular crowding is the hallmark of atypical hyperplasia. These atypical lesions are characterized by closely packed glands with little intervening stroma *without* evidence of stromal invasion.

Atypical endometrial hyperplasia may be confused with adenocarcinoma histologically, and because there is reasonable evidence that patients with hyperplasia, particularly atypical hyperplasia, have a higher than expected incidence of endometrial adenocarcinoma. The more atypical the hyperplasia, the greater the likelihood the patient will develop adenocarcinoma and the shorter the interval between the onset of hyperplasia and the diagnosis of adenocarcinoma.

ENDOMETRIAL CARCINOMA. Carcinoma of the endometrium may develop as a localized polypoid mass or as a diffuse lesion involving the endometrial surface. Characteristically it contains yellow areas of necrosis that often allow for macroscopic identification. Myometrial invasion may be evident grossly, as linear extensions beneath an endometrial mass, or as numerous nodules throughout the myometrium (Fig. 8–1). Carcinoma may extend into the cervix and be grossly visible.

Adenocarcinoma of the endometrium with or without squamous differentiation constitutes the most common epithelial malignancy of the endometrium, accounting for 85–95% of all carcinomas of the endometrium. Endometrial adenocarcinoma may grow in the form of well-

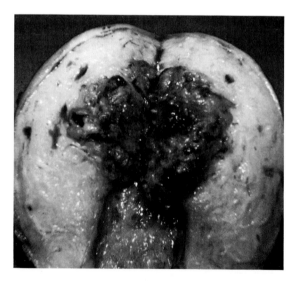

Fig. 8–1. Large uterus showing a polypoid adenocarcinoma of the endometrium. Deep myometrial invasion is evident.

developed glands, papillae, solid mass, sheets, and admixtures of these. The three-grade system adopted by the International Federation of Gynecology and Obstetrics (FIGO) is currently in use. In this system, grade 1 adenocarcinomas are those tumors which are composed entirely of glands and/or papillae. Grade 3 tumors comprise the poorly differentiated lesions growing predominantly as solid sheets of anaplastic cells. Grade 2 lesions have an intermediate pattern of growth, manifesting glandular elements with an admixture of the solid growth pattern (Fig. 8–2). Diagnostic problems for the pathologist arise at both extremes of the grading system: the very well-differentiated adenocarcinomas are difficult to distinguish from atypical hyperplasias and the very poorly differentiated carcinomas may resemble stromal sarcoma or undifferentiated neoplasia. In these cases the use of special stains and electron microscopy may be helpful. Since the prognosis and treatment of endometrial carcinoma will depend on the least differentiated area, a thorough microscopic evaluation is mandatory and the lesion should be designated by the most advanced grade. Other histologic features of prognostic significance are the depth of myometrial invasion, involvement of the endocervix, and histologic type of carcinoma. A histologic classification of primary endometrial carcinoma is shown in Table 8–4.

Adenocarcinoma of the endometrium frequently contains areas of squamous epithelium. Ng et al.[23] classified the tumors containing squamous elements into two categories: (1) adenoacanthoma, or adenocarcinoma with

TABLE 8–4. Histologic Classification of Endometrial Carcinoma.

Adenocarcinoma
  Endometrioid, with or without benign squamous differentiation
  Clear cell
  Mucinous
  Papillary, with or without psammoma bodies
  Ciliated
  Mixed
Squamous cell carcinoma
  In situ
  Invasive
Mixed adenosquamous cell carcinoma
Undifferentiated and anaplastic carcinoma

From Hendrickson MR, et al.[22]

squamous metaplasia, in which the squamous elements are benign; and (2) mixed adenosquamous carcinoma in which the squamous epithelium appears malignant. Silverberg and coworkers[24] found a marked tendency for the glandular elements in adenoacanthoma to be of low histologic grade and for those in mixed carcinoma to be poorly differentiated or anaplastic. Another important feature of mixed carcinomas was their tendency to invade the myometrium more frequently as evidenced in hysterectomy specimens.

In *adenoacanthomas* the squamous cells resemble those of mature or metaplastic squamous epithelium of the cervix and are usually found on the surface of the glandular tumor. In *adenosquamous* carcinoma the squamous elements resemble the various forms of squamous carcinoma of the cervix and demonstrate their malignant behavior by invading into the surrounding stroma. Keratin pearls may or may not be present. The glandular elements usually predominate but in some instances the squamous elements are the dominant feature. These tumors usually invade the myometrium extensively and show vascular invasion as well (Fig. 8–3). Ng et al.[23] reported that in 65% of adenosquamous carcinomas the metastatic lesions contained both glandular and squamous elements, 20% contained only glandular, 8% only squamous, and in 7% it was not possible to classify the metastatic cell type.

The presence of malignant squamous cells in endometrial carcinoma is associated with a poor prognosis. Silverberg et al.[24] reviewed 148 cases of endometrial cancer seen over a 15-year period: despite similar treatment regimens and in comparable clinical stages, the 5-year survival with pure adenocarcinoma was 56.3% compared to 35.3% for those with mixed adenosquamous carcinoma. Ng et al.[23] analyzed 542 cases of endometrial carcinoma seen over a period of 30 years and found an increasing frequency of adenosquamous carcinoma as compared with endometrial adenocarcinoma; they found that the mixed tumors occurred at an older age, had a shorter symptomatic period, and were more advanced at the time of diagnosis. The 5-year survival was less than 20%.

Clear cell carcinomas comprise no more than 5% of all endometrial carcinomas. The clear cell carcinomas have the same histologic fea-

Fig. 8–2. A Well-differentiated adenocarcinoma (grade 1) of the endometrium showing a predominantly glandular pattern with back-to-back glands and no intervening stroma. H & E; × 400.

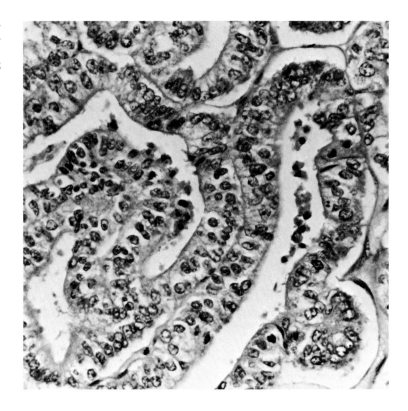

Fig. 8–2. B Moderately differentiated adenocarcinoma (grade 2) of the endometrium showing a mixture of solid and glandular components. H & E; × 400.

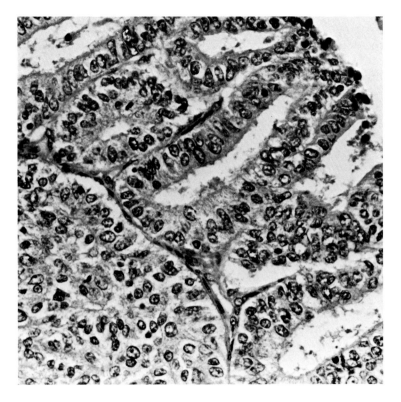

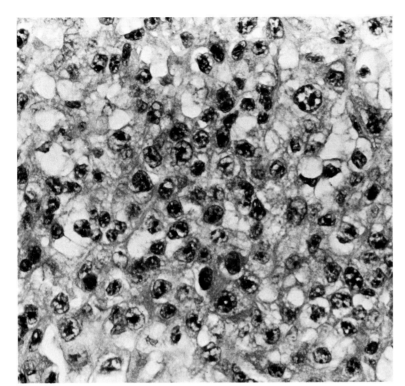

Fig. 8–2. C Poorly differentiated adenocarcinoma (grade 3) of the endometrium showing a predominantly solid pattern with pleomorphic nuclei. H & E; × 400.

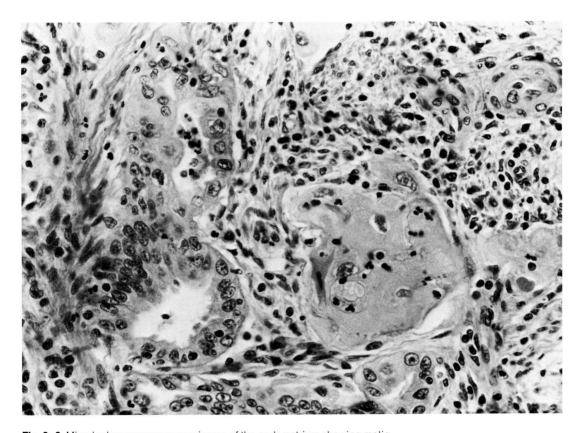

Fig. 8–3. Mixed adenosquamous carcinoma of the endometrium showing malignant glands and a separate malignant invasive squamous cell carcinoma. H & E; × 400.

tures as clear cell carcinomas arising in the ovary, cervix, and vagina. They are of mullerian origin and may have several histologic patterns. Clear and hobnail cells are present in varying proportions. The cells may grow, forming papillae, numerous small spaces or tubules, or may have a glandular configuration (Fig. 8–4). Often several patterns may be present in a tumor.

Clear cell carcinomas are very aggressive tumors. Christopherson et al.[25] and Kurman and Scully[26] have documented the poor prognosis of clear cell carcinomas. In Christopherson's study of 56 patients with clear cell carcinomas, only 35.7% survived 5 years. Even among patients with stage I disease, 5-year survival was only 44.2%.

Mucinous carcinomas of the endometrium are very rare. These tumors are indistinguishable from carcinomas arising in the cervix, ovary, or bowel. They are often well differentiated and composed of cells with bland nuclei and abundant, mucin-filled foamy cytoplasm.

Little information is available in the literature on the natural history of this type of endometrial tumor.

Papillary adenocarcinoma (with or without psammoma bodies) can arise primarily in the endometrium. This tumor, particularly when psammoma bodies are present, has a distinct tendency to invade the myometrium and to involve the myometrial lymphatics (Fig. 8–5). Extrauterine spread often mimicking ovarian carcinoma is also common in papillary adenocarcinoma of the endometrium. Christopherson and coworkers[27] reported 46 patients with papillary carcinoma of the endometrium; the median age at diagnosis was 63 years, and the survival rate was 51.1% at 5 years and 46.3% at 10 years. They concluded that this type of tumor appeared more aggressive with a higher death rate than the usual type of endometrial adenocarcinoma. Roberts and Lifshitz[28] recently reviewed the literature on papillary adenocarcinoma of the endometrium with psammoma bodies and added a case. Of nine cases

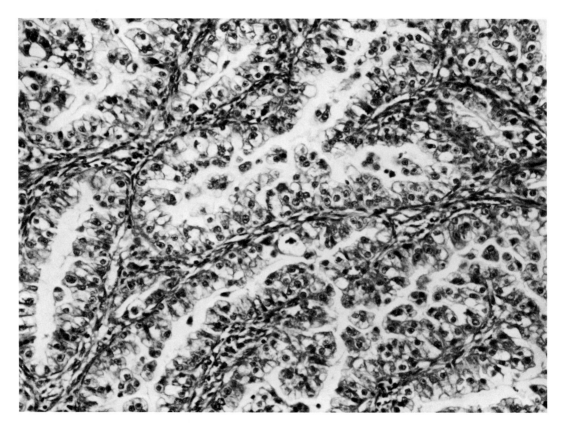

Fig. 8–4. Clear cell adenocarcinoma of the endometrium demonstrating a papillary and glandular configuration with the characteristic clear cells. H & E; × 200.

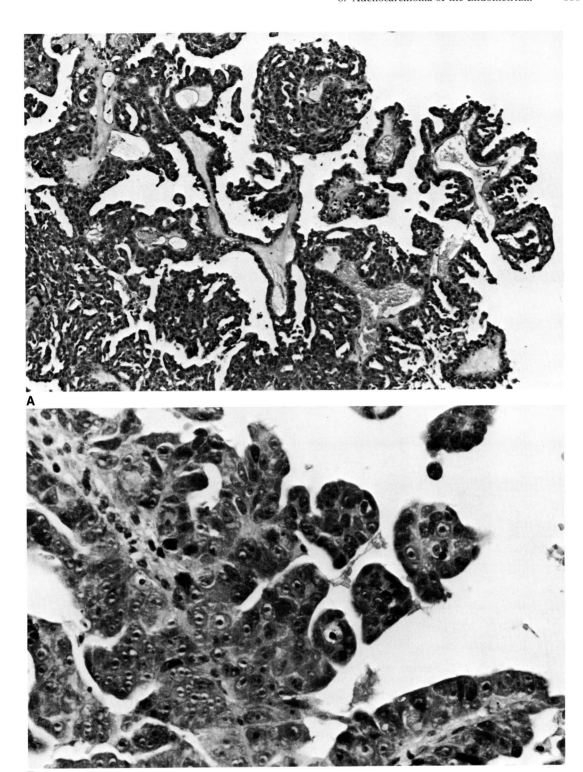

Fig. 8–5. A Papillary adenocarcinoma of the endometrium. Low power view demonstrating fibrovascular stalks and papillary formations. H & E; × 100. **B** Papillary adenocarcinoma of the endometrium. High power view demonstrating the characteristic pleomorphic nuclei with prominent nucleoli. H & E; × 400.

reported, seven were associated with deep myometrial invasion. Two patients died of disease, two had advanced disease at the time of the report, and the five remaining patients have had an average of 16 months follow-up.

Primary squamous cell carcinoma of the endometrium is rare and almost always found in elderly women. Fluhmann, in 1928,[29] established the criteria for the diagnosis of this entity. There must be *no* (1) coexisting endometrial adenocarcinoma; (2) connection between the endometrial tumor and the squamous epithelium of the cervix; or (3) primary squamous cell carcinoma of the cervix. The histogenesis of this tumor is controversial; it may originate from a focus of squamous metaplasia or from a "reserve cell" lying between the columnar epithelium and basement membrane.

White et al.[30] tabulated the salient clinical features of 18 reported cases of primary squamous cell carcinoma of the endometrium: the average age of the patients was 61 years, myometrial invasion or metastasis was present in 89%, and pyometra in 39% of the cases. The high incidence of pyometra was felt to be due to the effect of squamous cell tumor necrosis with inadequate uterine drainage. The prognosis of squamous cell carcinoma of the endometrium is very poor.[31] In Baggish and Woodruff's[32] series, none of the patients treated at the Johns Hopkins Hospital survived 5 years.

Squamous cell carcinoma in situ may be encountered in the endometrium, most often in association with squamous cell carcinoma in situ of the cervix. In rare instances the cervix, endometrium, fallopian tube, and surface of the ovary may all be involved with squamous carcinoma in situ.[33]

Clinical Staging

After the diagnosis of endometrial carcinoma has been established, a thorough diagnostic evaluation should be carried out and the disease staged before the institution of therapy. The current FIGO classification for endometrial carcinoma is shown in Table 8–5. This staging system reflects the natural history of endometrial carcinoma and classifies the disease from stage I to stage IV in groups of progressively worsening prognosis. This staging system is clinical and thus does not permit the use of surgical-pathologic data. A general physical and pelvic examination, as well as a fractional curettage, and endoscopic and radiographic studies should be performed. The abdomen should be examined for masses or

TABLE 8–5. Staging Classification of Endometrial Carcinoma (FIGO).

Stage 0:	Carcinoma in situ; histologic findings suspicious of malignancy (atypical adenomatous hyperplasia)
Stage I:	Carcinoma is confined to the corpus: A: The length of the uterine cavity is 8 cm or less B: The length of the uterine cavity is more than 8 cm The stage I cases should be subgrouped with regard to the histologic type of adenocarcinoma as follows: G_1: highly differentiated adenomatous carcinoma G_2: differentiated adenomatous carcinoma with partially solid areas G_3: predominantly solid or entirely undifferentiated carcinomas
Stage II:	The carcinoma involves the corpus and the cervix; histologic proof of endocervical involvement is available
Stage III:	The carcinoma has extended outside the uterus, but not outside the true pelvis; involvement may be with other genital structures, e.g., fallopian tubes and ovaries; it may involve the serosa of the bowel or rectum
Stage IV:	The carcinoma has extended outside the true pelvis or is obviously involved in the mucosa of the bladder or rectum; bullous edema as such does not permit allotment of a case to stage IV

organomegaly, presence of ascites, or metastases in the area of the umbilicus. The supraclavicular and inguinal lymph nodes should be palpated to detect suspicious lymphadenopathy. The external genitalia are rarely involved by endometrial cancer, but the anterior distal vagina is a fairly common site for submucosal metastases. On bimanual examination the uterine size, shape, and mobility as well as the condition of the paracervical, parametrial, and adnexal areas should be determined. Approximately 75% of cases will be stage I at the time of diagnosis (Table 8–6). These are subgrouped on the basis of histologic grade and length of uterine cavity measured from the external os to the uterine fundus. Adenocarcinoma in the endocervical curettings must be associated with normal endocervical glands and stroma to qualify as cervical extension and permit allotment of the disease to stage II. If there is a visible cervical lesion, cervical biopsies should be performed. Cervical conization is not recommended in the evaluation of a patient with endometrial cancer.

To complete the clinical staging a chest x-ray and an intravenous pyelogram should be obtained. Barium enema and sigmoidoscopy are recommended for patients over 65 years of age, or if the patient is symptomatic and/or the stool guaiac is positive. Bone and liver scans are not indicated unless specific symptomatology exists or laboratory tests are suggestive of metastatic disease. The finding of metastases in the vagina, paracervical or parametrial induration and nodularity, as well as the presence of adnexal mass allows a case to be staged as III. Extension of the disease to involve the mucosa of the bladder or rectum, or spread outside the pelvis, qualifies a patient for stage IV. The pelvic and paraaortic lymph nodes are the most frequent sites of lymphatic spread. Lung, liver, and bone constitute the most common metastatic sites of hematogenous spread. Some patients may present with ascites or clinical involvement of the inguinal or supraclavicular lymph nodes.

Prognostic Factors

Multiple factors have been identified that have significant prognostic value in endometrial carcinoma. The histologic differentiation of the tumor and uterine size are two factors that the FIGO classification has taken into consideration as substage categories within stage I. Although there is general agreement that the grade of tumor differentiation is an important prognostic factor, this is not true of uterine size. The depth of myometrial invasion, lymph node involvement, and malignant cells in peritoneal washings are important prognostic factors that cannot be determined preoperatively and therefore are not taken into consideration in the clinical FIGO staging system.

Histologic Differentiation. The degree of tumor differentiation has long been recognized as the single most important prognostic indicator in endometrial carcinoma limited to the corpus. Jones[35] correlated survival with tumor differentiation in 3990 patients from several reports. The survival decreases as the tumor loses its differentiation (Table 8–7). The degree of tumor differentiation also correlates well with the depth of myometrial invasion. Cheon[36] has shown that as the tumor becomes less differentiated, the depth of myometrial invasion increases.

The incidence of lymph node metastases also correlates closely with the degree of tumor differentiation. Lewis and coworkers[37] reported a series of 107 nonirradiated patients with stage I and II endometrial carcinoma, who underwent pelvic lymphadenectomies.

TABLE 8–6. Distribution of Endometrial Carcinoma by Stage.

STAGE	NUMBER OF PATIENTS	PERCENTAGE
I	10,699	73.8
II	1980	13.6
III	1355	9.3
IV	472	3.3

From Kottmeier H, Kolstal P.[34]

TABLE 8–7. Correlation Between Tumor Differentiation and 5-Year Survival Rate.

GRADE	NO. OF PATIENTS	SURVIVAL RATE
1	1558	81%
2	1515	74%
3	917	50%

Modified from Jones HW.[35]

Only 5.5% with grade 1 tumor had positive nodes, whereas 26% of patients with grade 3 lesions had nodal metastases.

UTERINE SIZE. Uterine size has long been thought to have prognostic significance. Jones[35] correlated uterine size and survival in stage I disease from nine reports in the literature totaling 1761 patients; he showed an 85.4% 5-year survival when the uterus was of normal size and 66.6% when it was enlarged. However, it should be pointed out that data in the recent literature fail to substantiate this correlation. Shah,[38] Nahhas,[39] Wade,[40] Malkasian,[41] and Austin[42] noted no prognostic significance of uterine size. A study from the Gynecologic Oncology Group[43] found a higher incidence of lymph node metastases in patients with large uteri as well as a good correlation with tumor grade (Table 8–8). It is however, recognized that all enlarged uteri are not due to cancer. A significant number of patients with endometrial carcinoma have an enlarged uterus secondary to leiomyomas or adenomyosis. Javert[44] examined the hysterectomy specimens of 100 patients with endometrial carcinoma and found the uterus to be enlarged in 54 cases, but only in eight was enlargement due to cancer.

STAGE OF DISEASE. The stage of endometrial carcinoma is a clear prognostic factor. The 5-year survival rate reported by FIGO from worldwide institutions is shown in Table 8–9. The significance of endocervical involvement is demonstrated by a worse prognosis than for the earlier lesions. Involvement of the uterine cervix opens new lymphatic pathways for dissemination and increases the likelihood of nodal metastases. The degree of cervical in-

TABLE 8–9. Five-year Survival in Endometrial Carcinoma.

STAGE	PATIENTS (%)	
I	7695/10,699	(71.9)
II	984/1980	(49.7)
III	416/1355	(30.7)
IV	44/472	(9.3)

From Kottmeier H, Kolsted P.[34]

volvement in endometrial carcinoma appears to have some prognostic value. Surwit and coworkers[45] reported that patients with stromal invasion of the cervix had a 3-year survival of 47%, whereas patients with involvement limited to the endocervical glands had a survival of 74%.

MYOMETRIAL INVASION. The depth of myometrial invasion is a valuable prognostic factor in endometrial carcinoma. Several publications have clearly demonstrated that as myometrial invasion increases, survival decreases. Jones[35] collected 910 patients from several reports in the literature, finding an 80.8% 5-year survival for patients with carcinoma limited to the endometrium. Patients with superficial myometrial invasion did as well as those with no invasion, but when deep myometrial invasion was present the survival dropped to 60.5% The depth of myometrial invasion correlates well with degree of tumor differentiation and survival (Table 8–10), as well as with pelvic and paraaortic lymph node metastases (Table 8–11). Lutz and coworkers[48] suggested that the proximity of the tumor to the uterine serosa is more important in determining prognosis than is the depth of myometrial invasion. Patients with tumors within 5 mm of uterine serosa had a 5-year survival of

TABLE 8–8. Stage and Grade by Pelvic and Aortic Node Metastases.

STAGE	PELVIC (%)	AORTIC (%)
IAG$_1$	1.7	1.7
IAG$_2$	9.3	6.9
IAG$_3$	22.2	16.6
IBG$_1$	3.2	0.0
IBG$_2$	11.1	2.7
IBG$_3$	45.0	40.0

From Creasman WT.[43]

TABLE 8–10. Five-year Survival in Relation to Histologic Grade and Myometrial Invasion.

MYOMETRIAL INVASION	TUMOR DIFFERENTIATION (%)			
	G$_1$	G$_2$	G$_3$	G$_4$
None	95	93	64	62
Superficial	92	72	50	50
Deep	33	37	25	14

Modified from Ng AB, Reagan JW.[46]

TABLE 8–11. Lymph Node Metastases vs. Depth of Myometrial Invasion for Clinical Stage I and Occult Stage II.

INVASION	PELVIC NODES (%)		AORTIC NODES (%)	
Endometrium only	1.3	(150)	1.7	(121)
Superficial muscle	2.7	(225)	0.6	(171)
Intermediate muscle	1.4	(74)	3.6	(55)
Deep muscle	28.4	(95)	17.1	(82)
Total	6.6	(544)	4.4	(429)

Number in parentheses is number of patients.
From Lewis GC, Bundy B.[47]

65%, whereas patients with tumors more than 10 mm from the serosa had a survival of 97%.

LYMPH NODE METASTASES. Lymph nodal involvement by endometrial carcinoma has been well documented. Morrow and coworkers[49] reviewed the literature on the subject and noted in a collected series of 369 patients with stage I endometrial carcinoma a 10.6% incidence of positive pelvic lymph nodes. When the cervix was involved (stage II) the lymph node involvement increased to 36.5%. Stallworthy[50] has also reported a 41% incidence of pelvic lymph node metastases in patients with cervical involvement.

The lymph node involvement in endometrial carcinoma correlates not only with the stage of the disease, but also with the degree of tumor differentiation and depth of myometrial invasion. In a prospective surgical-pathologic study of 206 patients with stage I endometrial carcinoma by the Gynecologic Oncology Group (GOG) Creasman[43] reported an excellent correlation between grade of tumor and pelvic and paraaortic lymph node metastases (Table 8–12). Analysis of over 500 patients with stage I and occult stage II endometrial carcinoma studied by the GOG shows that the likelihood of lymph node metastases also increases with depth of myometrial invasion

(Table 8–11). It is not clear that a significant number of patients with stage I endometrial carcinoma may have regional lymph node metastases.

PERITONEAL CYTOLOGY. The prognostic significance of positive peritoneal cytology in endometrial carcinoma has been recently recognized. Creasman and Rutledge[51] reported a 12% incidence of positive peritoneal cytology in endometrial carcinoma, although most of these patients did have gross metastatic disease outside the pelvis.

In stage I disease, Keettel et al.[52] reported a 12% incidence of positive peritoneal cytology. The prognosis of these patients is generally very poor. Szpak et al.[53] studied the peritoneal washings of 54 patients with stage I endometrial cancer, finding malignant cells in 12 (22%). These patients had similar tumor grades and depth of myometrial invasion as did patients with negative washings. In this study the number of malignant cells per 100 ml of washing fluid was quantitated. It is interesting to note that not all patients with positive washings had progressive disease or died of cancer. Only two of eight patients with fewer than 1000 malignant cells/100 ml of washing developed a recurrence, whereas all the patients with more than 1000 cells/100 ml of washing died of cancer despite the use of adjunctive radiation and progestin therapy.

Treatment

The optimal treatment of patients with adenocarcinoma of the endometrium still remains somewhat controversial despite three decades of accumulated experience in the management of this disease. As early as 1900, hysterectomy

TABLE 8–12. Endometrial Carcinoma Stage I: Grade vs. Nodal Metastases.

GRADE	PELVIC (%)	AORTIC (%)
G_1	2.2	1.1
G_2	10.1	5.0
G_3	34.2	28.9

From Creasman WT.[43]

TABLE 8–13. Five-year Survival by Treatment.

	SURGERY		IRRADIATION	
	No. of Patients	5-year Survival	No. of Patients	5-year Survival
Stage I	139	87%	130	69%
Stage II	33	70%	31	49%
Stages III and IV	20	69%	20	45%

From Bickenbach W, et al.[55]

became the therapy of choice in the treatment of endometrial cancer and continues to be the cornerstone of therapy. Heyman[54] in 1927 developed a technique of radium application with 5-year survival equal to that of operative treatment and challenged surgical therapy as the only modality of treatment. More recent studies comparing results by stage of disease have shown a clearcut advantage of surgery (Table 8–13). Radiation alone has been reserved for patients who cannot tolerate surgery or for palliation in patients with inoperable disease.

A variety of procedures including vaginal hysterectomy and radical hysterectomy with pelvic lymphadenectomy have been utilized in the surgical therapy of endometrial carcinoma. At present, the most common procedure employed is total abdominal hysterectomy with bilateral salpingo-oophorectomy. Vaginal hysterectomy has been employed because it is often shorter, less traumatic, and better tolerated by the obese and elderly patient who is a poor surgical risk. Pratt and coworkers[56] have demonstrated that excellent results can be obtained using vaginal hysterectomy in early, well-selected cases. In a series of 100 patients from the Mayo Clinic they reported a 5-year

survival of 84%. Most of the patients had well-differentiated lesions with minimal myometrial invasion and some were treated with postoperative radiation therapy. Although good results can be obtained in small, low grade lesions using the vaginal approach, there are several disadvantages which limit its usefulness in endometrial carcinoma. Ovarian metastases can occur in early lesions, and even in skillful hands the ovaries cannot always be removed vaginally. Neither can a thorough exploration of the abdominal cavity be performed or lymph nodes sampled.

Radical hysterectomy and pelvic lymphadenectomy for endometrial cancer was introduced by Meigs and Brunschwig. Jones[35] collected 376 patients from the literature with endometrial carcinoma treated with radical hysterectomy and pelvic lymphadenectomy showing an overall 5-year survival of 77% for all stages and 24% survival when the pelvic lymph nodes were positive, despite the fact that most of these patients were treated with postoperative radiation therapy. The morbidity associated with radical surgery in these obese and elderly patients is significant. Park[57] has reported a 24% incidence of major operative complications in patients undergoing "ex-

TABLE 8–14. Vaginal Vault Recurrence in Endometrial Carcinoma Stage I According to Treatment Method.

AUTHOR	SURGERY ONLY		SURGERY + RADIOTHERAPY	
Joelsson[59] (1973)			8/517	(1.5%)
Keller[60] (1974)	1/78	(1.3%)		
Homesley[61] (1976)	13/369	(3.5%)	1/61	(1.6%)
Lewis[62] (1977)	7/194	(3.6%)	4/380	(1%)
Bean[63] (1978)	1/107	(0.9%)	0/130	(0%)
Prem[64] (1979)	7/131	(5.3%)	1/63	(1.6%)
Piver[65] (1979)	4/53	(7.5%)	4/136	(2.9%)
Overall	33/932	(3.5%)	18/1287	(1.4%)

TABLE 8–15. Five-year Survival in Endometrial Carcinoma Stage I According to Tumor Grade and Treatment.

AUTHOR	G_1		G_2		G_3	
	S	S + RT	S	S + RT	S	S + RT
Frick[66] (1973)	78/88	78/86	7/10	25/36	3/5	9/14
Wharam[67] (1976)	80/82	14/14	63/69	60/69	5/9	15/26
Salazar[68] (1978)	96/100	111/114	80/89	461/510	20/32	170/221
Total	254/270	203/214	150/168	546/615	28/46	194/261
	(94%)	(94.8%)	(89.2%)	(88.7%)	(60.8%)	(74.3%)

S, surgery; RT, radiation therapy.

tended hysterectomy" for endometrial cancer. The fact that similar survival figures can be obtained with much less morbidity, even in stage II lesions, dictates against the use of radical hysterectomy and pelvic lymphadenectomy in endometrial carcinoma. Rutledge[58] reviewed the role of radical hysterectomy and pelvic lymphadenectomy in endometrial carcinoma and concluded that in stage I disease, this procedure had a limited role and probably was not indicated.

The results obtained with either surgery or radiation therapy have led to trials of combined treatment. For the last 30 years reports have appeared in the literature suggesting an increased survival when surgery is used in combination with some form of radiation therapy. Over the years it has become common to treat early endometrial carcinoma by intracavitary radium followed 4 to 6 weeks later by extrafascial abdominal hysterectomy. With this approach the incidence of vaginal vault recurrence has been reduced from 8 to 1% (Table 8–14).

More recently, data have appeared in the literature evaluating survival by tumor differentiation as well as by depth of myometrial invasion (Tables 8–15 and 8–16). These studies showed no difference in survival with grade 1

and 2 tumors treated with pre- or postoperative radiation. Earlier, recurrence in the vaginal cuff was attributed to operative spill through the cervical canal. A number of mechanical methods were introduced to occlude the cervix (suturing the external os, clamps, and so on) but all failed to gain acceptance. The risk of cuff recurrence is directly related to the degree of myometrial invasion, tumor differentiation, and endocervical involvement, factors known to be associated with an increased risk for lymphatic invasion. Pre- or postoperative irradiation to the vaginal vault and paracervical tissues is believed to decrease the local recurrence rate by virtue of eradicating tumor cells already present in lymphatic channels. This point of view has been well documented by Truskett[69] who reported the incidence of vaginal vault recurrence in patients treated with preoperative Heyman packing (without cervical or vaginal sources) to be the same as in patients treated by surgery only.

There is controversy regarding the treatment of patients with stage I grade 3 lesions. These patients have a high incidence of deep myometrial invasion and of lymph node metastases. Recurrences are also more frequent in these patients. Some clinics treat patients with stage IB with preoperative external radiation

TABLE 8–16. Five-year Survival in Endometrial Carcinoma Stage I According to Depth of Myometrial Involvement and Treatment.

RESIDUAL	SURGERY	SURGERY + RADIATION
No tumor	11/12 (96%)	27/28 (96.4%)
Endometrium + inner muscle	69/80 (86.2%)	49/64 (76.5%)
Middle or outer muscle	8/11 (77.7%)	36/44 (81.8%)

Modified from Frick HC II, et al.[66]

to deliver 4000–5000 rads to the whole pelvis, intracavitary radium, followed 4 to 6 weeks later by a total abdominal hysterectomy and bilateral salpingo-oophorectomy. In a retrospective study, Salazar and coworkers,[68] using preoperative external pelvic radiotherapy, reported a 5-year survival of 87% in 95 patients with stage I grade 3 endometrial cancer as compared with a 65% 5-year survival for 32 patients treated with surgery only.

Some institutions utilize preoperative radium only, either tandem and colpostats or Heyman packing plus vaginal ovoids, followed by a total abdominal hysterectomy and bilateral salpingo-oophorectomy. Underwood[70] has recommended that the hysterectomy be performed immediately after the radium is removed, and has shown this approach to be associated with favorable survival and low treatment morbidity.

The current trend in treating endometrial carcinoma stage I grade 3 is away from routine preoperative irradiation. This reflects a better understanding of the spread of endometrial carcinoma and the ready availability of high energy beam machines. Aalders,[71] in a prospective study randomizing patients to postoperative radiation therapy vs. no radiation therapy, found no difference in survival in grades 1 and 2. He recommended that external pelvic radiotherapy be administered only to patients with grade 3 lesions or those with deep myometrial invasion, a conclusion supported by Piver and associates.[65] In a nonrandomized study of 172 patients with stage I adenocarcinoma of the endometrium, Burrell et al.[72] found no difference in survival in patients with grade 3 lesion without myometrial invasion, whether they were treated with external radiotherapy or not.

The treatment of endometrial carcinoma should be based on a thorough evaluation of the prognostic factors as predictors of the potential spread of the disease. Radiation therapy for adenocarcinoma of the endometrium should be reserved primarily for patients with poor prognostic factors (deep myometrial invasion or lymph node metastases). Primary surgical approach will invariably reduce the number of cases receiving combination therapy and will eliminate the delay between diagnosis and surgical therapy. Paterson et al.[73] treated 140 patients with stage I endometrial

carcinoma with total abdominal hysterectomy and bilateral salpingo-oophorectomy. Adjunctive radiotherapy was administered only to patients with grade 3 lesions or those with greater than inner one-third myometrial invasion. Only 20.7% of patients required irradiation. There were no vaginal or pelvic recurrences and the 5-year survival was 93%. In the following paragraphs the current management of each stage of endometrial carcinoma is discussed.

STAGE I. The treatment of choice for endometrial carcinoma stage I (Fig. 8–6) is total abdominal extrafascial hysterectomy with bilateral salpingo-oophorectomy. The surgical procedure should be performed through a vertical incision to evaluate properly the extent of the disease. Once the peritoneal cavity has been entered, any fluid present in the pelvis should be collected. If none is present, 250–500 ml of normal saline solution should be used to irrigate the pelvic and abdominal cavity and then withdrawn with a bulb syringe. The fluid is submitted for cytologic evaluation. The abdominal contents are systematically explored with special attention to the liver, omentum, and retroperitoneal lymph nodes. Any suspicious lesions should be biopsied. The exploration should be performed in the least traumatic fashion. Removal of the adnexa is an integral part of the operation since they may contain microscopic metastases or may harbor a primary ovarian tumor. There is no therapeutic benefit in excising a margin of the vaginal cuff or in taking extraparametrial tissue.

Proper evaluation of the specimen by the pathologist is essential if optimal results are to be obtained. The degree of myometrial invasion, least differentiated areas of the tumor, and proximity of the tumor to the cervix need to be determined. Also, accurate study of the pelvic and paraaortic lymph nodes, adnexa, and peritoneal cytology is necessary. In most patients with stage I, grade 1 and 2, disease, subsequent radiation therapy should not be necessary unless there is significant myometrial invasion, cervical involvement, or adnexal metastases. If cancer cells are present in the peritoneal washings, adjunctive progestational therapy or intraperitoneal installation of chromic phosphate (^{32}P) can be considered.[74]

Postoperatively, patients with deep myome-

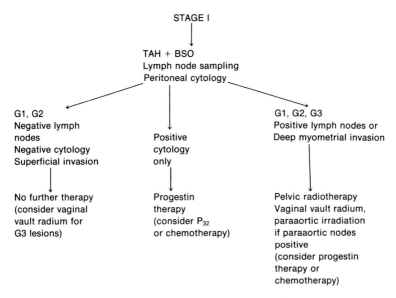

Fig. 8–6. Treatment of endometrial carcinoma.

trial invasion (over 50% of the uterine wall thickness), pelvic lymph node metastases, and/or spread to the adnexa are treated with whole pelvis irradiation, 4000–5000 rads administered in 5 to 6 weeks, and vaginal cuff radium. If the paraaortic lymph nodes are involved, extended field irradiation is employed. The use of adjunctive chemotherapy is currently being evaluated in this high risk group of patients.

STAGE II. The treatment of stage II endometrial carcinoma (Fig. 8–7) should encompass the likely metastatic sites. Current management consists of external radiation (4000–5000 rads, whole pelvis) and a single intracavitary radium and colpostat application, followed in 4 to 6 weeks by an extrafascial total abdominal hysterectomy and bilateral salpingo-oophorectomy with pelvic and paraaortic node sampling. Postoperatively, if me-

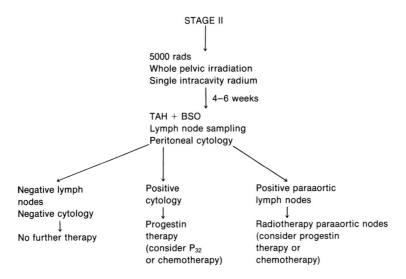

Fig. 8–7. Treatment of endometrial carcinoma.

tastases are present in the lymph nodes, progestational therapy or chemotherapy is recommended. Bruckman and coworkers[75] treated 40 patients with stage II endometrial carcinoma with radiotherapy followed by hysterectomy, obtaining an overall survival rate of 80%. Most of the failures were observed among patients with grade 3 disease. Cox and associates[76] studied 39 patients with stage II endometrial carcinoma treated with radiation therapy with and without subsequent hysterectomy. The 5-year survival with preoperative irradiation and abdominal hysterectomy was 89% as compared to 69% with radiation only. Several reports in the literature have also suggested improved prognosis with combination therapy (Table 8–17). Some authors advocate primary surgical therapy followed by irradiation to the pelvis and upper vagina if no visible disease is present in the cervix. Large prospective randomized trials are needed to evaluate this form of therapy.

STAGE III. The cornerstone of treatment for patients with endometrial carcinoma extending outside the uterine cavity but still confined to the pelvis is radiation therapy. With parametrial extension the disease is quite advanced and not suitable for hysterectomy. If there is regression of parametrial extension following radiotherapy, or if a stage III designation is based on vaginal metastases, an abdominal hysterectomy should be performed.

Patients classified as having stage III endometrial carcinoma on the basis of an adnexal mass should undergo primary surgery to determine the etiology of the mass. Occasionally an inflammatory adnexal mass or a primary ovarian malignancy will be found which can be effectively treated. If metastatic disease is found in the adnexa, pelvic irradiation should be administered postoperatively. Antoniades et al.[81] reported 37 patients with stage III endometrial carcinoma with three main patterns of spread: (1) downward into the vagina; (2) laterally into the parametrium and the pelvic wall; and (3) to the ovaries. Patients with ovarian extension had the best prognosis when treated by surgery followed by radiotherapy (30% recurrence rate). Patients with pelvic wall extension had the poorest prognosis (90% recurrence rate).

In a series of 26 patients with stage III endometrial carcinoma treated with a combination of radiation therapy and surgery, Bruckman[82] observed two distinct prognostic groups. Patients with disease confined to the ovary and/or fallopian tube had a 5-year survival of 80%, whereas patients with extension to the vagina or parametrial tissue had a survival of only 15%. Patients with extension of endometrial carcinoma to the parametrium or vagina usually have subclinical metastases beyond the pelvis. In these patients high dose, long-term progestin therapy or chemotherapy is recommended.

STAGE IV. The treatment of endometrial carcinoma presenting with distant metastasis should be individualized. For most of these patients the only suitable therapy is hormone or chemotherapy (see below). Surgery is warranted in cases with ascites or intraabdominal tumor amenable to reductive surgery. Hysterectomy when feasible may reduce tumor volume and prevent bothersome vaginal bleeding.

TABLE 8–17. Stage II Endometrial Carcinoma: Five-year Survival by Treatment Group.

AUTHOR	RADIOTHERAPY FOLLOWED BY HYSTERECTOMY	RADIOTHERAPY ONLY
Truskett[69] (1968)	4/5	1/6
Marcial[77] (1969)	6/7	0/1
Beiler[78] (1972)	9/10	2/3
Kottmeier[79] (1973)	22/27	56/105
Frick[66] (1973)	7/14	0/6
Homesley[80] (1977)	8/10	0/1
Total	56/73 (77%)	59/122 (48%)

Localized irradiation is of benefit in the palliation of bone or brain metastases.

Recurrent Endometrial Carcinoma

The interval between therapy for endometrial carcinoma and the first evidence of recurrence is usually short. Salazar[68] has reported that approximately 70% of failures are diagnosed within the first 2 years after treatment. However, there are some data to suggest that early-stage well-differentiated tumors tend to recur late, appearing 5 years or more after initial therapy. Treatment failures are usually secondary to extrapelvic metastases involving the lung, abdomen, liver, or bone. In nonirradiated cases the vaginal apex and pelvic side walls are important sites for treatment failure.

The treatment of recurrent endometrial carcinoma should be individualized according to the extent and location of metastases as well as previous treatment. Distant metastases should be treated with progestational therapy or chemotherapy. With metastases in the brain or bone, satisfactory palliation can be achieved with radiation therapy. Localized metastases in the vagina can be successfully treated with interstitial radium or intracavitary radium. Recurrences in the vaginal vault have been treated successfully with intravaginal radium application or external beam therapy.

Ultraradical pelvic surgery (pelvic exenteration) has been performed in patients with recurrent adenocarcinoma of the endometrium located in the center of the pelvis without demonstrable extrapelvic spread and not amenable to radiation therapy. Too few patients have been treated in this fashion to form any conclusions regarding the value of exenterative surgery in this disease. Pratt[83] reported that the results obtained with pelvic exenteration in properly selected patients are similar to those with pelvic exenteration for recurrent cervical cancer.

Hormonal Therapy

In 1961 Kelly and Baker[84] reported that patients with metastatic carcinoma of the endometrium responded to treatment with 17α-hydroxyprogesterone caproate. Since then, multiple reports have documented that progestational agents have a significant and established role in the treatment of advanced and recurrent endometrial carcinoma and may even produce long-term remission (Fig. 8–8). Treatment with progestational agents is especially attractive because of ease of administration, minimal side effects, and anabolic properties.

The most commonly used progestins are 17α-hydroxyprogesterone caproate, medroxyprogesterone, and megestrol acetate. A 1976 survey of gynecologic oncologists[85] revealed many different dose schedules for the administration of these agents. Adequate blood levels of this medication have not been determined. The general practice has been to start the patient with a loading dose followed by long-term maintenance. The recommended drug schedules are shown in Table 8–18. Deppe[86] has analyzed the reports of treatment of endometrial carcinoma with progestins finding an overall response rate of 39% (Table 8–19). In Kohorn's[85] review of the literature of the subject and a survey of the members of the Society of

TABLE 8–18. Hormone Therapy: Endometrial Carcinoma.

DRUG	LOADING DOSE	MAINTENANCE DOSE
Medroxyprogesterone (Depo-Provera)	1.2 g	400 mg/monthly
17α-Hydroxyprogesterone caproate (Delalutin)	1.0 g	100 mg/weekly
Megestrol acetate (Megace)	40–320 mg/day	Same

Fig. 8–8. A Chest roentgenogram showing bilateral lung metastases, 14 months after a total abdominal hysterectomy, bilateral salpingo-oophorectomy, and pelvic radio-therapy for adenocarcinoma of the endometrium.

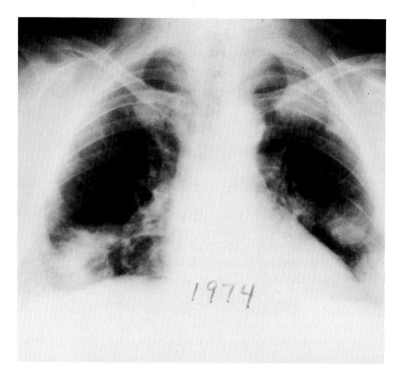

Fig. 8–8. B Chest roentgenogram 2 years after initiation of hormone therapy with Depo-Provera.

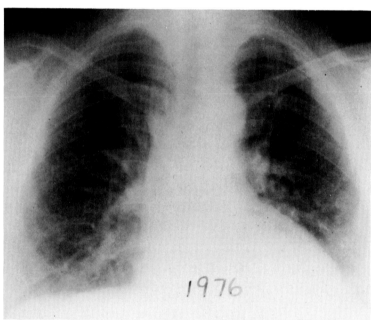

Gynecologic Oncologists the response rate was 33%. Patients with well-differentiated tumors responded better (30–50%) than did those with poorly differentiated tumors (0–15%). Duration of therapy was important. Best results were obtained with treatment regimens utilizing loading doses for at least 12 weeks. Abdominal metastases responded as well as

pulmonary lesions and patients with recurrent disease had a better response rate than did patients with persistent disease.

The mechanism of action of progestins in affecting remission in patients with endometrial carcinoma is just beginning to be understood. There is general agreement that the effect on the tumor is direct rather than

TABLE 8–19. Hormonal Agents in Endometrial Carcinoma.

DRUG	NO. OF PATIENTS	% RESPONSE
Hydroxyprogesterone	384	32
Medrogestone	56	49
Medroxyprogesterone	195	41
Megestrol	125	47
Tamoxifen	10	30

From Deppe G.[86]

mediated through the hypothalamic-pituitary axis. The histologic effect of progesterone in endometrial carcinoma has been well described from studies of serial biopsies in patients not amenable for surgery or radiation and from studies in which progestins were instilled directly into the uterine cavity. Histologically there is a decrease in the atypical character and pleomorphism of the glands with a decrease in mitotic figures and better differentiation of the glands. The cytoplasm becomes more granular and eosinophilic and secretory vacuoles appear. In well-differentiated tumors, the carcinoma is replaced by endometrial hyperplasia or by endometrial atrophy (Fig. 8–9).

During the last decade, the mechanism of action of estrogen and progesterone has been better clarified with the discovery of steroid receptors. Hormonal effects on end-organs are mediated by protein complexes formed by interaction of the steroids and the receptors. The introduction of techniques for detecting and measuring estrogen and progesterone receptors will help in the selection of patients for hormonal therapy. Receptors may be present or absent in endometrial carcinoma. The presence of progesterone receptors correlates with the histologic grade of the tumor. Well-differentiated tumors have a high frequency of progesterone receptors, whereas poorly differentiated tumors have a low frequency. Ehrlich and associates[87] have studied the cytoplasmic progesterone and estradiol receptors in normal and carcinomatous endometrium, finding that 84% of grade 1 tumors, 58% of grade 2, and 22% of grade 3 tumors have progesterone receptor binding protein.

It is the general belief that receptor data may correlate with clinical findings of responsiveness to progesterone in patients with advanced or recurrent endometrial cancer. Ehrlich[87] and Pollow[88] have demonstrated a correlation of clinical response to progestins with histologic

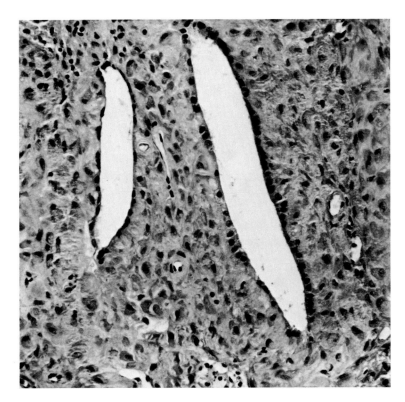

Fig. 8–9. Endometrial tissue from a patient who had a well-differentiated adenocarcinoma of the endometrium treated with Megace. The glands are atrophic and the surrounding stroma shows a marked decidual reaction. H & E; × 200.

grade in patients with endometrial carcinoma. When no progesterone receptor was detectable response was unlikely. Responses were frequent when significant progesterone receptor was measured. Ehrlich,[87] Creasman,[89] and Martin[90] noted an excellent correlation between receptor content and response to progestin therapy: 90% response in 20 patients with receptor-positive tumors as compared to 7.1% response in 31 patients whose tumors were negative for progesterone receptors. If these findings are substantiated, receptor analysis will become routine in the selection of progesterone or chemotherapy for patients with advanced or recurrent endometrial carcinoma.

Gurpide[91] demonstrated that progestins lower the levels of estrogen receptors in normal endometrium and in endometrial carcinoma. Antiestrogens such as Tamoxifen, a nonsteroidal drug, would block the proliferative stimulus of estrogen by interacting with the receptor without being hormonally active. Based on this concept, Swenerton[92] postulated that Tamoxifen might be helpful in the treatment of patients with advanced endometrial carcinoma. He administered Tamoxifen, 10 mg orally twice daily, on a continuous basis to 12 patients with recurrent endometrial carcinoma, observing a 30% response rate in ten evaluable patients. Bont[93] treated 17 patients with persistent or recurrent endometrial carcinoma with Tamoxifen, observing a 50% objective remission rate. These observations support the concept that antiestrogens and progestins can be effective through separate steroid receptor mechanisms. Clinical trials with Tamoxifen in the treatment of advanced or recurrent endometrial carcinoma are currently underway.

Nonhormonal Chemotherapy

The role of chemotherapy in the treatment of adenocarcinoma of the endometrium has not been well evaluated because of the demonstrated response of these tumors to surgery, radiotherapy, and progestins. Donovan[94] reviewed the literature of chemotherapy in 1974 and identified 15 agents that had been used in 126 patients with an overall response rate of 26%. 5-Fluorouracil (5-FU) and cyclophos-

phamide were the most frequently studied drugs inducing an objective response in 24% and 28% of the patients, respectively (Table 8–20).

Adriamycin has been evaluated in endometrial carcinoma by the Gynecologic Oncology Group (GOG).[95] Among 43 patients with advanced endometrial carcinoma there were 11 complete and five partial responders for an overall response rate of 37.2%. The response rate was not influenced by previous therapy, tumor differentiation, or site of metastases.

Another drug of interest in the management of endometrial carcinoma is cis-platinum. Several reports of small series in the literature confirm activity in endometrial carcinoma in 20–30% of the patients treated. These patients have previously failed surgery, radiotherapy, progestins, and other chemotherapy regimens.[96] In a report of the GOG[97] the response induced with high dose platinum (100–120 mg/M^2) was better than with a lower dose (50 mg/M^2). In a recent study, Deppe[98] reported a 30% response rate in 13 patients treated with cis-platinum who had prior intensive treatment with other agents. Further studies with cis-platinum as the first agent in endometrial carcinoma are required before its real value in this disease can be determined.

The recent trend in the treatment of advanced or recurrent adenocarcinoma of the endometrium is the use of combination chemotherapy. Muggia[99] treated 11 patients with advanced endometrial carcinoma with a combination of adriamycin and Cytoxan given intravenously every 21 days, obtaining an objective response rate of 62%. Koretz and coworkers[100] employed a three-drug combination of cis-platinum, adriamycin, and cyclophosphamide in seven patients, obtaining a

TABLE 8–20. Single Agents in Endometrial Carcinoma.

DRUG	RESPONSE
5-Fluorouracil	25%
Cyclophosphamide	28%
Chlorambucil	9%
Nitrogen mustard	27%
6-Mercaptopurine	20%
Adriamycin	37%
cis-Platinum	30%

TABLE 8–21. Combination Chemotherapy in Endometrial Carcinoma: Uncontrolled Studies.

AUTHOR	COMBINATION	NO. OF PATIENTS	RESPONSE (%)
Muggia[99] (1977)	CTX + ADR	11	62.5
Koretz[100] (1980)	DDP + ADR + CTX	7	57.1
Bruckner[101] (1977)	CTX + ADR + 5 − FU + MPA	7	57.
Cohen[102] (1977)	MLP + 5 − FU + MPA	33	51.
Deppe[103] (1981)	CTX + ADR + 5 − FU + MGA	29	44.
Piver[104] (1980)	MLP + 5 − FU + MPA	11	54.

CTX, cyclophosphamide; ADR, adriamycin; DDP, cis-platinum; 5-FU, 5-fluorouracil; MPA, medroxyprogesterone acetate; MGA, Megestrol acetate; MLP, Melphalan.

57% response rate. Because of the small number of patients treated with these combination regimens no definite conclusions can be drawn. Some investigators have added progestin to combination chemotherapy regimens without apparent benefit (Table 8–21).

Only two controlled prospective trials have evaluated the efficacy of combination chemotherapy in patients with advanced and recurrent endometrial carcinoma. The GOG compared the efficacy of melphalan, 5-FU, and megestrol acetate with cyclophosphamide, adriamycin, 5-FU, and megestrol acetate. There was no difference in response between the two treatment regimens and the overall objective response was about 35%. The Eastern Oncology Group[105] has randomized patients with advanced endometrial carcinoma to a regimen of cyclophosphamide, adriamycin, and megestrol acetate, either with or without 5-FU, obtaining a response rate of 27% and 16%, respectively. From the available reports in the literature it seems that the superiority of combination regimens over single agent adriamycin has not been established. Further prospective randomized trials are underway to evaluate combination chemotherapy vs. single agent therapy in this disease.

REFERENCES

1. American Cancer Society. Cancer facts and figures. 1982:16.
2. Weiss NS, Szekely DR, Austin DF. Increasing incidence of endometrial cancer in the United States. N Engl J Med. 1976; 294:1259–1262.
3. Ziel HK. Estrogen's role in endometrial cancer. Obstet Gynecol. 1982; 60:509–515.
4. Morrow CP, Townsend DE. Cancer of the uterine corpus. In: Morrow CP, Townsend DE, eds. Synopsis of gynecologic oncology. New York: Wiley, 1981:133–155.
5. Wynder EL, Escher GC, Mantal N. An epidemiologic investigation of cancer of the endometrium. Cancer. 1966; 19:489–520.
6. Armstrong B, Doll R. Environmental factors and cancer incidence and mortality in different countries, with special reference of dietary practices. Int J Cancer. 1975; 15:617–665.
7. Gusberg SB, Frick HC. Cancer of the endometrium: diagnosis and histogenesis. In: Gusberg SB, Frick HC, eds. Corscaden's gynecologic cancer. Baltimore: Williams & Wilkins, 1970:363.
8. Silverberg SG, Makowski EL, Endometrial carcinoma in young women taking oral contraceptives. Obstet Gynecol. 1975; 46:503–506.
9. Smith DC, Prentice R, Thompson DJ, et al. Association of exogenous estrogen and endometrial cancer. N Engl J Med. 1975; 293:1164–1167.
10. Ziel HK, Finkle WD. Increased risk of endometrial carcinoma among users of conjugated estrogens. N Engl J Med. 1975; 293:1167–1170.
11. Mack TM, Pike MC, Henderson BE, et al. Estrogens and endometrial cancer in a retirement community. N Engl J Med. 1976; 294:1262–1267.
12. McDonald TW, Annegers JF, O'Fallon WM, et al. Exogenous estrogen and endometrial carcinoma: case control and incidence study. Am J Obstet Gynecol. 1977; 127:572–580.
13. Antunes CMF, Stolley PD, et al. Endometrial cancer and estrogen use. Report of a large

case control study. N Engl J Med. 1979; 300:9–13.

14. Christian L: Oestrogens and endometrial cancer: A point of view. Clin Obstet Gynecol. 1977; 4:145–167.

15. Gordon J, Reagan JW, Finkle WD, et al. Estrogen and endometrial carcinoma. An independent pathology review supporting original risk estimate. N Engl J Med. 1977; 297:570–571.

16. Smith DC, Prentice RL, Bauermeister DE. Endometrial carcinoma: Histopathology, survival, and exogenus estrogens. Gynecol Obstet Invest. 1981; 12:169–179.

17. Jick HJ, Watkins RN, Hunter JR, et al. Replacement estrogens and endometrial cancer. N Engl J Med. 1979; 300:218–222.

18. Koss LG, Schreiber K, Oberlander SG, et al. Screening of asymptomatic women for endometrial cancer. Obstet Gynecol. 1981; 57:681–691.

19. Anderson DG, Eaton CJ, Galinkin LJ, et al. The cytologic diagnosis of endometrial adenocarcinoma. Am J Obstet Gynecol. 1976; 125:376–383.

20. Hathcock EW Jr, Williams GA, Engelhardt S. Office aspiration curettage of the endometrium. Am J Obstet Gynecol. 1974; 120:205–213.

21. Hofmeister FJ. Endometrial biopsy: Another look. Am J Obstet Gynecol. 1974; 118:773–777.

22. Hendrickson MR, Kempson RL. Epithelial neoplasms: Endometrial carcinoma. In: Hendrichson MR, Kempson RL, eds. Surgical pathology of the uterine corpus. Philadelphia: Saunders, 1980:333–388.

23. Ng AB, Reagan JW, Storaasli JP, et al. Mixed adenosquamous carcinoma of the endometrium. Am J Clin Pathol. 1973; 59:765–781.

24. Silverberg SG, Bolin MG, DeGiorgi LS. Adenoacanthoma and mixed adenosquamous carcinoma of the endometrium. A clinicopathologic study. Cancer. 1972; 30:1307–1314.

25. Christopherson WM, Alberhasky RC, Connelly PJ. Carcinoma of the endometrium. I. A clinicopathologic study of clear-cell carcinoma and secretory carcinoma. Cancer. 1982; 49:1511–1523.

26. Kurman RJ, Scully RE. Clear cell carcinoma of the endometrium. An analysis of 21 cases. Cancer. 1976; 37:872–882.

27. Christopherson WM, Alberhasky RC, Connelly PJ. Carcinoma of the endometrium. II. Papillary adenocarcinoma. A clinical pathological study of 46 cases. Am J Clin Pathol. 1982; 77:534–540.

28. Roberts JA, Lifshitz S. Papillary adenocarci-

noma of the endometrium with psammoma bodies. J Iowa Med Soc. 1982; 72:196–199.

29. Fluhmann CF. Squamous epithelium in the endometrium in benign and malignant conditions. Surg Gynecol Obstet. 1928; 46:309–316.

30. White AJ, Buchsbaum HJ, Macasaet MA. Primary squamous cell carcinoma of the endometrium. Obstet Gynecol. 1973; 41:912–919.

31. Lifshitz S, Schauberger CW, Platz CA, et al. Primary squamous cell carcinoma of the endometrium. J Reprod Med. 1981; 26:25–27.

32. Baggish MS, Woodruff TD. The occurrence of squamous epithelium in the endometrium. Obstet Gynecol Surv. 1966; 22:69–115.

33. Voet RL, Waisman J, Ballon SC. Intraepithelial epidermoid carcinoma of the cervix, endometrium, and a fallopian tube. Gynecol Oncol. 1979; 8:349–352.

34. Kottmeier H, Kolstad P, eds. Annual report on the results of treatment in carcinoma of the uterus, vagina and ovary, Vol. 16. Stockholm: FIGO, 1976.

35. Jones HW. Treatment of adenocarcinoma of the endometrium. Obstet Gynecol Surv. 1975; 30:147–169.

36. Cheon HK. Prognosis of endometrial carcinoma. Obstet Gynecol. 1969; 34:680–684.

37. Lewis B, Stallworthy JA, Cowdell R. Adenocarcinoma of the body of the uterus. J Obstet Gynaecol Br Commonw. 1970; 77:343–348.

38. Shah CA, Green TH. Evaluation of current management of endometrial carcinoma. Obstet Gynecol. 1972; 39:500–509.

39. Nahhas WA, Lund CJ, Rudolph JH. Carcinoma of the corpus uteri. Obstet Gynecol. 1971; 38:564–570.

40. Wade ME, Kohorn EI, Morris JMc. Adenocarcinoma of the endometrium: evaluation of preoperative irradiation and factors influencing prognosis. Am J Obstet Gynecol. 1967; 99:869–876.

41. Malkasian GD. Carcinoma of the endometrium. Effect of stage and grade on survival. Cancer. 1978; 41:996–1001.

42. Austin JH, MacMahon B. Indicators of prognosis in carcinoma of the corpus uteri. Surg Gynecol Obstet. 1969; 128:1247–1252.

43. Creasman WT. Surgical treatment of endometrial carcinoma. In: Buchsbaum HJ, ed. Gynecology and obstetrics, Vol. 4. Hagerstown, Md.: Harper & Row, 1981.

44. Javert C, Renning E. Treatment of endometrial adenocarcinoma. Am J Roentgenol. 1956; 75:508–514.

45. Surwit EA, Fowler WC, Rogoff EE, et al. Stage II carcinoma of the endometrium. Int J Radiat Oncol Biol Phys. 1979; 5:323–326.

46. Ng AB, Reagan JW. Incidence and prognosis of endometrial carcinoma by histologic grade and extent. Obstet Gynecol. 1970; 35:437–443.

47. Lewis GC, Bundy B. Surgery for endometrial cancer. Cancer. 1981; 48:568–574.

48. Lutz MH, Underwood PB, Kreatner A, et al. Endometrial carcinoma. A new method of classification of therapeutic and prognostic significance. Gynecol Oncol. 1978; 6:83–94.

49. Morrow CP, DiSaia PJ, Townsend DE. Current management of endometrial carcinoma. Obstet Gynecol. 1973; 43:399–406.

50. Stallworthy JA. Surgery for endometrial cancer in the bonney tradition. Ann R Coll Surg Engl. 1971; 48:293–305.

51. Creasman WT, Rutledge FR. The prognostic value of peritoneal cytology in gynecologic malignant diseases. Am J Obstet Gynecol. 1971; 110:773–781.

52. Keettel WC, Pixley EE, Buchsbaum HJ. Experience with peritoneal cytology in the management of gynecologic malignancies. Am J Obstet Gynecol. 1974; 120:174–182.

53. Szpak CA, Creasman WT, Vollmer RT, et al. Prognostic value of cytologic examination of peritoneal washings in patients with endometrial carcinoma. Acta Cytol. 1981; 25:640–646.

54. Heyman J. Radiological or operative treatment of cancer of the uterus. Acta Radiol. 1927; 8:363–366.

55. Bickenbach W, Lockmuller H, Dirlich G, et al. Factor analysis of endometrial carcinoma in relation to treatment. Obstet Gynecol. 1967; 29:632–636.

56. Pratt JH, Symmonds RE, Welch JS. Vaginal hysterectomy for carcinoma of fundus. Am J Obstet Gynecol. 1964; 88:1063–1071.

57. Park RC, Patow WE, Petty WM, et al. Treatment of adenocarcinoma of the endometrium. Gynecol Oncol. 1974; 2:60–70.

58. Rutledge F. The role of radical hysterectomy in adenocarcinoma of the endometrium. Gynecol Oncol. 1974; 2:331–347.

59. Joelsson I, Sandri A, Kottmeier HL. Carcinoma of the uterine corpus. A retrospective survey of individualized therapy. Acta Radiol. (Suppl.) 1973; 334:3–63.

60. Keller D, Kempson RL, Levine G, et al. Management of the patient with early endometrial carcinoma. Cancer. 1974; 33:1108–1116.

61. Homesley HD, Boronow RC, Lewis JL. Treatment of adenocarcinoma of the endometrium at Memorial-James Ewing Hospitals, 1949–1965. Obstet Gynecol. 1976; 47:100–105.

62. Lewis GC, Mortel R, Nelson HS. Endometrial cancer. Therapeutic decision and the staging process in "early" disease. Cancer. 1977; 39:959–966.

63. Bean HA, Bryant AJ, Carmichael JA, et al. Carcinoma of the endometrium in Saskatchewan, 1966 to 1971. Gynecol Oncol. 1978; 6:503–514.

64. Prem KA, Adcock LL, Okagaki T, et al. The evaluation of a treatment program for adenocarcinoma of the endometrium. Am J Obstet Gynecol. 1979; 133:803–813.

65. Piver MS, Yazigi R, Blumenson L, et al. A prospective trial comparing hysterectomy, hysterectomy plus vaginal radium, and uterine radium plus hysterectomy in stage I endometrial carcinoma. Obstet Gynecol. 1979; 54:85–89.

66. Frick HC II, Munnell EW, Richart RM, et al. Carcinoma of the endometrium. Am J Obstet Gynecol. 1973; 115:663–676.

67. Wharam MD, Phillips TL, Bagshaw MA. The role of radiation therapy in clinical stage I carcinoma of the endometrium. Int J Radiol Oncol Biol Phys. 1976; 1:1081–1089.

68. Salazar OM, Feldstein ML, DePapp EW, et al. The management of clinical stage I endometrial carcinoma. Cancer. 1978; 41:1016–1026.

69. Truskett ID, Constable WC. Management of carcinoma of the corpus uteri. Am J Obstet Gynecol. 1968; 101:689–694.

70. Underwood PB, Lutz MH, Kreutner A, et al. Carcinoma of the endometrium: Radiation followed immediately by operation. Am J Obstet Gynecol. 1977; 128:86–98.

71. Aalders J, Abeler V, Kolstad P, et al. Postoperative external irradiation and prognostic parameters in stage I endometrial adenocarcinoma. Obstet Gynecol. 1980; 56:419–427.

72. Burrell MO, Franklin EW, Powell JL. Endometrial cancer. Evaluation of spread and follow-up in 189 patients with stage I or stage II disease. Am J Obstet Gynecol. 1982; 144:181–185.

73. Paterson E, Spratt D. Tomkiewicz Z, et al. Management of stage I carcinoma of the uterus. Obstet Gynecol. 1982; 59:755–758.

74. Creasman WT, DiSaia PJ, Blessing J, et al. Prognostic significance of peritoneal cytology in patients with endometrial cancer and preliminary data concerning therapy with intraperitoneal radiopharmaceuticals. Am J Obstet Gynecol. 1981; 141:921–929.

75. Bruckman JE, Goodman RL, Murthy A, et al. Combined irradiation and surgery in treatment of stage II carcinoma of endometrium. Cancer. 1978; 42:1146–1151.

76. Cox JD, Komaki R, Wilson JF, et al. Locally advanced adenocarcinoma of the endometrium. Results of irradiation with and without

subsequent hysterectomy. Cancer. 1980; 45:715–719.

77. Marcial VA, Tome JM, Ubinas J. The combination of external irradiation and curietherapy used preoperatively in adenocarcinoma of the endometrium. Am J Roentgenol Radium Ther Nucl Med. 1969; 105:586–595.

78. Beiler DD, Schmutz DA, O'Rourke TL. Carcinoma of the endometrium: Radiation and surgery versus surgery alone. Radiology. 1972; 102:159–164.

79. Kottmeier HL. Corpus et colli. What is this disease? What is the treatment? Clin Obstet Gynecol. 1973; 16:276–285.

80. Homesley HD, Boronow RC, Lewis JL. Stage II endometrial adenocarcinoma. Memorial Hospital for Cancer, 1949–1965. Obstet Gynecol. 1977; 49:604–608.

81. Antoniades J, Brady LW, Lewis GC. The management of stage III carcinoma of the endometrium. Cancer. 1976; 38:1838–1842.

82. Bruckman JE, Bloomer WD, Marck A, et al. Stage III adenocarcinoma of the endometrium. Two prognostic groups. Gynecol Oncol. 1980; 9:12–17.

83. Pratt JH. Surgical treatment of recurrent endometrial carcinoma. In: Lewis GC, ed. New concepts in gynecology oncology. Philadelphia: Davis, 1966:261.

84. Kelly RM, Baker WH. Progestational agents in the treatment of carcinoma of the endometrium. N Engl J Med. 1961; 264:216–222.

85. Kohorn EJ. Gestogens and endometrial carcinoma. Gynecol Oncol. 1976; 4:398–409.

86. Deppe G. Chemotherapeutic treatment of endometrial carcinoma. Clin Obstet Gynecol. 1982; 25:93–99.

87. Ehrlich CE, Young PC, Cleary RE. Cytoplasmic progesterone and estradiol receptors in normal, hyperplastic, and carcinomatous endometria. Therapeutic implications. Am J Obstet Gynecol. 1981; 141:539–546.

88. Pollow K, Robel P, Vihko R. Steroid receptors and the human endometrium. In: Richardson GS, MacLaughlin DT, eds. Hormonal biology of endometrial cancer. VICC Technical Report. Geneva: 1978.

89. Creasman WT, McCarty KS Sr, McCarty KS Jr. Clinical correlation of estrogen, progesterone binding proteins in human endometrial adenocarcinoma. Obstet Gynecol. 1980; 55:363–370.

90. Martin PM, Rolland P, Gammette M, et al. Estradiol and progesterone receptors in normal and neoplastic endometrium. Correlations between receptors, histopathologic examina-

tions, and clinical responses under progestin therapy. Int J Cancer. 1979; 23:321–329.

91. Gurpide E. Hormones and gynecologic cancer. Cancer. 1976; 38:503–508.

92. Swenerton KD. Treatment of advanced endometrial adenocarcinoma with tamoxifen. Cancer Treat Rep. 1980; 64:805.

93. Bonte J, Ide P, Billiet G, et al. Tamoxifen as a possible chemotherapeutic agent in endometrial adenocarcinoma. Gynecol Oncol. 1981; 11:140–61.

94. Donovan JF. Nonhormonal chemotherapy of endometrial adenocarcinoma. Cancer 1974; 34:1587–1592.

95. Thigpen JT, Buchsbaum HJ, Mangan C, et al. Phase II trial of adriamycin in the treatment of advanced or recurrent endometrial carcinoma. A Gynecologic Oncology Group study. Cancer Treat Rep. 1979; 63:21.

96. Seski JC, Edwards CL, Herron J, et al. Cisplatin chemotherapy for disseminated endometrial cancer. Obstet Gynecol. 1982; 59:225–228.

97. Thigpen T, Shingleton H, Homesley H, et al. Cisplatin in the treatment of advanced or recurrent cervix and uterine cancer. In: Prestayko AW, Crooke ST, Coster SK, eds. Cisplatin: current status and new developments. New York: Academic Press, 1980.

98. Deppe G, Cohen CJ, Bruckner HW. Treatment of advanced endometrial adenocarcinoma with cisdichlorodiamine platinum (II) after intensive prior therapy. Gynecol Oncol. 1980; 10:51–54.

99. Muggia FM, Chia G, Reed LJ, et al. Doxorubicin-cyclophosphamide. Effective chemotherapy for advanced endometrial adenocarcinoma. Am J Obstet Gynecol. 1977; 128:314–319.

100. Koretz MM, Ballon S, Friedman MA, et al. Platinum, adriamycin, and cyclophosphamide in advanced endometrial carcinoma. Proc Am Assoc Cancer Res Am Soc Clin Oncol. 1980; 21:784.

101. Bruckner HW, Deppe G. Combination chemotherapy of advanced endometrial adenocarcinoma with adriamycin, cyclophosphamide, 5-fluorouracil, and medroxyprogesterone acetate. Obstet Gynecol. 1977; 50:10s–12s.

102. Cohen CJ, Deppe G, Bruckner HW. Treatment of advanced adenocarcinoma of the endometrium with melphalan, 5-fluorouracil, and medroxyprogesterone acetate. A preliminary study. Obstet Gynecol. 1977; 50:415–417.

103. Deppe G, Jacobs AJ, Bruckner HW, et al. Che-

motherapy of advanced and recurrent endometrial carcinoma with cyclophosphamide, doxorubicin, 5-fluorouracil, and megestrol acetate. Am J Obstet Gynecol. 1981; 140:313–316.

104. Piver MS, Lele S, Barlow JJ. Melphalan, 5-fluorouracil, and medroxyprogesterone acetate in metastatic or recurrent endometrial carcinoma. Obstet Gynecol. 1980; 56:370–372.

105. Horton J, Elson P, Gordon P, et al. A comparison of combination therapies for advanced endometrial cancer. Proc Am Assoc Cancer Res Am Soc Clin Oncol. 1981; 22:664.

Urinary Tract Disorders 9

Robert C. Corlett

As with most other organ systems, the lower urinary tract is more often a target for disease or altered physiology in the elderly than in the younger individual. Changes in vesical function with age are not limited to females, but this discussion will be limited to women in the postmenopausal age group.

The appearance of new problems (or the exacerbation of preexisting ones) may be broadly considered to be secondary to one of two separate factors: (1) the process of aging itself and (2) the diminished estrogen levels associated with cessation of ovarian function. Clinically, the symptom complex caused by either of these two processes may be identical (e.g., incontinence, nocturia, frequency). However, the pathophysiology, clinical and urodynamic findings, and therapy may be different. For ease of discussion the negative influences of these two inexorable developments will be considered separately, although they can, and usually do, occur simultaneously.

Normal Physiology

A brief discussion of the normal neurophysiology of micturition and continence is warranted to better appreciate the changes occurring in the menopausal female.

The intricate interplay between the sympathetic and parasympathetic systems in promoting normal micturition and storage of urine is discussed in detail in the excellent review article by Mahony et al.[1] and will be discussed only superficially.

The organization of the micturition reflex is extremely complex and involves several central reflex centers as well as numerous peripheral influences of both a facilitatory and inhibitory nature. The act of voiding is a reflection of the sum of all neural influences acting on the pontine and sacral reflex centers.

CONTINENCE. Continence, or storage of urine, utilizes at least four different reflex arcs. The first two, termed the "sympathetic stabilizing reflexes," are activated by detrusor stretch receptors in response to increasing intramural tension resulting from increasing intravesical volume. The first reflex inhibits detrusor contractility (i.e., the property of accommodation), whereas the second increases the tone of the internal sphincter. Beta sympathetic receptors are involved in the first and alpha receptors in the second. The third reflex inhibits bladder activity by the activation of tension receptors in the striated muscle of the pelvic floor; the fourth is activated by increasing mural tension in the bladder neck resulting in greater tone of the striated external sphincter.

MICTURITION. The fifth and sixth reflexes are concerned with the initiation of micturition. These are activated by diaphragmatic and abdominal wall contraction and by the increasing mural tension as the bladder fills, respectively. The urethrodetrusor inhibitory reflex (seventh reflex) causes relaxation of the internal sphincter during the entire voiding phase of micturition; the eighth reflex sends inhibitory impulses to the pudendal nucleus with resultant relaxation of the striated external sphincter. There are at least four other reflexes concerned with the coordinated act of micturition. It should be apparent that overactivity or functional failure of any of these integral reflexes may manifest as a disorder of the lower urinary tract.

Aging Changes

Decline in the integrity of the neuromuscular system is a normal accompaniment of age. Various age-related degenerative changes have been described in the sensory and autonomic ganglia. The deep tendon reflexes (DTR) become increasingly sluggish with age and may ultimately disappear. The loss of DTRs begins at about age 50; by age 80 few people have intact ankle jerks.[2] The blunting of abdominocutaneous reflexes, prolongation of pupillary reaction time, diminishment of olfactory, gustatory, and auditory sensations, and a progressive loss of vibratory sensation (approximately half of those individuals over 80 will have lost these sensations in the lower extremity) are some of the neurologic changes which are a direct result of the aging process.

The range of ocular motion is frequently limited in all directions and generalized age-related weakness of striated musculature is widely recognized. In all muscles studied there is an increase in interstitial connective tissue.[2] In general the conditioned and unconditioned responses are of much smaller magnitude in the elderly than in the normal young adult.[3]

CONTINENCE. Considering, first, the neurophysiology of storage (or continence), one can appreciate that a decline in either the sympathetic, parasympathetic, or somatic (via the pudendal nerves) nervous system can upset the delicate homeostasis between continence and incontinence. For example, a "slowdown" of the sympathetic stabilizing reflexes (first and second reflexes) allows detrusor irritability (or loss of accommodation) and loss of the appropriate increase in urethral resistance in response to an increasing intravesical volume. Would this type of incontinence be considered neurogenic or anatomic? Would the therapy be medical or surgical? Tanagho[4] has shown that in the normal continent individual an in-

crease in the urethral pressure profile accompanies an increasing vesical volume. However, the incontinent female does not demonstrate this compensatory change. The third reflex relies on an intact pelvic floor for activation of detrusor inhibitory fibers, but what happens in the elderly female with no pubococcygeal tone whatever? Similarly, the fourth reflex is useless in the absence of healthy pelvic floor striated muscle.

MICTURITION. On the other end of the spectrum are disorders of voiding associated with impairment in the finely coordinated integral reflexes. Partial failure of urethral or pelvic floor relaxation during micturition may cause inefficient voiding with subsequent development of increased intravesical pressure, increased residual urine, recurrent bacteriuria, overflow incontinence, and so forth. These may manifest with a myriad of symptom complexes including hesitancy, frequency, nocturia, a feeling of incomplete voiding, and postvoid dribbling. These changes can, of course, occur in the woman who has suffered a neurologic accident but may also occur in the (seemingly) neurologically intact patient. Thus, with prolongation in latency periods, degenerative changes in autonomic ganglia, and so on, one can have a situation that clinically mimics either bladder instability or true stress incontinence or both.

Estrogen Deficiency

The empiric distinction made in this chapter between postmenopausal changes due to senescence and those due to estrogen deprivation may be more apparent than real. The human female is somewhat unique among mammals in that much of her total life span exists after cessation of menses. She may have one-third of her life yet ahead of her at this point, whereas in the mouse, monkey, and rat only 10–15% of the total life span occurs in the menopausal period.[5]

In the human female, reproduction may serve as a biologic model for aging. Decreased steroidal production by the ovaries results in the senscent changes of the secondary sexual organs. The decline in production of these sex steroids, principally 17β-estradiol, which begins several years prior to menopause, is responsible for subtle changes which cannot be readily separated from the alterations resulting from aging.

The clinical symptomatology of estrogen deficiency is varied and not limited to the genital system. In the brain there is a reduced ability to provide certain enzymes necessary for proper transmission of nerve impulses. In addition, estrogen receptor concentrations in the brain were observed to diminish with aging.[5]

Embryologically, the lower urinary tract and reproductive tract have similar origin. Estrogen receptors have been demonstrated in the urethra.[6] Although no receptors have yet been demonstrated in the bladder, there are a number of clinical observations which suggest a steroid responsiveness by the bladder.

Studies of urethral pressures reveal this to be an age-related phenomenon. Plante and Susset[7] found the maximum urethral pressure to be significantly lower in a group of women over age 70 when compared to younger women. They felt that a loss of urethral compliance occurs resulting in loss of urethral elasticity. This increased urethral rigidity was worsened if there had been prior "significant urogynecologic operations."[8] Tanagho concurred and stated, "in women, vaginal urethral dissection inevitably damages the striated external sphincter."[9] This may occur as a consequence of urethral or periurethral fibrosis, which probably develops to varying degrees in cases involving dissection of the anterior vaginal wall.

Edwards and Malvern[10] also found an inverse relationship between age and urethral pressure profile, which may be expressed as:

amplitude (in cmH_2O) =
$$92 - \text{patient's age (in years)}$$

As one might expect, an organ which demonstrates estrogen receptors and a change in physiologic parameters associated with a state of declining estrogen production should respond to the administration of estrogens. Faber and Heidenreich,[11] treating stress incontinence, and Smith,[12] treating atrophic urethritis, achieved excellent results using estrogen replacement. A significant rise in the urethral pressure profile was demonstrated by Faber and Heidenreich in 95% of patients following estrogen treatment for 2–4 months (Fig. 9–1). Estrogen treatment causes a proliferation of the atrophic urethral epithelium, which can be demonstrated by cytology. Lack of formal maturation of the squamous epithelium from estrogen deficiency can convert the entire distal urethra to a rigid, inelastic tube. Eventually, the thin, friable epithelium may take on the same inflamed, ulcerative appearance of the vagina in the more commonly recognized senile vaginitis. With time, stricture

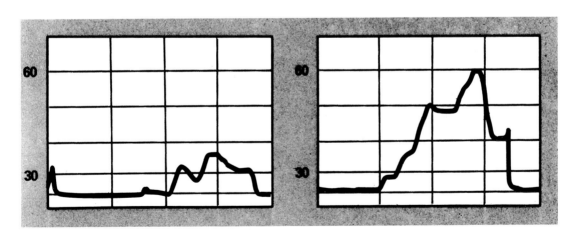

Fig. 9–1. *Left:* Urethral pressure profile on a menopausal patient before topical estrogen treatment. *Right:* After treatment. Note the significant improvement in maximal pressure as well as functional length. Reproduced with permission from Corlett RC Jr. Gynecologic Urology: Parts I and II. In: Kistner RW, et al., eds. Current problems in obstetrics and gynecology. Copyright © 1978 by Year Book Medical Publishers, Inc., Chicago.)

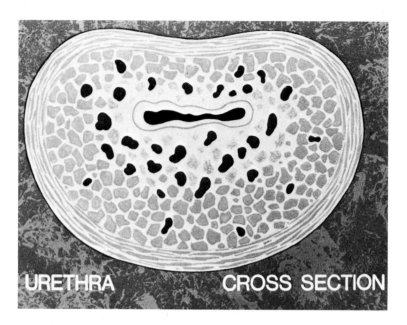

Fig. 9–2. A cross-section of the female urethra in the reproductive years reveals a rich venous network between the mucosa and muscularis. This erectile tissue has a washerlike effect in maintaining a water-tight closure of the urethra and contributes significantly to the resting urethral pressure. This vascular network may become atrophic in the menopausal female, and this, combined with the thinning of the urothelium, contributes to poor apposition of the urethral lumen and diminished urethral pressure. These estrogen-dependent changes result in urinary incontinence which can be resolved medically.

formation develops. In addition to its proliferating effect on the urothelium, estrogen increases the vascularity of the urethra and thus enhances the vascular sleeve surrounding the urethra (Fig. 9–2).

Clinical Presentation

The potential magnitude of the problem can be inferred from the 1980 census, which showed 30 million women over the age of 50 in the population. Surveys estimate the percentage of incontinent geriatric patients in hospitals at between 25 and 50%. Surveys of outpatients reveal a slightly lower incidence of reported incontinence (13–42%).[13,14]

Incontinence is not even the most common urologic symptom in postmenopausal women. In Brocklehurst's text on geriatrics, nocturia was reported at 61 to 67% in three different series.[13] Other symptoms surveyed include frequency (daytime) (23–35%), scalding (13%), and difficulty in voiding (3–7%). Bacteriuria is

age-related and in the menopausal female may be as high as 10%.[15]

INCONTINENCE. Incontinence may result from a number of different pathologic processes. It may be due to the process of aging itself, as a result of weakened compensatory neurologic reflexes with or without associated urethral and pelvic floor atrophy. Probably the most common cause of significant urinary incontinence, especially in the elderly postmenopausal woman, is an unstable bladder. Brocklehurst and Dillane, using cystometrography, demonstrated a high incidence of uninhibited neurogenic bladder in elderly continent women.[16] Nearly all of the women with known neurologic lesions had abnormal cystometrograms, and of the neurologically intact group, 15 of 24 demonstrated an abnormal cystometrogram—as defined by uninhibited detrusor contractions, reduced capacity, or elevated residual urine. They state, "it appears that a poorly functioning bladder is a common accompaniment of old age even among those who are not suffering from incontinence."

These functional changes may produce, in addition to urinary incontinence, symptoms of nocturia, enuresis, frequency, and urgency.

Stress urinary incontinence is also common in the menopausal female. Assuming clinical and urodynamic findings supporting that diagnosis, and assuming no other findings of depressed bladder functions, the problem may be approached in the usual fashion. Pubococcygeal exercises have reportedly been successful in the management of stress incontinence,[17] but in this author's experience they are curative only in milder cases. To be most efficacious, a regular exercise routine should be started in the reproductive years—before urinary incontinence has developed. The appropriate exercise may be taught by having the patient perform a squeeze maneuver during a digital examination. The patient is instructed to exercise twice daily and to progress to at least 100 contractions per session.

Surgical Management. Surgery for stress incontinence in the elderly female must be selective. Difficulties with impaired voiding and urinary retention are more common in the elderly patient following surgery. The extent of correction of the anatomic defect should take into consideration the patient's degree of activity. Unlike the 40-year-old jogger or tennis player, the 68-year-old retired woman may require less elevation of the bladder neck for comparable results. Otherwise, as with the case illustrated in Fig. 9–3, outflow obstruction can develop. This may respond to internal urethrotomy or urethral dilatation, but not always. The clinical picture, the patient's age, and her activity should dictate the type of surgical procedure selected.

Nonsurgical Management. The other treatment modality, in addition to Kegel's exercises, which should be considered prior to surgery is estrogen replacement. Either oral estrogen or local application of estrogen cream is helpful.[18,19] Reduction in symptoms results from improved apposition of the urethral wall and the increased urethral tone associated with improved vascularity.

Other medications with adrenergic effects may be utilized to improve urethral pressure. Such drugs as Ornade, Ephedrine, and Tofranil can be used for this purpose, but in the author's experience they have not proven very helpful in the patient with a stable bladder. Additionally, many patients have medical

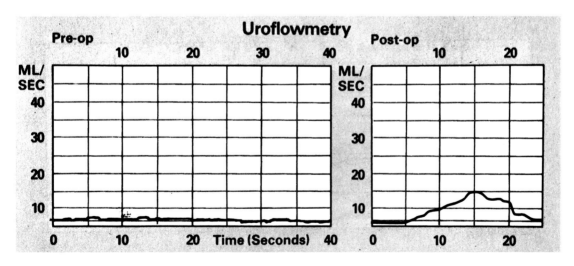

Fig. 9–3. The flow rate on the left was obtained in a menopausal female 1 year following a Marshall-Marchetti-Krantz procedure. The graph on the right was obtained several months following an internal urethrotomy. The peak flow rate normally exceeds 18 ml/s and in this instance was increased threefold following urethrotomy. The symptoms of frequency, nocturia, urgency, and dribbling all improved significantly as well. Reproduced with permission from Corlett RC Jr. Gynecologic urology: Parts I and II. In: Kistner RW, et al., eds. Current problems in obstetrics and gynecology. Copyright © 1978 by Year Book Medical Publishers, Inc., Chicago.)

problems such as hypertension which limit the use of these drugs.

OVERFLOW INCONTINENCE. Overflow incontinence is another form of urinary incontinence which is found with greater frequency in the aged female. Outflow obstruction may be functional (as a result of dyscoordinated micturition) or anatomic, but either can result in the sequence of increased intravesical pressure, bladder decompensation, increased residual urine, bacteriuria, and trabeculation. Brocklehurst[13] studied 25 autopsy specimens from patients 74–102 years old. The majority showed trabeculation which was due partly to hypertrophy of the detrusor bundles and partly to loss of supporting elastic tissue. The elderly patient is much more susceptible to adverse drug reactions; therefore if overflow incontinence, poor flow rate, or elevated residual urine are present, a careful drug history should be obtained to rule out the use of any medication which might have anticholinergic properties. Dopamine, Ornade, Phenergan, and Tofranil are but a few of the drugs with strong secondary anticholinergic effects that may cause urinary retention in the susceptible individual.

URETHRAL SYNDROME. The urethral syndrome is a condition in which symptoms of disturbed micturition (burning, frequency, hesitancy, nocturia, and urgency) are found in association with sterile urine cultures. This is not a single entity, but probably represents several different conditions with similar presentations. Lipsky[20] performed a urodynamic evaluation on a group of 43 women with the urethral syndrome. He demonstrated outflow obstruction in over half the patients. Two types of obstruction were noted. The first, found mainly in menopausal women, was a narrowing of the distal segment of the urethra. The second type of obstruction was seen in younger women and was a result of incomplete relaxation of the external sphincter. The main criterion for obstruction was peak flow rate, with values less than 15 ml/s considered obstructive. The flow rate varies inversely with age and this must be kept in mind when assessing specific values. Abrams and Torrens[21] give the following norms:

Men	< 40 years	> 22 ml/s
Men	40–60	> 18 ml/s
Men	> 60	> 13 ml/s
Women	< 50	> 25 ml/s
Women	> 50	> 18 ml/s

In recording flow rates, we have found that voided volumes of 200 ml are acceptable, but the coefficient of variation was lowest when the volume was in excess of 300 ml.[22] In addition to peak flow the curve should demonstrate a rapid increase in rate so that the maximum level is reached within the first one-third of the total voiding time.

Postmenopausal women with obstruction may be treated satisfactorily with oral estrogen and either external urethroplasty or urethral dilation. Schleyer-Saunders treated 300 women with mixed urinary symptoms (including dysuria and incontinence).[23] He used only hormone implants and reported improvement in 70%. However, he further categorized his results into good (30%) and fair (40%). Smith, who has written extensively on the subject, observed that when symptoms were present for less than 12 months, estrogen treatment alone (Premarin, 0.6 mg daily for 3 weeks out of 4 for a total of 3 months) was often successful.[12] But if symptoms were more prolonged (greater than 1 year), then urethral dilation was added to hormone replacement for optimal results.[12]

Internal urethrotomy may be utilized in place of urethral dilation (Fig. 9–4). It is felt by some to have a more prolonged effect. Stanton's group achieved good success in menopausal patients with obstruction, using the Otis urethrotome. They noted, however, greater improvement in those patients with bladder instability in addition to obstruction (demonstrated by uroflowmetry).[24]

In those patients responding to estrogen treatment alone, improvement was noted as early as 1 week following institution of therapy. Patients remained symptom free for 6 weeks to 4 months after discontinuation of treatment, but then symptoms returned with progressive severity. In view of the temporary nature of recovery following short-term treatment, it would seem reasonable to treat indefinitely. It may well be that lower doses given less frequently will suffice for the prevention of the

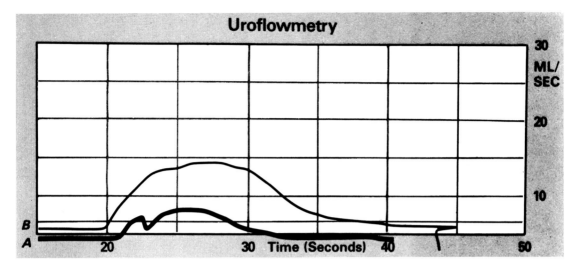

Fig. 9–4. The lower flow rate was obtained from a 62-year-old female complaining of frequency, hesitancy, urgency, dysuria, and nocturia. Urethral dilation and antimicrobial therapy were ineffectual. She obtained transient improvement of all symptoms on a regimen of estrogen cream, but not until she had undergone an internal urethrotomy with the Otis urethrotome did she obtain significant relief of all symptoms. In addition, her peak flow rate improved from 7 to 14 ml/s, as seen in the upper flow rate taken 1 year later. Reproduced with permission from Corlett RC Jr. Female patient. 1979; 4:30–34.

atrophic changes discussed above; whereas once the estrogen deficiency has proceeded unchecked to the point of anatomic changes in the lower urinary tract, a larger, more frequently administered regimen will be required.

The present medicolegal climate and the lay press coverage of the reported relationship between endometrial carcinoma and hormone replacement therapy in the postmenopausal female have forced the gynecologist into a posture of benign neglect. The FDA has required warning labels on estrogen products since 1977 which advise of an increased risk of up to 15-fold for the development of endometrial carcinoma. The agency strongly recommends short courses of therapy (less than 1 year) if estrogen is required for treatment of vasomotor symptoms. This approach, however, cannot be expected to have any long-lasting, beneficial effects on the menopausal woman with bladder symptoms. These patients require prolonged, if not indefinite, estrogen replacement. Greenblatt[25] disagrees sharply with the approach advocated by the FDA and others, since he has extensive experience with long-term, balanced hormone replacement.

Summary

Dysfunction of the lower urinary tract is a common problem in the aging female and cannot always be approached in the usual fashion. The presenting symptom complex is variable, and similar symptoms may result from different pathophysiologic processes. Adequate hormone replacement therapy, a pubococcygeal exercise program, and enlargement of the outflow tract with dilation or urethrotomy when indicated have been underutilized in the treatment of menopausal problems. Parasympathomimetric agents and anticholinergic drugs may have a role, but their use must be tempered by the increased drug sensitivity found in the elderly individual.

REFERENCES

1. Mahony D, Laferte R, Blais D. Integral storage and voiding reflexes. Urology. 1977; 9:95–106.
2. Johnson W. The older patient. New York: Hoeber, 1960:467–512.
3. Welford AT, Birren JE. Behavior, aging and the nervous system. Springfield, Ill.: Thomas, 1965:326–352.

4. Tanagho E, Miller E, Meyers F, Corbett HR. Observation on the dynamics of the bladder neck. Br Urol. 1966; 38:72–84.

5. Eskin BA. Aging and the menopause. In: Eskin BA, ed. The menopause, comprehensive management. Masson, 1980:73–92.

6. Lindskog M, Sjogren C, Ulsten U, Anderson K. Estrogen binding sites in nuclear fractions from the rat urogenital tract. Presented at 10th Annual Meeting of the International Continence Society. Los Angeles, 1980.

7. Plante P, Susset J. Studies of female urethral pressure profile. I. The normal urethral pressure profile. J Urol. 1980; 123:64–69.

8. Susset J, Plante P. Studies of female urethral pressure profile. II. Pressure profile in female incontinence. J Urol. 1980; 123:70–74.

9. Tanagho E, Miller E. Functional consideration of urethral sphincter dynamics. J Urol. 1973; 109:273–278.

10. Edwards L, Malvern J. The urethral pressure profile. Theoretical considerations and clinical application. Br J Urol. 1974; 46:325–335.

11. Faber P, Heidenreich J. Treatment of stress incontinence and estrogen in postmenopausal women. Urol Int. 1977; 32:221–223.

12. Smith P. Postmenopausal urinary symptoms and hormonal replacement therapy. Br Med J. 1976; 2:941.

13. Brocklehurst JC. The bladder. In: Brocklehurst JC, ed. Textbook of geriatric medicine and gerontology. London: Churchill Livingstone, 1973:298–370.

14. Ouslander JG, Kane RL, Abrass IB. Urinary in continence in elderly nursing home patients. JAMA. 1982; 284:1194–1198.

15. Corlett RC. Urologic problems in menopause. Female Patient. 1979; 4:30–34.

16. Brocklehurst JC, Dillane JB. Studies of the female bladder in old age. I. Cystometrograms in nonincontinent women. Gerontol Clin. 1966; 8:285–305.

17. Kegel A. Stress incontinence of urine in women: physiologic treatment. J Int Coll Surg. 1956; 25:487.

18. Schief I, Tulchinsky D, Ryan K. Vaginal absorption of estrone and 17β-estradiol. Fertil Steril. 1977; 28:1063–1066.

19. Rigg L, Hermann H, Yen SC. Absorption of estrogen from vaginal creams. N Engl J Med. 1978; 298:195–197.

20. Lipsky H. Urodynamic assessment of women with urethral syndrome. Eur Urol. 1977; 3:202–208.

21. Abrams P, Torrens M. Clinical urodynamics, Urol Clin North Am. 1979; 6:71–79.

22. Corlett R, Roy S. Carbon dioxide uroflowmetry. J. Urol. 1979; 122:512–514.

23. Schleyer-Saunders E. Hormone implants for urinary disorders in postmenopausal women. J Am Geriatr Soc. 1976; 24:337–339.

24. Stanton S, Hilton P, Cardoza L, Annan, H. Internal urethrotomy in the management of impaired voiding in the female. Presented at the 10th Annual Meeting of the International Continence Society. Los Angeles, 1980.

25. Greenblatt R, Nezhat C, Karpas A. The menopausal syndrome: hormone replacement therapy. In: Eskin BA, ed. The menopause, comprehensive management. New York: Masson, 1980:151–172.

Surgery in the Postmenopausal Woman 10

Félix Krauer

Epidemiology

Between 1950 and 1975 the population of persons aged 65 or more in the United States increased by 50%.[1] These persons represent 12% of the total population. Similar observations have been made in European countries. The total population of Switzerland, for example, has doubled between 1900 and 1975. The number of persons over 65 years of age increased during the same period by 275% and the over-80 age group by 550%.[2] In West Germany, the total population increased by 7% between 1963 and 1967, whereas the number of persons aged over 100 years showed an increase of 40%.[3]

The average life-expectancy of a 70-year-old Swiss woman is about 13 years and at age 80 about 7 years. The corresponding figures for women in the United States are reported to be approximately 15 years and 9 years, respectively.[1,4] In terms used in oncology this means that a 70-year-old person has a 75% chance of still being alive after 5 years and a 47% chance of surviving 10 years. At 80 years of age the average 5-year survival is still around 47% and the 10-year survival approximately 14%. At 90 years of age the 5-year survival drops to approximately 17% and the 10-year survival to only 1%.[5]

In an average gynecologic unit, about 30% of the beds are occupied by women over 60 years of age and some 20% of all gynecologic operations are performed on this group of patients (Table 10–1). Improvements in medical technology, anesthesiology, and surgical technique facilitate the decision for undertaking surgical treatment in older women without compromising the outcome.[6–9]

In actuality, there is no reason to categorize a 60-year-old woman as old. Eighty years of age would be more adequate because in this group geriatric aspects are predominant.[10a,10b] This category of patients might represent up to 7% of women over 60 years of age who undergo gynecologic surgery.[11]

Indications for Gynecologic Surgery

The great number of different indications for gynecologic surgery in younger women is in contrast to the rather uniform situation in geriatric patients. In over 80% of the latter, the preoperative diagnosis is breast cancer, genital prolapse with or without urinary incontinence, or genital cancer. Genital prolapse is the main indication (approximately 50% of all surgical indications) followed by genital carcinoma (30%) and benign gynecologic tumors (15%) in this group of women.[12] When breast cancer is included in these statistics, it may be the most important surgical problem in the old woman (Tables 10–2 to 10–4).[13]

BREAST CARCINOMA. One out of two women aged over 70 years self-diagnoses breast cancer. One out of two already has axillary lymph node metastases. When women over age 70 years are screened by medical personnel, breast cancer is detected at a stage when only 25% of the patients have axillary

TABLE 10–1. Age Distribution of Gynecologic Inpatients (University Hospitals of Geneva and Basel).

	INPATIENTS	MAJOR OPERATIONS		MINOR OPERATIONS
		Geneva (1978–1980)	Basel (1978–1979)	Geneva (1978–1980)
All ages	9086	1825	1379	5668
Age 70–79	343	135	105	119
Age ≥80	96	29	16	51
Totals for patients aged 70 years or older	439	164	121	170

lymph node metastases.[14] The mean tumor size in older patients is usually somewhat smaller at the time of diagnosis than in younger women and corresponds to an early UICC (Union International Contre le Cancer) stage T2.[15]

Women with stage T2 breast cancer have a 5-year survival of approximately 50% after adequate treatment. Therefore, it seems justified to include old women with a life expectancy of 5–10 years in a treatment schedule which is not different from that applied to young patients, provided that the treatment itself does not have an incomparably high morbidity or mortality rate.

Before undertaking surgical treatment of breast cancer one must realize that sometimes adjuvant treatment is necessary. Adjuvant chemotherapy is usually impossible in patients over 80 years of age, but hormonal treatment and local radiotherapy are undoubtedly well tolerated.

GENITAL CARCINOMA. Endometrial carcinoma is often diagnosed in an early operable stage in older women. Surgery, as the treatment of first choice, can therefore be considered. Pelvic lymphadenectomy, however, should be performed only if further therapy, such as pelvic or abdominal radiotherapy, is planned. An abdominal hysterectomy and bilateral salpingo-oophorectomy have low postoperative morbidity and mortality rates even in very old patients.

With cancer of the *ovary*, surgical treatment is much more controversial, since the diagnosis is often made in advanced stages III and IV. The indication for surgical treatment is rarely obvious, since in these advanced stages and for this age group, short-term survival is only about 10%. Modern adjuvant chemotherapy which might improve the survival rate is impossible because toxic side-effects are too common.

Vulvar cancer is detected, unfortunately, rather late in older patients and is therefore sometimes unsuitable for surgical treatment. In operable stages, according to the criteria applied to younger women, there is no doubt that surgery should be considered. One should give preference to radical vulvectomy and even adjuvant radiotherapy is possible in this age group.

Cervical cancer is a rather exceptional diagnosis in geriatric patients. Treatment modalities are not standardized, but surgery (as it is used in younger patients) and radiotherapy (as

TABLE 10–2. Indications for Major Operations in 77 Patients Aged 80 Years or Older.

DISEASE PROCESS	INCIDENCE
Breast carcinoma	40%
Genital prolapse and incontinence	30%
Genital carcinoma	25%
Other gynecologic diseases	5%

From Krauer F. Unpublished data.

TABLE 10–3. Indications for Major Operations in 38 Patients Aged 70 Years or Older with Benign Disease.

INDICATION	INCIDENCE
Genital prolapse	80%
Fibroids	8%
Ovarian tumors	8%
Atypical endometrial hyperplasia	3%

From Krauer F. Unpublished data.

TABLE 10–4. Major Operations in 96 Patients Aged 80 Years or Older.

OPERATION	NO. OF PROCEDURES	
Laparotomy	3	
Abdominal hysterectomy	6	20%
Adnexectomy	10	
Vaginal hysterectomy	15	
Vaginal repair	21	43%
Urethral suspension	5	
Vulvectomy	6	5%
Mastectomy (Patey)	30	32%

From Krauer F. Unpublished data.

TABLE 10–5. Changes in Cardiac Functions with Age.

	AGE (YEARS)		
	25	80	Δ(%)
Heart rate (beats/min)	70	67	−5
Stroke volume (ml)	80	60	−25
Cardiac output (liter/min)	5.5	4.0	−30
Maximum heart rate (beats/min)	200	145	−30
Maximum cardiac output (liter/min)	16	9	−50
Mean transit time (s)	19	29	+50

a complementary treatment) may have their place in the treatment of invasive cervical cancer. Wertheim operations are undoubtedly possible even in patients over the age of 80 years, but more often a palliative treatment such as hemostatic or analgesic radiotherapy must be chosen because of the advanced stage of the cancer.

In general, surgery should be appropriate to the stage and performed in a manner consistent with that for a younger patient. Local tumor control and surgical reduction of the tumor mass often improve the quality of life for the geriatric patient for several years.[1,16–19]

BENIGN GYNECOLOGIC LESIONS. Genital prolapse, urinary incontinence, and benign tumors are not so problematic for the gynecologic surgeon. The surgical intervention is generally easy, and the question of survival does not have to be taken into consideration as for malignant disease.

Genital prolapse is often pronounced, and surgical correction is indicated because urinary retention or incontinence, as well as pain and discomfort are often associated. Benign tumors, mostly ovarian cysts, are diagnosed from pain or abdominal swelling, and surgical treatment is indicated. Occasionally, ovarian cancer in an early stage is detected at the time of surgery and can be treated successfully.

Risk Factors

Surgical treatment is less life threatening in elderly patients than it was 20 or 40 years ago. It still carries a significant hazard however, and the jeopardy undoubtedly increases with age. The extent of surgical stress is limited by the functional reserve capacity of the patient's organ system. Such capacity diminishes physiologically with age[20] and can be modified by many diseases.

PHYSIOLOGIC DECLINE IN VITAL ORGAN FUNCTIONS WITH AGE.

Cardiovascular Functions. With age, the heart has a tendency to become smaller. The aorta and the coronary arteries lose their elasticity and show signs of arteriosclerosis. The cardiac valves become more rigid. These morphologic changes modify in different ways the hemodynamic performance of an old heart (Tables 10–5 and 10–6).[21–25]

The stroke volume diminishes and, as a consequence, the cardiac output decreases by about 30% when compared to a 25-year-old person. The reserve capacities, which are the maximum heart rate and the maximum cardiac output, are strongly reduced. The reduction in cardiac output (−1% per year after the age of 50) is greater than would be expected as a consequence of the decreased basal metabolic rate of the total organism (−0.3 to −0.4% per year). There is not only a reduction but also a redistribution of the cardiac output. The kidneys, for instance, are much more affected than other organs. The renal blood flow is reduced by about 50%, whereas hepatic or cere-

TABLE 10–6. Consequences of the Age-related Changes in Cardiac Functions.

Reduction of peripheral tissue perfusion
Decreased velocity of blood flow
Redistribution of the reduced cardiac output
Reduction of cardiac reserves (30–50%)

bral blood flow decreases by only some 10–15%. In some areas the blood supply might become so impaired as to jeopardize the normal metabolism of certain organs.

The reduction in peripheral tissue perfusion seems to be a significant limiting factor for the maximal working capacity of an older person. Even under resting conditions one often finds a slight metabolic acidosis, although compensated. Under working or stress conditions, such an acidosis may become rapidly aggravated and fatal if not diagnosed early and treated immediately. The decreased velocity in blood flow also helps to explain the higher incidence of thromboembolic postoperative complications in the elderly patient.

Considering other possibilities than age which may alter the cardiac output (such as shock, heavy blood loss, high body temperature, and anemia), and keeping in mind that all could arise simultaneously, it is obvious that the cardiac functions of the old patient may suddenly decompensate. An accumulation of risk factors must therefore be avoided.

Respiratory Functions. Deformation and loss of elasticity of the thoracic cage is a normal occurrence in elderly persons. Also the movements of the diaphragm are reduced, and these factors, together with a loss of alveolar elasticity, explain the increase in pulmonary dead space, compliance, and residual volume. The functional respiratory volume therefore decreases, as does the maximal expiratory volume per second and the maximal ventilation per minute. To this reduction of alveolar ventilation is added a diminution of pulmonary blood perfusion due to age-associated vascular alterations. The ventilation/perfusion ratio is disturbed and one notices a decrease in the blood oxygen saturation, the blood oxygen partial pressure (pO_2) and a slight respiratory alkalosis associated with a moderate hypoventilation (Tables 10–7 and 10–8).[26–28]

The decrease in oxygen uptake amounts to about −15%. This is more than would be expected from the mere decrease in the basal metabolic rate, which at the age of 80 years is about −10 to −11%. The fall of the arterial pO_2 to values of approximately 75–80 mmHg causes an oxygen deprivation in peripheral tissues and favors anaerobic metabolism with all its consequences.

TABLE 10–7. Changes in Pulmonary Functions with Age.

	AGE (YEARS)		
	25	70	Δ(%)
Vital capacity (liter)	3.7	3.0	−20
Breathing frequency (breaths/min)	12	16	+25
Maximum tidal volume (liter)	1.7	0.6	−65
Maximum breathing capacity (liters/min)	135	65	−50
Functional residual capacity (liters)	2.6	3.4	+30
Pulmonary resistance (cmH$_2$O/liter/sec)	1.9	2.8	+47
Compliance (ml/cmH$_2$O)	140	110	−25

Looking at the oxygen dissociation curve (Fig. 10–1), it becomes obvious that an 80-year-old woman lives under conditions comparable to those of a person breathing air with an oxygen concentration of only 18% instead of the normal 21%. Her ventilatory reserves are reduced by approximately 50% and she remains close to the danger point of an arterial pO_2 of approximately 60 mmHg. A slight impairment of the pulmonary gas exchange or a mild acidosis (as one might expect from the reduced peripheral tissue perfusion) may lead to decompensation of the ventilatory capacity.

Intra- and postoperative spontaneous breathing is therefore hazardous. Assisted ventilation during anesthesia, and generous oxygen supply afterward and for a prolonged period, are prerequisites for the maintenance of undisturbed aerobic metabolism.

Renal Functions. One often observes a moderate dehydration in older people due essentially to a reduced water intake. Urinary tract infections are quite common, particularly in persons suffering from lower urinary tract obstruction or incomplete bladder voiding with

TABLE 10–8. Consequences of the Age-related Changes in Pulmonary Functions.

Increased ventilation of dead space
Diminished alveolar ventilation
Decreased oxygen uptake (−15%)
Decreased arterial pO_2 (75–80 mmHg)
Reduction of ventilatory reserves (~50%)

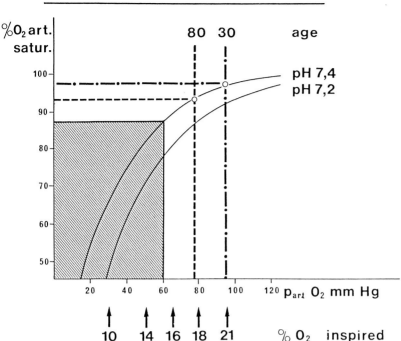

Fig. 10–1. Oxyhemoglobin dissociation curve. See text for explanation.

residual urine. The so-called age-associated changes in renal functions may therefore be due to pathologic processes involving the urinary tract and kidneys. Nevertheless, the renal functions in patients over 70 years of age show characteristic alterations. Renal blood flow, glomerular filtration rate, tubular maximal reabsorption rate, maximal diuresis, and maximal concentration capacity are all seriously decreased (Fig. 10–2; Table 10–9).[29–34]

From the practical point of view, probably the most important consequence of this decline in renal function is the lower elimination rate of drugs. The overall incidence of side-effects of drugs is about seven times higher in old persons than in younger ones. The most frequent complication arises from digitalis therapy, a drug which also has a low therapeutic ratio.[34–36] Drug therapy must therefore be modified and adapted to the reduced renal function in order to avoid drug accumulation.

Water and electrolyte balance are rarely disturbed in gynecologic patients, even in elderly ones. Parenteral postoperative nutrition does not normally pose problems, provided that a fluid overload is avoided, a mistake which, however, easily happens. A sufficient (i.e., rather high) urine output should be maintained to enable the total elimination of average daily waste products. This high urinary volume is necessary because of the decreased renal concentration capacity.

GENERAL RISK FACTORS. All gynecologic operations in older patients entail a high risk. This becomes even more evident when one employs a checklist, such as the one designed by Lutz[37] for use in general surgery and modified by Börner[38] for gynecologic surgery. Thus, a detailed preoperative checkup and diagnosis are essential. In this context, two aspects should be considered: (1) the patient's general condition; and (2) the underlying surgical disease.

Exact characterization and measurement of preexisting risk factors make it easier to justify

TABLE 10–9. Consequences of the Age-related Decline in Renal Functions.

Lower renal elimination rate of drugs and metabolites
Oliguria
Water retention
Electrolyte imbalance (?)
Reduced total renal capacity (~50%)

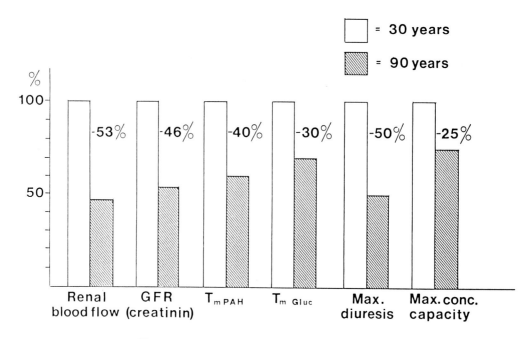

Fig. 10–2. Changes in renal function with age.

the need for surgical intervention. It is important to know whether the patient can stand a certain surgical stress. It should be noted that intra- and postoperative complications are particularly frequent in patients with preexisting cardiovascular or bronchopulmonary disease. The most frequent cause of postoperative mortality in geriatric patients is pulmonary embolism.

It is an exception that a gynecologic surgical intervention causes a fatal aggravation of a pre-existing disease if this has been correctly diagnosed and treated before surgery.

Investigations concerning the underlying gynecologic disease must be done in addition to the general checkup. In the case of breast disease or genital prolapse, these procedures are usually easy and without discomfort. Much more delicate are the questions to be resolved in the case of urinary incontinence or an intraabdominal process, especially when there is a suspicion of malignancy.

An exhaustive preoperative diagnostic procedure is indicated only if therapeutic consequences can be determined. Generally, a few uncomplicated diagnostic examinations are preferred to a multitude of sophisticated investigations. A difficult differential diagnosis is rare in older patients, and functional tests of an organ or organ system, where an active physical and intellectual collaboration of the patient is necessary, are bound to fail. The experience of the surgeon associated with a few efficient clinical and laboratory tests provide the easiest and most convenient method of appreciating the patient's condition. Examinations which are only done to document a clinically evident situation are unnecessary and only of academic value.

Diagnostic surgical interventions have to be considered very carefully. Dilatation and curettage (D & C) as well as biopsy, exploratory laparotomy, and laparoscopy are known to be associated with fatal complications if not performed with the same precautions as any major gynecologic surgical intervention.[39,40]

Postoperative Morbidity

The frequency of postoperative complications in older patients is comparable to that in younger women (15–20%).[10a–11] This is, however, true only if the preexisting risk factors have been detected and reduced or eliminated by adequate preoperative treatment (Table 10–

TABLE 10–10. Postoperative Morbidity After
Major Surgery in 77 Patients Aged 80 Years or
Older.

DISORDER	INCIDENCE
Pneumonia	2
Cardiac decompensation	2
Thromboembolism	4
Psychotic syndrome	1
Diabetic decompensation	1
Urinary infection (uncomplicated)	13
Anemia (<10 g-% Hb)	2
Signs of overdigitalization	2

From Krauer F. Unpublished data.

10). The characteristics of postoperative complications are, however, different. In geriatric patients the most frequent complications are thromboembolism, cardiovascular complications, postoperative hypoxia and acidosis, and fever or pelvic infection.

As a consequence of this observation, the following prophylactic measures will be discussed: (1) prophylactic anticoagulation; (2) prophylactic antibiotics; (3) prophylactic digitalization; (4) prophylactic intestinal stimulation; and (5) essentials of surgical technique.

Age, varicosity, and cancer, a characteristic triad of old patients, favor postoperative thrombosis and embolism. Lethal postoperative pulmonary embolisms are described even after such so-called minor surgical interventions as breast biopsy and D & C.[40–45]

Age is no longer, in our opinion, a contraindication for anticoagulation. Several methods are available today which lower the incidence of fatal pulmonary embolism.[44–50]

1) Low-dose subcutaneous heparin, 5000-U two or three times per day starting 2–7 h before the operation and administered for at least 7 days or until full mobilization of the patient.
2) Low-dose subcutaneous heparin, 2500-U twice daily, combined with dihydroergotamine, 0.5 mg twice daily, for 7–10 days.
3) Perioperative intravenous infusions of high molecular dextran 500-ml three times during the first and second days.

It is possible that these prophylactic measures may increase the perioperative blood loss or favor postoperative incidental hemorrhage.[51] It is therefore necessary to pay particular attention to hemostasis, and a generous use of drains is recommended.[52] Reintervention for postoperative hemorrhage is particularly jeopardizing in elderly patients and must be avoided by using a subtle surgical technique.

It has been shown that the frequency of postoperative pelvic or abdominal wall infections can be drastically reduced using different systems of drainage.[52,53] General prophylactic antibiotics do not improve the postoperative infectious morbidity in gynecologic surgery and should therefore be restricted to a few particular situations, such as urinary tract infections which have not been treated prior to the operation, in patients who need postoperative bladder drainage, or if the intestine was accidentally injured and preoperative bowel preparation has not been performed.

There is no doubt that patients with cardiac insufficiency must be treated with digitalis before surgery can be discussed.[54,55] Prophylactic digitalization in patients without cardiac insufficiency is, however, a subject for discussion.[56–58] Overdigitalization and hypokalemia are frequent in older patients; therefore, the use of digitalis is justified only in the presence of clinically manifest cardiac insufficiency. If prophylectic digitalization is not used, however, postoperative cardiac failure must be diagnosed in a very early stage and treated rapidly and adequately.[55,59]

Postoperative ileus or subileus in older patients is rare after gynecologic operations. Bowel movements are, however, often delayed by 2 or 3 days. Oral alimentation should therefore start somewhat later than in younger patients. Any kind of bowel stimulation (e.g., parasympathicomimetics, enema) is an unnecessary, sometimes even dangerous trauma to the older patient and does not accelerate postoperative recovery.[13]

The postoperative morbidity or mortality is only marginally related to the kind of operation performed and is comparable to that in younger women. When performing a surgical correction for genital prolapse, there is no difference in the postoperative outcome whether a vaginal hysterectomy is added to the repair or not.[12] Even additional urethral suspension procedures do not increase postoperative morbidity.[13] With respect to breast surgery, the low morbidity is well known either after simple or modified radical mastectomy and axillary lymphadenectomy.[13] A more conservative surgical approach to breast cancer in older patients therefore seems unjustified, particularly since postoperative regional radiotherapy, if indicated, is also well tolerated[14] and adjuvant hormonal therapy may be more efficient after complete surgical treatment.

Without going into details of surgical techniques, it is important to respect a few particulars when operating on older patients. The surgical team must be backed up by an intensive care–type infrastructure since all interventions in older patients are high risk operations. With respect to the surgery itself, one should be aware that time and blood loss are probably the most critical factors which influence the postoperative outcome. The operation should not last more than 3 h and hemostasis must be meticulous—operative blood loss must be rapidly and adequately compensated since even small changes in the circulatory blood volume are badly tolerated.

Postoperative Mortality

The average mortality rate is 7–8% for women over the age of 60, independent of the type of operation or the underlying surgical disease.[12] Eighty percent of the deaths occur during the first 4 weeks after operation. During this period of time, the mortality rate averages 6%. If the patient's age is taken in consideration, it becomes evident that the mortality rate does

TABLE 10–12. Postoperative Mortality According to Type of Operation.

OPERATION	LITERATURE REVIEW[a]	PERSONAL SERIES[b]
Prolapse	2%	0%
Breast surgery	2.5%	0%
Vulva surgery	5%	0%
Laparotomy	14%	3%

[a] From Jaluvka U.[12] N = 6658, including 261 patients 80 years of age or older.
[b] From Krauer F. Unpublished data. N = 77 patients 80 years of age or older.

not change much up to the age of 80 years. The higher rate of 13.8% after age 80 can be explained by the fact that many operations for advanced cancers are included in this group (Table 10–11).

Laparotomies have the highest morbidity and mortality rates even if one considers only the cases without cancer. Exploratory laparotomies, seldom indicated in geriatric surgery, and operations for benign genital tumors show a postoperative mortality of about 5%. This percentage is not influenced by the radicality of the intervention. It makes no difference, for instance, if a bilateral salpingo-oophorectomy is performed alone or associated with an abdominal total hysterectomy (Table 10–12).[12,16]

An overall mortality rate of 14% after laparotomies reported in the literature[12] may probably be explained by the fact that many urgent laparotomies, and laparotomies for inoperable abdominal cancer are included in these statistics. It is well documented that these procedures have a postoperative mortality rate

TABLE 10–11. Postoperative Mortality After Major Gynecologic Surgery in Different Age Classes.

	AGE (YEARS)		MORTALITY
Literature review[a]	60–64		6.0
	65–69		7.8
	70–74		8.7
	75–79		8.9
	≥80	(N = 261)	13.8
	Overall	(N = 6658)	7.7
Personal series[b]	≥80	(N = 77)	3.0

[a] From Jaluvka V.[12]
[b] From Krauer F. Unpublished data.

TABLE 10-13. Postoperative Mortality According to Underlying Disease.

	LITERATURE REVIEW[a]	PERSONAL SERIES[b]
Extragenital disease	13.6%	1.5%
Gynecologic cancer	12.1%	1.5%
Gynecologic disease (nontumoral)	6%	0%
Benign gynecologic tumors	5%	0%
Prolapse	2%	0%

[a] From Jaluvka V.[12] N = 6658, including 261 patients 80 years of age or older.
[b] From Krauer F. Unpublished data. N = 77 patients 80 years of age or older.

TABLE 10–14. Postoperative Mortality According to Site of Cancer.

SITE	MORTALITY (%)
Abdominal carcinoma	50
Ovarian carcinoma	25
Cervical carcinoma	12
Endometrial carcinoma	10
Vulvar carcinoma	7
Breast carcinoma	2.5

TABLE 10–16. Major Operations for Benign Disease in 38 Patients Aged 70 Years or Older.

OPERATION	NO. OF PATIENTS
Vaginal hysterectomy with repair	24
Colpohysterectomy	1
Repair alone	2
Abdominal hysterectomy + bilateral salpingo-oophorectomy	7
Abdominal hysterectomy alone	3
Laparotomy	1

From Krauer F. Unpublished data.

which is three to six times higher than for elective surgery.[9] In cancer patients, the postoperative mortality rate can rise up to 50%. Moreover, the cancer localization must be considered when evaluating the mortality rate. It is obvious that abdominal carcinoma is associated with a much higher postoperative mortality than vulvar or breast cancer, for example (Tables 10–13 and 10–14).

Diagnostic exploratory laparoscopies, which are often used in young women, are contraindicated in older patients. The pneumoperitoneum and the Trendelenburg position compulsory for pelvic inspection may cause fatal cardiovascular complications during the procedure. Laparotomies are preferred under such circumstances.

Long-term Follow-up After Gynecologic Surgery for Benign Disease of Cancer

Our series of 58 patients aged 70 years and older operated for various *benign* diseases has been reevaluated 1–3 years after surgical treatment to determine whether the patients had

TABLE 10–15. Number of Patients 70 Years of Age or Older Undergoing Surgery for Benign Disease.

	NO. OF PATIENTS
Minor operations	20
Major operations	
Abdominal	11
Vaginal	27
Anesthesia	
General	51
Epidural	7

Personal series. N = 58.
From Krauer F. Unpublished data.

any therapeutic benefit. The patients were interviewed and a gynecologic examination was performed to verify the anatomic results (Tables 10–15 and 10–16). About 95% of all patients were entirely satisfied and did not express any complaints. In approximately 85% the anatomic result was also judged to be normal (Tables 10–17 and 10–18).[60]

In attempting to determine the benefit of surgical treatment for gynecologic or breast *cancer* in another series of 33 patients, we noticed after a limited 1- to 4-year postoperative follow-up an overall mortality of 27% (nine of 33). Only one patient did not die from cancer (pulmonary embolism). This mortality rate compares well with the 5-year overall mortality rate of 47% as published by Lewis in 1968.[61] The best results were obtained with surgery for breast cancer where only two of 20 patients died during the follow-up period. With respect to the other cancers, three of seven endome-

TABLE 10–17. Morbidity After Surgery for Benign Disease.[a]

NATURE OF MORBIDITY AFTER MAJOR SURGERY[b]	INCIDENCE (%)
Urinary infections (uncomplicated)	60
Fever (>38°C) or abscess	20
Fractured femor (N = 1), mechanical ileus (N = 1), acute psychotic syndrome (N = 2)	12
Anemia (<10 g-% Hb)	8
Total (N = 23)	60

N = 58 patients 70 years of age of older.
[a] Postoperative mortality after major surgery (up to 6 months postoperative) was 0%.
[b] No complications ensued after minor surgery. (N = 20).

TABLE 10–18. Postoperative Follow-up (1–3 Years) After Major Surgery for Benign Disease. (38 Pat. Aged > 70 Y.)*

	SUCCESS		
	Total	Partial	FAILURE
Patient's personal evaluation (N = 36)	89%	3%	8%
Doctor's evaluation (plus gynecologic exam) (N = 31)	78%	16%	6%

FAILURES	INCIDENCE
Recurrent urinary stress/incontinence	2 patients
Urgency/incontinence	1 patients
Recurrent cystourethrocele (asymptomatic)	2 patients

N = 38 patients 70 years of age or older.
From Krauer F. Unpublished data.

trial cancer patients and three of three ovarian cancer patients did not survive during the period of observation. The three vulvar cancer patients did survive during the follow-up period. All survivors were able to live a normal life without being handicapped by their disease or by posttreatment sequelae.[62]

Summary

Gynecologic surgical treatment in geriatric patients is possible for a wide range of indications without an unacceptably high morbidity or mortality rate. With respect to cancer patients over 80 years of age, the major goal of surgery is probably the local control of tumor manifestations and improvement of the quality of life. The long-term survival is secondary but must always be kept in mind when selecting the type of surgical intervention. Cancer should be operated whenever possible according to the rules valid for younger women, i.e., according to the tumor stage. On the other hand, one must realize that a 75 year old woman has statistically a much higher probability of dying of heart disease or of a stroke than of cancer (ratio 5 : 1).

Surgery for genital displacement yields gratifying results in geriatric patients. The therapeutic benefit is guaranteed, and all types of interventions bear very low risks. Disabling situations can easily be corrected and the quality of life may be greatly improved even without heroic surgery.

Provided that the patient's general risk factors are diagnosed and treated preoperatively, the indication for gynecologic surgery is evident, the intervention is performed under optimal conditions, and the patient's collaboration is guaranteed, major gynecologic surgery in women over the age of 80 years is justified and beneficial.

REFERENCES

1. Pierson RL, Figge PK, Buchsbaum HJ. Surgery for gynecologic malignancy in the aged. Obstet. Gynecol. 1975; 46:523.
2. Statistisches jahrbuch der Schweiz. Berne: 1977.
3. Franke H. Gesundheitszustand und klinische Beobachtungen bei den Hundertjährigen der Bundesrepublik Deutschland. Schweiz Rundschau Med. 1977; 66:1149.
4. Paillat F. Evolution démographique et sénescence. In: Martin E, Junod J-P, eds. Abrégé de gérontologie. Berne: Huber, 1977:56.
5. Rohner A. Chirurgie du vieillard. In: Martin E, Junod J-P, eds. Abrégé de gérontologie, 2nd ed. Berne: Huber, 1977:443–450.
6. Berle P, Steinborn H, Thomsen K. Forschritte und Wandel in der geriatrischen operativen Gynäkologie. Geb Frauenheilk. 1976; 36:237.
7. Börner P, Heidenreich W, Majewski A. Zunehmende Individualisierung der Therapie des Endometriumkarzinoms. Geb Frauenheilk. 1977; 37:142.
8. Börner P. Risikoklassifizierung und Risikoabwägung als Voraussetzung zur Operation von Risikopatientinnen. Geb Frauenheilk. 1977; 37:897.
9. Kraas R, Berger HG, Schwermann R, Athanasiadis S. Das Operationsrisiko bei Abdominaleingriffen im Alter, in Abhängigkeit von der Operationsvorbereitung. Vortrag auf der 120. Tagung der Vereinigung Nordwestdeutscher Chirurgen, Hamburg, 1978.
10a. Krauer F. La chirurgie gynécologique chez les octogénaires. Congrès Suisse de Gynécologie et Obstétrique, Montreux, 1979.
10b. Krauer F. La chirurgie gynécologique chez les octogénaires. Indications—sélection—limites. Gynäk Rdsch 1979; 19(Suppl. 2):66.
11. Magnin G, Delafosse B, Raudrant D, et al. Le risque opératoire chez la femme âgée. In: Société Française de Gynécologie, eds. Pathologie

génitale de la femme au 3ème âge. Paris: Masson, 1979.

12. Jalůvka V. Surgical geriatric gynecology. Basel: Karger, 1980.

13. Richter R, Krauer F, Käser O. Gynäkologische Operationen bei alten Frauen. Gynäkologe. 1980; 13:198–204.

14. Levy P, Krauer F, Junod J-P. La femme âgée et le cancer du sein: quelle attitude adopter. Gynäk Rdsch 1979; 19(Suppl. 2):83.

15. Schäfer P. Cancer du sein: Corrélation entre facteurs épidémiologiques et facteurs pronostiques de la tumeur. Méd Hyg. 1979; 37:4417.

16. Julůvka V. Grössere gynäkologische Operationen bei 80 jährigen und älteren Frauen. Arch Gynäk. 1977; 222:73.

17. Kucera H, Michalica W, Weghaupt K. Geriatrische Gynäkologie unter besonderer Berücksichtigung maligner Tumoren. Fortschr Med. 1979; 87:919.

18. McKeithen WS. Major gynecologic surgery in the elderly female 65 years of age and older. Am J Obstet Gynecol. 1975; 123:59.

19. O'Leary J, Symmonds LE. Radical pelvic operations in geriatric patients. A 15-year review of 133 cases. Obstet Gynecol. 1966; 28:745.

20. Cole WH. Medical differences between the young and the aged. J Am Geriatr Soc. 1970; 18:589.

21. Brandfonbrenner M, Landowne M, Shock NW. Changes in cardiac output with age. Circulation. 1955; 12:557.

22. Franke H. Altern und Alter: Das Herz im Alter. Ciba-Revue, 1981, p. 3.

23. Harris R. Cardiac changes with age. In: Goldmann R, Rockstein M, eds. The physiology and pathology of human aging. New York: Academic Press, 1975.

24. Landowne M, Brandfonbrenner M, Shock NW. The relation of age to certain measures of performance of the heart and the circulation. Circulation. 1955; 12:567.

25. Strandell T. Circulatory studies on healthy old men. Acta Med Scand. 1964; Suppl. 414:1.

26. Bates DV, Macklen PT, Christie RV. Respiratory function in diseases: Predicted values for pulmonary function tests in women, 2nd ed. Philadelphia: Saunders, 1971:94.

27. Campbell JC. Detecting and correcting pulmonary risk factors before operation. Geriatrics. 1977; 32:54.

28. Press P. Maladies du système respiratoire. In: Martin E, Junod J-P, eds. Abrégé de gérontologie. Berne: Huber, 1977:209–221.

29. Davis DF and Shock NW. Age changes in glomerular filtration rate, effective renal plasma flow, and tubular excretory capacity in adult males. J Clin Invest. 1950; 29:496.

30. Delachaux A. Maladies rénales et urologiques. In: Martin E, Junod J-P, eds. Abrégé de gérontologie, 2nd ed. Berne: Huber, 1977:231–237.

31. Goldmann R, and Rockstein M. The physiology and pathology of human aging. New York: Academic Press, 1975.

32. Lindeman RD. Age changes in renal function. In: Goldman R, Rockstein M, eds. The physiology and pathology of human aging. New York: Academic Press, 1975.

33. Møcholm-Hansen J, Kampmann J, Laursen H. Renal excretion of drugs in the elderly. Lancet. 1970; 1:1170.

34. Triggs EJ, Nation RL. Pharmacokinetics in the aged: A review. J Pharmacokinet Biopharmaceut. 1975; 3:387.

35. Evered DC, Chapman C. Plasma digoxin concentrations and digoxin toxicity in hospital patients. Br. Heart J. 1971; 33:540.

36. Ewy GA, Kapadia GG, Yao L, Lullin M. Digoxin metabolism in the elderly. Circulation. 1969; 39:449.

37. Lutz H, Klose R, Peter K. Die Probelmatik der präoperativen Risikoeinstufung. Anästh Inform. 1976; 17:342.

38. Börner P, Böhme U, Zimmerman P, Majewski U. Der Einfluss allgemeiner Operations-risiken auf die Operationsindikationen gynäkologischer Karzinome. Geb Frauenheilk. 1980; 40:205.

39. Jalůvka V. Probelaparotomie im geriatrischgynäkologischen Operationsgut. Geb Frauenheilk. 1977; 37:317.

40. Krauer F. Is age a limiting factor for gynecological surgery? XXVIth Annual Meeting of the Society of Pelvic Surgeons, Basel, 1976.

41. Ballard RM, Bradley-Watson PJ, Johnstone FD, et al. Low doses of subcutaneous heparin in the prevention of deep vein thrombosis after gynecologic surgery. J Obstet Gynaecol Br Commonw. 1973; 80:469.

42. Beneke G. Frequenz thromboembolischer Erkrankungen im Alter. In: Marx R, Thies HA, eds. Alter und Blutgerinnung. Stuttgart: Schattauer, 1970.

43. McCarthy T-G, Queen J, Johnstone FD, et al. A comparison of low-dose subcutaneous heparin and intravenous dextran 70 in the prophylaxis of deep venous thrombosis after gynaecological surgery. J Obstet Gynaecol Br Commonw. 1974; 81:486.

44. Schorr DM, Gruber UF. Prophylaxe thromboembolischer Komplikationen in der operativen Gynäkologie. Geb Frauenheilk. 1977; 37:291.

45. Walsh JJ, Bonnar J, Wright FW. A study of pulmonary embolism and deep leg-vein thrombosis after major gynaecological surgery using

labelled fibrinogen. Phlebography and lung scanning. J Obstet Gynaecol Br Commonw. 1974; 81:311.

46. Ardelt W, Dittrich A, Bolze H. Medikamentöse Thromboembolieprophylaxe in der operativen Gynäkologie. Geb Frauenheilk. 1974; 34:664.

47. Hohl M, Lüscher KP, Gruber UF. Nebenwirkungen bei perioperativer Thromboembolieprophylaxe. Gynäkologe. 1978; 11:45.

48. Hohl MK, Lüscher KP, Tichy J, et al. Prevention of postoperative thromboembolism by dextran 70 or low-dose heparin. Obstet Gynecol. 1980; 55:479.

49. Hohl MK, Luscher KP, Annaheim M, Gruber UF. Dihydroergotamine and heparin or heparin alone for the prevention of postoperative deep vein thromboembolism in gynecology. Arch Gynecol. 1980; 230:15.

50. Schander K. Der heutige Stand der Thromboembolie-prophylaxe in der Geburtshilfe und Gynäkologie. Gynäkologe. 1978; 10:198.

51. Kindermann G. Operative Probleme der Gynäkologie bei der älteren Frau. Klinikarzt. 1976; 6:136.

52. Swarts WH, Tanaree P. T-tube suction drainage and/or prophylactic antibiotics. A randomized study of 451 hysterectomies. Obstet Gynecol. 1976; 47:665.

53. Hirsch HA. Postoperative Komplikationen nach vaginalen Hysterektomien und Inkontinenzoperationen. Gynäk Rdsch. 1979; 19(Suppl. 1):76.

54. Deutsch S, Dalen JE. Indications for prophylactic digitalization. Anaesthesiology. 1969; 30:648.

55. Neuhaus K. Präoperative Abklärung und Behandlung gynäkologischer Patientinnen. Geb Frauenheilk. 1977; 37:367.

56. Börner P, Böhme U, Wehrle KP, Zimmerman P. Präventive Therapie allgemeiner Risiken von gynäkologischen Operationen. Geb Frauenheilk. 1978; 38:1.

57. Gahl K, Lichtlen P. Präoperative Störungen der Herzfunktion: Erkennung, Bedeutung und Behandlung im Hinblick auf allgemeinchirurgische Eingriffe. In: Pichlmayer R, ed. Postoperative Komplikationen, Prophylaxe und Therapie. New York: Springer-Verlag, 1976.

58. Jahrmärker H. Digitalistherapie. New York: Springer-Verlag, 1975.

59. Dettli L. Arzneimitteldosierung bei Niereninsuffizienz. In: Koller F, Nagel GA, Neuhaus K, eds. Internistische Notfallsituationen. Stuttgart: Thieme. 1976:241.

60. Cottagnoud C. Personal communication, 1982.

61. Lewis ACW. Major gynecological surgery in the elderly. A review of 305 patients. J Int Fed Gynecol Obstet (Napoli). 1968; 6:244.

62. Krauer F. Geriatric gynecological surgery. Chicago: Society of Pelvic Surgeons. 1981.

Psychobiologic Aspects of the Menopausal Syndrome

11

Meir Steiner

Menopause is associated with major endocrinologic, biochemical, physiologic and psychologic changes. All women who live beyond the age of 60 years experience this period of transition from the reproductive to the nonreproductive stage of life, of which the most striking feature is the cessation of menstruation. For some women this transition is accompanied by somatic and psychologic symptoms and illness usually referred to as the *menopausal syndrome*. This chapter will discuss the present state of clinical and psychoneuroendocrine knowledge in the disorders regarded as *menopausal psychiatric syndromes* (MPS). In order to avoid confusion the relevant terminology as recommended by the WHO Scientific Group will be used[1]:

1) The term *menopause* is defined as the permanent cessation of menstruation resulting from loss of ovarian follicular activity.
2) *Surgical menopause* refers to the procedure of bilateral oophorectomy, with or without hysterectomy.
3) *Perimenopause* (or *climacteric*) includes the period immediately prior to the menopause (when endocrine, biologic, and clinical features of approaching menopause are already obvious) and at least 12 months after the menopause.
4) *Postmenopause* begins after a period of 12 months of spontaneous amenorrhea has been observed.
5) *Premenopause* includes the whole of the reproductive period prior to the menopause.

Clinical Considerations

The diagnostic criteria and classification of menopausal psychiatric syndromes or symptoms have been reconsidered many times over the past century. Classically the symptomatology has been divided artificially into three groups[2,3]:

1) *Vasomotor symptoms* (autonomic nervous system imbalance): the most frequent and characteristic presenting symptoms are hot flushes and night sweats.
2) *Emotional symptoms* (psychogenic): disturbing psychologic alterations such as diminished energy and drive, fluctuations in mood, irritability, tension, apprehension, headaches, loss of libido, insomnia, and dysphoria are just a few of a long list of symptoms cited as being associated with the climacteric.
3) *Musculoskeletal symptoms* (and other features related to metabolic changes): these include the "objective" signs of aging such as skin and breast atrophy, senile vaginitis, hirsuitism, thrombosis, degenerative arthropathy, and osteoporosis.

It is immediately obvious that such a catalog of complaints represents an "incomprehensible nadir of well being"[3] in the formerly well-balanced woman.

It also is well known that MPS have been invariably linked with depression. Most of the characteristics of *major depressive disorders* (*with or without melancholia*) and other depressive states (nonendogenous), as described in the *Diagnostic and Statistical Manual of Mental Disorders, 3rd ed.* (DSM-III) of the American Psychiatric Association,[4] can usually be found in depressed menopausal women.

Any physical or psychologic stress may precipitate a depression in a predisposed individual, but it is often difficult, and sometimes impossible, to differentiate among factors that may have caused the depression, may only have triggered it, or may be coincidentally related to its onset.[5] Thus, the challenge facing psychiatrists is to evaluate first the specificity of the menopausal syndrome.[6]

The only specific pathophysiologic changes that are universally recognized as occurring in relation to menopause are the presence of hot flushes, night sweats, and atrophic vaginitis, all of which seem to be associated with postmenopausal estrogen deficiency. However, the specificity of menopausal or postmenopausal psychiatric illness, in particular depression, is controversial. Several well-established epidemiologic studies have indicated that women preponderate among depressives.[7] It was believed that this preponderance (a ratio of at least 2:1 for depression in women when compared to men) can mainly be attributed to an increase in susceptibility of women to depression in the menopausal years. Thus a distinct clinical entity, namely *involutional melancholia,* became part of the official nomenclature.[8,9] In the *Diagnostic and Statistical Manual of Mental Disorders, 2nd ed.* (DSM-II) of the American Psychiatric Association,[10] involutional melancholia is defined as:

> . . . a disorder occurring in the involutional period and characterized by worry, anxiety, agitation, and severe insomnia. Feelings of guilt and somatic preoccupations are frequently present and may be of delusional proportions. This disorder is distinguishable from manic depressive illness by the absence of previous episodes . . . and it is distinguished from psychotic depressive reaction in that the depression is not due to some life experience.

Further studies failed to support the distinctiveness of postmenopausal depression. The prevalence of depression in women during menopausal years was found to be similar to the risk for depression during other times of the life span.[11–13] In addition, it has also been shown recently that depressed women who are in the menopausal years do not have a distinct symptom pattern, and do not exhibit an absence of previous episodes or absence of life-stress precipitants.[14] The evidence thus far supports the decision to exclude involutional melancholia, as currently defined, from the DSM-III.[4] Nevertheless, the menopause coincides with an age period which shows the peak incidence of hospital admissions for depression,[15] and therefore the coincidental presence of psychiatric morbidity and the menopause has to be kept constantly in mind.

Physiologic Factors

There is compelling evidence that altered neuroregulation can change behavior.[16] Gonadal steroid hormones are known to influence the central nervous system (CNS) and affect behavior and are considered as possible CNS neuroregulators. These hormones are partial determinants of certain sexually dimorphic behaviors, interacting with psychologic, sociocultural, and other biologic factors. Areas of research which have focused on this interaction include the role of testosterone and agression in men,[17] mood and the menstrual cycle,[18,19] and mental disorders associated with childbearing in women,[20] to name just a few.

Menopause, in an oversimplified statement, is regarded as the inevitable consequence of the natural atresia of ovarian follicles and is thus associated with a reduction of estrogen secretion. The mechanism of the biologic clock which initiates the onset of neuroregulatory changes leading toward menopause in unknown. It is believed that the process begins in the brain with a switch from a cyclic to a noncyclic schedule of hypothalamic secretion of neurotransmitter substances. A chain of events then leads to a change in programing along the hypothalamic-pituitary-gonadal (HPG) axis. An ensuing steady state of gonadotropin secretion, which results in an elevation particularly of the follicle stimulating hormone (FSH), but also of the luteinizing hormone (LH), causes ovarian noncyclicity. Ovarian function diminishes, cyclic ovulation and menstrual bleeding disappear, and with further passage of time ovarian function diminishes and the blood levels of *ovarian estrogen* decrease to only very small, barely detectable, amounts.[21] The phasic changes of the various hormones along the HPG axis during the perimenopause and postmenopausal years are described in detail in Chapter 1.

The incidence of the menopausal syndrome in surgical menopause (sudden onset of "ovarian insufficiency") is reported to be very high. It includes vasomotor symptoms experienced as hot flushes, sweating, vertigo, headache, and fatigue, as well as insomnia, depression, decrease in libido, and irritability.[22] These same symptoms accompany the onset of "natural" menopause in an estimated 25% of women.[23] In some of the earlier reports MPS have been labeled as pure *estrogen deficiency disorders*. Eisdorfer and Raskind[24] reviewed the published evidence regarding this syndrome and reached the conclusion that, if it occurs, only the vasomotor symptoms can be attributed to estrogen insufficiency. More recent studies attempt to establish a more detailed psychoendocrine profile of the symptomatic climacteric.

The symptomatic climacteric in contrast to the asymptomatic counterpart has been characterized in a recent study by high FSH and LH and low prolactin (PRL) values. The symptomatic women in this study were described as having anxiety and depression of various kinds, whereas the asymptomatic women had high FSH, lower LH, and lower estrogen values, and higher PRL levels.[25] It has also been hypothesized that postmenopausal dysphoria may occur when high PRL levels are associated with low estrogens, whereas postmenopausal irritability may occur when high PRL levels are associated with low progesterone.[19] Direct clinical testing of this idea has not yet been performed.

Two independent studies have shown a clear temporal relationship between pulsatile release of LH and initiation of menopausal hot flushes.[26,27] Pulsatile release of LH is known to involve also pulsatile luteinizing releasing factor (LRF) secretion. These observations suggest that menopausal flushes are a manifestation of a classical estrogen-withdrawal syndrome mediated through functional changes in estrogen receptor sites, linked to the control of LRF pulsatile secretion. LRF is, at least in part, under the control of catecholaminergic central activity, but the link to the catecholamine hypothesis of depression is still missing.

As already mentioned, postmenopausal depressed women have a symptom profile similar to the depressive profile during other times of the life span. In addition, some of the newly introduced neuroendocrine biologic markers for melancholia have also been applied to the menopause. The results of two of these studies, i.e., (1) the overnight modified dexamethasone suppression test for melancholia and (2) the growth hormone (GH) response to hypoglycemia, have both failed to show any menopausal specificity. Postmenopausal melancholic women show the same degree of abnormality on these tests when compared to all other groups of melancholic patients.[28,29] These findings are consistent with the hypothesis of diminished functional catecholaminergic activity in depressed patients. The stimulation of GH release by clonidine has also been suggested as a test of the postsynaptic alpha-receptor sensitivity of depressed patients. Two recent pilot studies have shown a reduced GH response to clonidine in postmenopausal depressed women similar to the response observed in other melancholic patients.[30,31] In these studies the number of postmenopausal females was very small. A more recent study has shown that even in postmenopausal females, where GH responses to clonidine are universally low, the maximal GH response is less in postmenopausal depressed patients than in postmenopausal controls.[32]

The significance of the ovarian hormones for adrenergic brain processes awaits further elucidation. Aging is known to be associated with a decline in brain catecholamines and their biosynthetic enzymes.[33] Aging is also associated with an increase in brain monoamine oxidase (MAO)[34]—a major enzyme involved in the catabolic pathway of the catecholamines. It has been suggested that this age-related decline in catecholamines, coupled with hypoestrogenism, alters the sensitivity of the catecholaminergic system in postmenopausal women.[35] It is noteworthy that several of the hormonal states claimed to be associated with high MAO activity have also been associated with depressive episodes.[36]

Recent evidence also indicated that catecholestrogens are not only metabolic end products, but possess potent biologic and endocrine activities of their own.[37] It is assumed that catecholestrogens are a major estrogenic constituent of brain and various endocrine tissues, occurring in concentrations that exceed those of their parent compounds.[38] The catecholestrogens probably act at the level of the hypothalamic-pituitary axis and as such may have an important role in psychoneuroendocrine regulation.

To date we assume that steroid hormones act on the CNS, and that they may cause changes in neural structure, function, and chemistry. Studies of direct vs. indirect, short- vs. long-term, and cellular vs. subcellular effects are all under way. What still remains to be seen is whether any of these neurochemical events are essential, relevant, or even sufficient for the observable changes in behavior.

Psychologic Aspects

Menopause acts to a greater or lesser extent as a stress which may induce or precipitate any form of psychologic disturbance in the predisposed woman. Changes in body image, activation of unconscious intrapsychic conflicts, and the emotional reorganization required are all part of the normal adjustments made during this period of transition.

Menopause represents the loss of the ability to reproduce. In the "normal" emotional life of women the reproductive ability is intimately related to femininity, the loss of which represents a blow to feminine self-esteem. In addition, with the menopause, the impact of aging is forced upon women more abruptly, representing more of a psychologic trauma than in the case of men who experience a more gradual and less obvious loss of reproductive capacity.[39]

Many women have been observed to engage in increased activity during the perimenopause.[40] This "thrust of activity" seems to have the effect of a psychologic defense mechanism. The success or failure of these adaptive devices depends upon the circumstances of each individual woman's past and current life. The well-adjusted woman may react to the menopause with heightened interests and activities along lines accepted in her environment. Other women with different premenopausal person-

ality traits or characteristics might use defense mechanisms which are identified as being less acceptable, less effective, or even considered as reflecting an impairment in critical judgment. The more extreme forms of psychopathology, i.e., the utilization of the least effective defenses, then lead to the development of several recognizable symptom clusters. These may include extreme anxiety, panic attacks, psychosomatic complaints, and most commonly dysphoria; occasionally complete denial of reality may even lead to a psychotic episode.

As stated by Donovan[39]:

> "Women who have been able to accept and thereby to satisfy normal feminine drives, women who have established emotionally rewarding relationships through their lives, and women who experience the psychological losses related to the menopause in a state of relative emotional security, are less threatened by the inevitable loss.

As mentioned previously there are no psychologic symptoms specific to menopause.[41] These symptoms of the climacteric are general and include, among others, tension, nervousness, irritability, fatigue, anxiety, insomnia, and depression. The most commonly linked symptom to menopause has always been depression. In discussing the term depression, it is crucial to distinguish whether one is referring to mood, symptom, or syndrome.

In recent years it has been suggested that one way of differentiating between the depressive syndromes is to classify them as endogenous or nonendogenous. It has been stated already that the incidence of endogenous depression (melancholia, "biologic" depression) increases with age but has no special association with menopause.[11] Nonendogenous depressive syndromes previously referred to as neurotic or reactive and most recently known as *dysthymic disorder*[4] seem to have a greater claim for specificity around the menopause. Traditional psychodynamic concepts have emphasized the role of object loss as the paradigm for symptom formation in the affective disorders.[42,43] One such specific loss has been explored in postmenopausal depressed women and referred to as *the empty nest syndrome*.[44] This has been defined as the temporal association of clinical depression with the cessation of childrearing, the departure of children, and the marriage of children. Women described as suffering from this type of depression share a common inability to deal successfully with termination of childrearing and have difficulty in adjusting to their status as childless mothers. The existing quality of the relationship between the woman and her husband is obviously of particular significance. There is evidence that the departure of children is most traumatic to mothers in homes in which couples found little satisfaction in each other and have relied primarily on their children for the fulfillment of their emotional needs.[45]

The state of the marriage itself has an influential impact on the symptomatology of the menopause. The more proximate reason for marital breakdown at this stage is the departure of the children, revealing a longstanding absence of companionship, affection, or sexual interest, but a woman going through menopause and divorce at the same time is much more likely to develop an anxiety and/or depressive reaction.[6]

SURGICAL MENOPAUSE. The psychologic implications of surgical menopause are somewhat more complex. It is well known that hysterectomy, with or without oophorectomy, belongs to the group of surgical interventions that has a high incidence of depressive reactions.[46] Here the woman has to cope with an acute onset of menopause, the aftermath of the hysterectomy, and the anxiety related to her prognosis (especially in cases where the primary reason for surgical intervention is neoplastic in nature).

DIAGNOSTIC CRITERIA. The diagnostic criteria and classification of the more severe forms of mental illness when associated with menopause seem not to differ from the diagnostic spectrum observed at any other period in life. Nevertheless, at least in some cases, when the mental disorder appears at the time of the menopause it assumes a special significance. Such is the case in paranoid delusional reactions or in the morbid jealousy syndromes.[47] In these clinical pictures the menopausal woman incorporates her difficulties in dealing with the changes in her life into a delusional belief. She is preoccupied, for example, with finding "evidence" that her husband is unfaithful to her: she will follow him, question

him, and create an almost unbearable situation for herself and her family. In some of these women there is a history of a preexisting paranoid trait, but in others the clinical syndrome appears initially during the perimenopause.

As to *minor* psychologic and somatic symptomatology, there is now accumulated evidence that they are increased among perimenopausal women.[48,49] A recent study confirmed this elevation in symptoms around the time of the climacteric, but it also showed that this was mainly due to an increase in stressful life events and less related to menopause itself.[50]

Thus, whether the menopause per se is associated with lessened resistance to psychogenic stress is as yet an unresolved issue.

Psychosocial Factors

Critics of the conventional clinical approach argue that the menopausal syndrome is a social role foisted on middle-aged women in western societies.[51] The factors that are of possible relevance have been recently reviewed.[1] These include (1) the psychosocial significance of menstruation and cross-cultural differences in the stigma of menstruation; (2) the psychosocial significance of childlessness; (3) changes in social status, socioeconomic level, and role of postmenopausal women; and (4) attitudes of husbands to their postmenopausal wives.

One obvious way of resolving this controversy would be to study perimenopausal women in different societies. As yet there are few studies comparing attitudes and reactions to the menopause in different cultures. The results of one study in lower-class Indian women indicate that hot flushes, night sweats, and insomnia seem to be clearly associated with the menopause and that they experience this transition as being more stressful than do western women.[52] In another study, women from a particular and relatively affluent Indian caste reported fewer perimenopausal complaints than women in the United States.[53] Social class, working and socioeconomic status, and other cultural and demographic variables have all been linked to differences in severity of menopausal symptoms,[54–56] but these studies have a number of methodologic weaknesses, i.e., they rely heavily on impressions.

One study that clearly stands out in its format, comprehensiveness, and methodology is the study by Maoz and his colleagues.[57,58] Their basic model was to compare five ethnic groups of women in Israel, who formed a continuum from most traditional (rural, Arabs) to most modern (urban, European), and assess psychosexual history, social roles, symptoms of menopause, attitudes toward climacteric (including "perception of menopause" and "image of menstruation"), and degree of physical and mental well being. The results indicate the importance of ethnic considerations in shaping psychic and psychosomatic symptomatology related to the menopause. One of many clear messages to be learned from this study is that menopause is not perceived universally as a loss. To some women, depending on their sociocultural background, menopause is only a relative loss, to others it is even a gain. It would be interesting to investigate other populations in different parts of the world with similar instruments. If some cultural differences determine perimenopausal symptoms, it is important to further investigate this field before health care priorities can be properly evaluated.

Sexuality During the Menopause

Unfortunately, sexuality of the menopausal woman has historically been subject to ignorance, myth, and misconception.[59] Much of the blame can be dated back to early writings of psychiatrists themselves. Benedek[60] wrote that women have a biologic need for pregnancy and motherhood and that the loss of reproductive function leads to *desexualization*. She believed that menopause is a process in which the integrative strength of the personality diminishes.

Deutsch[40] wrote extensively about the meaning of menopause and described the process as "narcissistic mortification," "organic decline," and "partial death." Some of these beliefs seem to relate to society's emphasis on reproductive ability and are still present even among teachers of medical students.[61]

Decrease in libido as a presenting symptom has been documented in up to 25% of postmenopausal women.[62] This has not been always associated with atrophic vaginitis or other physiologic changes of aging which are known to cause some problems during coitus. What is being measured and how libido is quantified have not been clarified, however.

Sexual behavior has to be viewed along several orthogonal dimensions—libido, drive, or desire being only one of them. Of equal importance are the dimensions of sexual response, sexual activity, and the sexual partner. Masters and Johnson[63] have shown that responses in all four phases of the sexual response cycle (excitement, plateau, orgasm, and resolution) are decreased with aging. For some as yet undetermined reason, this diminished response is even more pronounced in women who reach menopause through surgery.[64]

Perimenopausal changes in sexual behavior depend largely on the individual's history and the levels of activity and response of the partner. The notion that sexual activity declines perimenopausally is misleading. Some menopausal women experience increased and new sexual interests. For some women the freedom from fears of pregnancy leads not only to renewed sexual interest but also to an increase in the experience of pleasure and satisfaction in a sexual relationship.

Thus, the psychologic and physiologic experience of menopause, ethnic and sociocultural background, and previous life experience (and misconceptions) are major contributing factors in determining the quality of the sexual relationship during the middle years.

Treatment

Treatment for severe mental disorders associated with the menopause is essentially the same as for other reactive, affective, psychotic, or organic psychiatric disorders. Indications for specific treatments follow the same guidelines as for similar nonmenopausal episodes. Thus major and minor tranquilizers, antidepressants, lithium, and electroconvulsive therapy are used as indicated.

The belief that the menopausal syndrome is a state of chronic estrogen deficiency has led to an enormous proliferation of suggested remedies. Specialized menopause clinics are involved in service and research investigating the best form of hormone replacement therapy (HRT).

To review the subject of HRT is beyond the scope of this chapter; the topic is addressed elsewhere in this volume. Unfortunately the risk/benefit aspects of these interventions are far from being resolved. Titles of articles such as "A prospective, controlled trial of six forms of HRT given to postmenopausal women"[65] only exemplify the controversy surrounding this topic. Nevertheless, what seems to be of significance here is the claim made by several researchers that HRT, especially estrogens, have a specific psychologic effect. A profound euphoric or "mental tonic" effect of estrogen administration on postmenopausal women has been described. Many of these studies are difficult to interpret because of methodologic shortcomings.[66,67] Somewhat stronger evidence was found in support of a positive effect of estrogen treatment in more recent studies.[68–70] However, the high placebo effect in most of the controlled studies and the extreme differences in benefit/risk factors between short- and long-term HRT need further clarification.

When the effects of HRT on specific symptoms are studied the results are even less promising. The effect of estrogen on sleep, mood, and anxiety[71] and depression[72] was found to be little different than the effects of placebo. When general well being, as a result of estrogen therapy, is reported,[73] this "mental tonic" effect is likely to stem from relief of primary menopausal difficulties such as hot flushes, night sweats, and vaginal atrophy.[74] For these primary acute symptoms short-term symptomatic therapy with estrogens seems to be appropriate. As to the recommendations for estrogen therapy for severe, chronic, and persistent depression in perimenopausal women,[75] there is general agreement now that these were premature.[76]

Estrogens nevertheless are still prescribed indiscriminately and hailed as a panacea for mid-life distress. Opposition to this practice is now growing. The WHO Scientific Group[1] recently concluded that menopause is part of the normal aging process which in itself does not require therapeutic intervention. The WHO Scientific Group did not recognize the health status of women during this period as being a simple endocrine-deficiency state which could

or should be corrected by attempting to recreate for each woman a premenopausal hormonal environment.

Future Research

The least convincingly related symptoms to hormonal menopausal changes are the associated psychologic disturbances. A major difficulty, identified by several reviewers in this field, is the inconsistency in the nomenclature used to describe psychologic symptoms and complaints related to the menopause.

One suggested area of research has been to create a language, an "international menopausal index,"[77] as the first step in enhancing our understanding of the problem. The advantages of common definitions, nomenclature, and standardized parameters of climacteric changes are obvious and numerous.

1) Improvement of communication between multidisciplinary team members involved in the caretaking of the menopausal woman.
2) Expanded ability to compare data within and across nations, thus increasing understanding of the sociocultural significance of the menopause in different settings.
3) Feasibility of exact registration of research methods and results, especially where different or similar therapeutic approaches are utilized.

Any further research which will attempt to link physiologic, endocrine, or biochemical changes to menopausal psychologic disturbances will depend on these phenomenologic classificatory parameters. To date even when further research into the effects of HRT is being discussed these issues are completely neglected.[78,79]

With the establishment of a "menopausal index" it is conceivable that three major menopausal subgroups will emerge: (1) "normal" menopause—with an identifiable psychopathology; (2) nonspecific "general" psychiatric disturbances—only temporally linked to the menopause by coincidence or as a general stress reaction; and (3) specific menopausal psychiatric syndromes. The nonspecific psychiatric disturbances presumably follow patterns and present with biologic markers similar to those observed during other times of the life span. As to the specific MPS, these occur with different intensity and the line between normal and pathologic manifestations is very thin. It is suggested that changes should be monitored at multiple levels of behavioral and neuroendocrine systems. As in other areas of medical research a suitable animal could be studied as a model for disorders in the human climacteric. Preliminary results in nonhuman menopausal primates[80] and in middle-aged rats[81] are encouraging.

Two concepts must be borne in mind when future research into the physiology of MPS is discussed. In the first place, menopausal psychologic distress is not a unitary phenomenon. Several different and possibly distinct disorders are included, sharing with each other only the fact that the onset of the disorder coincides with the hormonal event.

Secondly, it must be remembered that the symptoms observed in MPS do occur at other times in the person's life, do not occur in all women, and do occur in men.[82,83] The physiology of the menopause is thus not a cause in itself of any of the symptoms, but rather must be regarded as a contributing or triggering factor acting upon an underlying predisposition. It is only with a systematic conceptual approach allowing for the possibility of multiple etiologies, including an interrelationship between various predisposing physiologic, psychosocial, and sociocultural factors, that new explanations of menopause will arise.

REFERENCES

1. Report of a WHO Scientific Group. Research on the menopause. WHO Techn Rep Ser. 1981; 670:3–120.
2. Utian WH. Current status of menopause and postmenopausal estrogen therapy. Obstet Gynecol Surv. 1977; 32:192–204.
3. Studd J, Chakravarti S, Oram D. The climacteric. Clin Obstet Gynaecol. 1977; 4:3–29.
4. DSM-III. Diagnostic and statistical manual of mental disorders, 3rd ed. Washington, D.C.: The American Psychiatric Association, 1980.
5. Lehmann HE. Affective disorders in the aged. Psychiatr Clin North Am. 1982; 5:27–44.
6. Dominian J. The role of psychiatry in the menopause. Clin Obstet Gynaecol. 1977; 4:241–258.
7. Weissman MM, Klerman GL. Sex differences and the epidemiology of depression. Arch Gen Psychiatry. 1977; 34:98–111.
8. Milici PS. The involutional death reaction. Psychiatr Q. 1950; 24:775–781.
9. Barnett J, Lefford A, Pushman D. Involutional melancholia. Psychiatr Q. 1953; 27:654–662.
10. DSM-II. Diagnostic and statistical manual of mental disorders, 2nd ed. Washington, D.C.: The American Psychiatric Association, 1968.
11. Adelstein AM, Downham DY, Stein Z, et al. The epidemiology of mental illness in an English city. Soc Psychiatry. 1968; 3:47–59.
12. Hallstrom T. Mental disorder and sexuality in the climacteric. In: Forssman H, ed. Reports from the Psychiatric Research Centre, St. Jorgen's Hospital, University of Goteborg, Sweden. Stockholm: Scandinavian University Books, 1973.
13. Winokur G. Depression in the menopause. Am J Psychiatry. 1973; 130:92–93.
14. Weissman MM. The myth of involutional melancholia. JAMA. 1979; 242:742–744.
15. Spicer CC, Hare SA, Slater E. Neurotic and psychotic forms of depressive illness. Br J Psychiatry. 1973; 123:53–54.
16. Barchas JD, Akil H, Elliott GR, et al. Behavioral neurochemistry: neuroregulators and behavioral states. Science. 1978; 200:964–971.
17. Rubin RT, Reinisch JM, Haskett RF. Postnatal gonadal steroid effects on human behavior. Science. 1981; 211:1318–1324.
18. Steiner M, Carroll BJ. The psychobiology of premenstrual dysphoria: review of theories and treatments. Psychoneuroendocrinology. 1977; 2:321–335.
19. Carroll BJ, Steiner M. The psychobiology of premenstrual dysphoria: the role of prolactin. Psychoneuroendocrinology. 1978; 3:171–180.
20. Steiner M. Psychobiology of mental disorders associated with childbearing. An overview. Acta Psychiatr Scand. 1979; 60:449–464.
21. Money J. Endocrine influences and psychosexual status spanning the life cycle. In: van Praag HM, ed. Handbook of biological psychiatry, Part III. Brain mechanisms & abnormal behavior. New York: Marcel Dekker, 1980.
22. Chakravarti S, Collins WP, Newton JR. Endocrine changes and symptomatology after oophorectomy in premenopausal women. Br J Obstet Gynaecol. 1977; 84:769–775.
23. Chakravarti S, Collins WP, Forecast JD, et al. Hormonal profiles after the menopause. Br Med J. 1976; 2:784–786.
24. Eisdorfer C, Raskind M. Aging, hormones and human behavior. In: Eleftheriou BE, Sprott RL, eds. Hormonal correlates of behavior, Vol. 1. New York: Plenum Press, 1975:369–394.

25. Sonnendecker EWW, Polakow ES, Gerdes L. Psycho-endocrine differences and correlations in symptomatic and asymptomatic climacteric women—the possible role of prolactin. SA Med J. 1981; 60:661–665.
26. Tataryn IV, Meldrum DR, Lu KH, et al. LH, FSH and skin temperature during the menopausal hot flash. J Clin Endocrinol Metab. 1979; 49:152–154.
27. Casper RF, Yen SSC, Wilkes MM. Menopausal flushes: a neuroendocrine link with pulsatile luteinizing hormone secretion. Science. 1979; 205:823–825.
28. Carroll BJ. The dexamethasone suppression test for melancholia. Br J Psychiatry. 1982; 140:292–304.
29. Gruen PH, Sachar EJ, Altman N, et al. Growth hormone responses to hypoglycemia in post-menopausal depressed women. Arch Gen Psychiatry. 1975; 32:31–33.
30. Matussek N, Ackenheil M, Hippius H, et al. Effect of clonidine on growth hormone release in psychiatric patients and controls. Psychiatr Res. 1980; 2:25–36.
31. Checkley SA, Slade AP, Shur E. Growth hormone and other responses to clonidine in patients with endogenous depression. Br J Psychiatry. 1981; 138:51–55.
32. Siever LJ, Uhde TW, Silberman EK, et al. Growth hormone response to clonidine as a probe of noradrenergic receptor responsiveness in affective disorder patients and controls. Psychiatr Res. 1982; 6:171–183.
33. McGeer E, McGeer PL. Neurotransmitter metabolism in the aging brain. In: Terry RD, Gershon S, eds. Neurobiology of aging. New York: Raven Press, 1976:389–403.
34. Robinson DS, Nies A, Davis JN, et al. Ageing, monoamines, and monoamine-oxidase levels. Lancet. 1972; 1:290–291.
35. Halbreich U, Asnis G, Ross D, et al. Amphetamine-induced dysphoria in postmenopausal women. Br J Psychiatry. 1981; 138:470–473.
36. Klaiber EL, Kobayashi Y, Broverman DM, et al. Plasma monoamine oxidase activity in regularly menstruating women and in amenorrheic women receiving cyclic treatment with estrogens and a progestin. J Clin Endocrinol Metab. 1971; 33:630–637.
37. Davies JJ, Naftolin F, Ryan KF, et al. The affinity of catechol estrogens for estrogen receptors in the pituitary and anterior hypothalamus of the rat. Endocrinology. 1975; 97:554–557.
38. Paul SM, Axelrod J. Catechol estrogens: presence in brain and endocrine tissues. Science, 1977; 197:657–659.
39. Donovan JC. Psychologic aspects of the menopause. Obstet Gynecol. 1955; 6:379–384.
40. Deutsch H. The psychology of women. New York: Grune & Stratton, 1945.
41. Rosenthal MB. Psychological aspects of menopause. Primary Care. 1979; 6:357–364.
42. Freud S. Morning and melancholia. In: Collected papers, Vol. 4. London: Hogarth Press, 1946:152.
43. Abraham K. Notes on the psycho-analytical investigation and treatment of manic-depressive insanity and allied conditions. In: Selected papers of Karl Abraham. London: Hogarth Press, 1968: 137–156.
44. Deykin EY, Jacobson S, Klerman G, et al. The empty nest: psychosocial aspects of conflict between depressed women and their grown children. Am J Psychiatry. 1966; 122:1422–1426.
45. Luckey EB, Bain JK. Children—a factor in marital satisfaction. J Marr Fam. 1970; 32:43–44.
46. Steiner M, Aleksandrowicz DR. Psychiatric sequelae to gynecological operations. Isr J Psychiatr Relat Sci. 1970; 8:186–192.
47. Langfeldt G. The erotic jealousy syndrome. Acta Psychiatr Scand (Suppl). 1961; 36(Suppl 151):7–68.
48. Ballinger CB. Psychiatric morbidity and the menopause: clinical features. Br Med J. 1976; 1:1183–1185.
49. Wright AL. On the calculation of climacteric symptoms. Maturitas. 1981; 3:55–63.
50. Cooke DJ, Greene JG. Types of life events in relation to symptoms at the climacterium. J Psychosom Res. 1981; 25:5–11.
51. Townsend JM, Carbone CL. Menopausal syndrome: illness or social role—a transcultural analysis. Cult Med Psychiatry. 1980; 4:229–248.
52. Sharma VK, Saxena MSL. Climacteric symptoms: a study in the Indian context. Maturitas. 1981; 3:11–20.
53. Flint MP. Transcultural influences in perimenopause. In: Haspels AA, Musaph H, eds. Psychosomatics in perimenopause. Lancaster: MTP Press, 1979:41–56.
54. Polit DF, LaRocco SA. Social and psychological correlates of menopausal symptoms. Psychosom Med. 1980; 42:335–345.
55. Flint MP, Garcia M. Culture and the climacteric. J. Biosoc Sci (Suppl). 1979; 6:197–215.
56. van Keep PA, Kellerhals JM. The ageing woman. Acta Obstet Gynecol Scand (Suppl). 1975; 51:17–27.
57. Maoz B, Antonovsky A, Apter A, et al. The perception of menopause in five ethnic groups in Israel. Acta Obstet Gynecol Scand. 1977; 65:69–76.
58. Datan N, Antonovsky A, Maoz B. A time to reap: the middle age of women in five Israeli

subcultures. Baltimore: Johns Hopkins University Press, 1981.

59. Gruis ML, Wagner NN. Sexuality during the climacteric. Postgrad Med. 1979; 65:197–207.

60. Benedek T. Climacterium: a developmental phase. Psychoanal Q. 1950; 19:1–27.

61. Klaus H. The menopause in gynecology: a focus for teaching the comprehensive care of women. J Med Educ. 1974; 49:1186–1189.

62. Moore B, Gustafson R, Studd JWW. Experience of a national health service menopause clinic. Curr Med Res Opin. 1975:42–56.

63. Masters WH, Johnson V. Human sexual response. Boston: Little, Brown, 1966:223–248.

64. Zussman L, Zussman S, Sunley R, et al. Sexual response after hysterectomy-oophorectomy: recent studies and reconsideration of psychogenesis. Am J Obstet Gynecol. 1981; 140:725–729.

65. Lind T, Cameron EC, Hunter WM, et al. A prospective controlled trial of six forms of hormone replacement therapy given to postmenopausal women. Br J Obstet Gynecol. (Suppl). 1979; 3:1–29.

66. Kupperman HS, Wetchler BB, Blatt MH. Contemporary therapy of the menopausal syndrome. JAMA. 1959; 171:1627–1637.

67. Wilson RA, Wilson TA. The fate of non-treated postmenopausal women: a plea for the maintenance of adequate estrogen from puberty to the grave. J Am Geriatr Soc. 1963; 11:347–362.

68. Utian WH. Mental tonic effect of estrogen therapy in postmenopause. The Family, 4th International Congress of Psychosomatic Obstetrics and Gynecology, Tel Aviv. Basel: Karger, 1975:520–524.

69. Fedor-Freybergh P. The influence of estrogens on the well being and mental performance in climacteric and postmenopausal women. Acta Obstet Gynecol Scand (Suppl). 1977; 64:2–61.

70. Lauritzen C, van Keep PA. Proven beneficial effects of estrogen substitution in the postmenopause—a review. Front Hormone Res. 1978; 5:1–25.

71. Thomson J, Oswald I. Effect of estrogens on the sleep, mood and anxiety of menopausal women. Br Med J. 1977; 2:1317–1319.

72. Schneider MA, Brotherton PL, Hailes J. The effect of exogenous estrogens on depression in menopausal women. Med J Aust. 1977; 2:162–163.

73. Durst N, Maoz B. Changes in psychological well being during menopause as a result of estrogen therapy. Maturitas. 1979; 1:301–315.

74. Wood C. Menopausal myths. Med J Aust. 1979; 1:496–499.

75. Klaiber EL, Broverman DM, Vogel W, et al. Estrogen therapy for severe persistent depressions in women. Arch Gen Psychiatry. 1979; 36:550–554.

76. Coope J. Is estrogen therapy effective in the treatment of menopausal depression? J Roy Coll Gen Pract. 1981; 31:134–140.

77. Jaszmann LJB. The value of the different parameters in the assessment of extragenital symptoms in the climacteric woman. The Family, 4th International Congress of Psychosomatic Obstetrics and Gynecology, Tel Aviv. Basel: Karger, 1975:507–510.

78. Kay CR. Logistics of study on hormone therapy in the climacteric. Postgrad Med J. 1978; 54(Suppl. 2):92–94.

79. Wiseman RA. Future research—potentially rewarding areas for investigation. Postgrad Med J. 1978; 54(Suppl. 2):95–99.

80. Hodgen GC, Goodman AL, O'Connor A, et al. Menopause in rhesus monkeys: model for study of disorders in the human climacteric. Am J Obstet Gynecol. 1977; 127:581–584.

81. Wilkes MM, Lu KH, Hopper Br, et al. Altered neuroendocrine status of middle-aged rats prior to the onset of senescent anovulation. Neuroendocrinology. 1979; 28:255–261.

82. Henker FO. Sexual, psychic and physical complaints in 50 middle-aged men. Psychosomatics. 1977; 18:23–27.

83. Steiner BW, Satterberg JA, Muir CF. Flight into femininity: the male menopause? Can Psychiatr Assoc J. 1978; 23:405–410.

Menopause and Sleep 12

Veronica A. Ravnikar, Isaac Schiff, and
Quentin R. Regestein

Menopausal women commonly complain of insomnia. However, this symptom is very difficult to study since it is intermingled with a number of complaints: vasomotor flushes, irritability, anxiety, poor memory, and depression. We can speculate that all of these symptoms are somehow interrelated. It is well established that menopausal females have low levels of estrogen and elevated gonadotropins, and, in fact, pituitary luteinizing hormone (LH) secretion correlates with menopausal flushing.[1–3] A decrease in plasma levels of LH, however, has been described in postmenopausal women with unipolar depression when compared with age-matched controls.[4] Urinary estrogen excretion is also lower in postmenopausal women who have unipolar depression.[5] Whether the altered pituitary hormonal secretion in the menopause is related to changes in hypothalamic peptide hormones such as LHRH, which in turn can affect behavior, is worth consideration. The purpose of this chapter is to tabulate all the current research in this area as it relates to sleep disturbances in the menopause.

The methods used to study sleep disturbances objectively are electroencephalograms, electrodermal recordings of hot flushes, assay of coincident hormonal determinations, and psychometric testing.

Stages of Sleep

Dement and Kleitman[6,7] defined five polygraphic stages of sleep: stages 1 through 4 are referred to as NREM sleep; and an additional stage, rapid eye movement (REM) sleep. Polygraphic records consist of simultaneous electroencephalogram (EEG), eye movement (EOG), and chin electromyographic (EMG) patterns. A graphic description of the entire sleep cycle pattern monitored by simultaneous EEG, EOG, EMG, and EKG is depicted in Figs. 12–1 to 12–6.

In stage 1 sleep awareness stops; this is a threshold stage lasting about 15 min. At this time, body temperature falls slightly, the respiration and heart rates slow, and muscles relax. A typical recording of the EEG would show low voltage fast activity and fragmented background or "alpha" rhythm (Fig. 12–3). Subsequently, the individual traverses to stage 2 sleep, characterized by short bursts of "spindle" activity (Fig. 12–4): a 12–14 cycle/sec activity named for its resemblance to spindles. Stages 3 and 4, also termed deep sleep, follow about one-half hour after sleep begins. The EEG trace is no longer that of low voltage activity, but rather displays slower frequency and higher amplitude patterns known as delta waves which resemble a tidal ebb and flow of electric potential (Fig. 12–5).

Subsequently, the process starts reversing from stage 3 to stage 2, and then to REM sleep. This is described as rapid eye movement sleep or paradoxical sleep since at this time the eyes dart back and forth under closed eyelids (Fig. 12–6); respiratory rate, heart rate, and blood pressure become variable, much as during wakefulness. The muscles of the trunk and limbs are mostly limp but the muscles of the face twitch in brief episodes. The EEG recording looks like stage 1 sleep. There is an increase in blood flow to the brain and body temperature rises. Awakened from REM sleep, the subject usually recalls a dream; awakened from

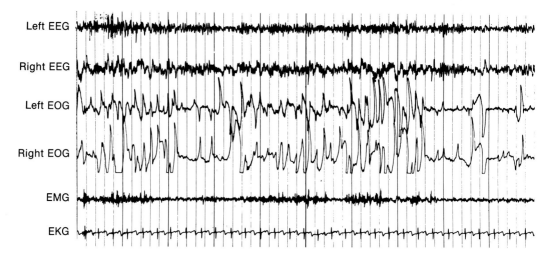

Fig. 12–1. Awake stage. Alpha rhythm admixed with low voltage fast pattern. Eye movement is continuous, and muscle activity is seen in bursts. For Figs. 12–1 to 12–6, the first trace represents left EEG; second trace, right EEG; third trace, left EOG; fourth trace, right EOG; fifth trace, EMG; sixth trace, EKG. Each figure shows 20 s. (Figures 12–1 to 12–8 reprinted with permission of Contemporary Ob/Gyn, Medical Economics Co. From Ravnikar VA. Hormone therapy for menopausal sleep problems? Contemporary Ob/Gyn 1982, 20:72–93.)

deep sleep the subject might recall nothing, or vague perceptions, like a color. REM sleep initially lasts only 5–15 min. The cycle is then repeated: REM to stage 2 and back again, with perhaps a brief appearance of deep sleep prior to stage 2 and a short, unremembered waking period after REM periods. In one night there are approximately five complete 90-min cycles. The first 4 h of an 8-h sleep contain most of the 60–90 min of stage 3 and 4 sleep obtained.

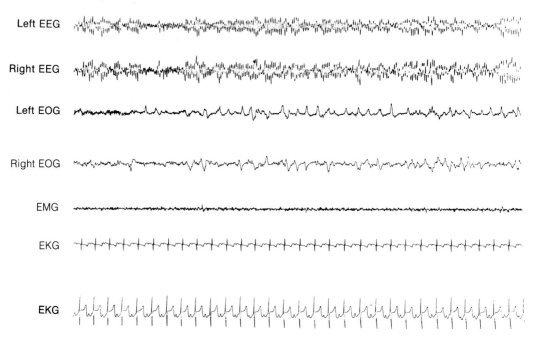

Fig. 12–2. Awake but calm. Alpha rhythm appears throughout EEG leads. Eye movements are slow.

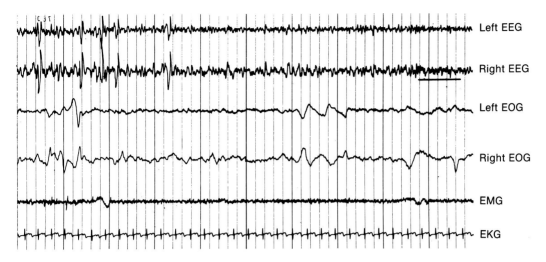

Fig. 12–3. Stage 1—drowsy. Fragmenting alpha rhythm underlined.

REM periods lengthen the longer an individual sleeps. During the last 3 h of sleep stages 3 and 4 disappear, and REM sleep periods may last 20–40 min. Depriving anyone of REM sleep causes increased REM sleep on subsequent nights, known as REM rebound.

The cycle of sleep described refers to uninterrupted sleep. At menopause, however, many women complain of frequent wakenings. Such wakenings are often associated with hot flushes. Menopausal patients who complain of frequent insomnia also complain of excitability, irritation, and depression. They also complain of lessened memory function. Since experimental REM sleep deprivation causes memory impairment, patient complaints about memory may be related to a loss of REM sleep.

Electrodermal recordings of hot flush episodes during sleep have also been done. Flushes are recorded by elevated finger temperatures which appear after the subjective vasomotor sensation, decreased skin resistance over the forehead due to sweating, and increased heart rate during a hot flush episode. These indirectly indicate activity of the sympathetic nervous system.[8–11] Combining both hot flush data and polygraphic recordings of sleep allows a detailed evaluation of the relationship between hot flush episodes and insomnia with frequent nocturnal awakening.

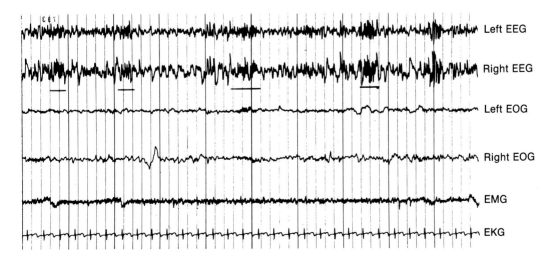

Fig. 12–4. Stage 2—medium sleep. EEG spindles underlined.

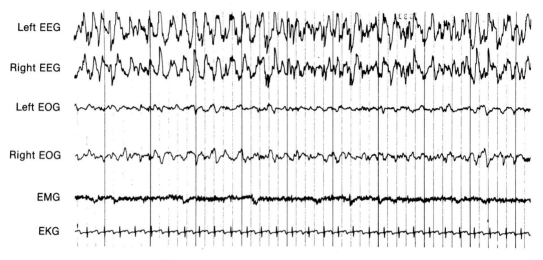

Left EEG

Right EEG

Left EOG

Right EOG

EMG

EKG

Fig. 12–5. Stage 4—deep sleep. EEG slow waves, 1–3 cycles/s, dominate entire record in high amplitudes. By contrast, stage 3 would have more than 20% but less than 50% slow waves.

Hormonal Levels and Sleep

Objective measurements of LH and FSH can be made before and after hormonal treatment to indirectly indicate the target organ effects of the absorption of exogenous hormone.[12] Furthermore, fluctuations in hormonal levels can be determined via assays on plasma samples periodically obtained from in-dwelling catheters.

Sleep-related fluctuations of human growth hormone (GH), prolactin, and gonadotropins (LH, FSH) have been identified. Little data, however, are available on the changes in circadian (daily) and ultradian (shorter than daily) cycles in the menopause.

Human growth hormone is secreted only during slow wave sleep. Furthermore, the peak secretion occurs only during the first few hours of sleep. Thereafter, sleep inhibits GH release. The initial, main period of slow wave sleep is followed by REM sleep; it has been implied that GH may actually trigger REM sleep and improve memory functioning. Secretion of GH induced by stress (e.g., hypoglycemia) depends on central nervous system (CNS) cate-

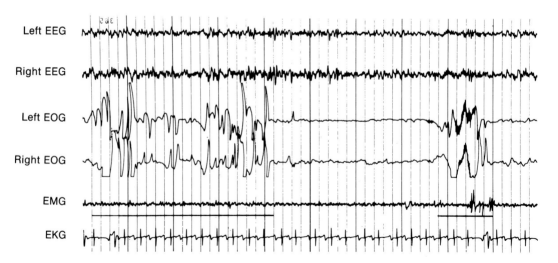

Left EEG

Right EEG

Left EOG

Right EOG

EMG

EKG

Fig. 12–6. REM stage. EEG resembles stage 1. Bursts of rapid eye movements are present, with muscle twitch above left underline.

cholamines,[13] and GH responses to hypoglycemia appear to be blunted in menopausal depressed patients, who have lower levels of CNS catecholamines.[14]

Prolactin levels also rise during sleep. Large secretory pulses of prolactin occur, resulting in progressively higher prolactin levels as sleep proceeds. The highest concentration in the early morning hours is followed by a precipitous drop when the individual awakens. There is some suggestion that prolactin secretion may be closely related to REM/NREM cyclicity, since both are regulated by similar neurotransmitters.

Normal cycling females show a decrease in LH secretion during the first 3 h of sleep.[16] In prepubertal males and females, however, there is a striking release of this hormone during the onset of sleep.[17] In adults, LH spikes are higher during REM periods when compared to other intervals.[18] Recent studies have correlated the association of LH spikes with menopausal vasomotor flushes.[1–3] However, objectively recorded hot flushes have been reported in patients with pituitary insufficiency, making LH spikes an unlikely explanation for flushes.[19] Nevertheless, LH spike releasing hormone (LHRH) frequency and amplitude is also increased in awake menopausal patients with hot flushes compared to those who do not have hot flushes.[20]

Cortisol is also secreted in pulses more toward the early morning hours.[21] Opening the eyes in the morning produces a prompt rise in cortisol.[22] Estradiol and testosterone secretion also occurs in pulses during the night with heightened activity in the morning.[23]

The different secretory patterns of GH and prolactin, which are highest during sleep, compared with cortisol and LH, which are higher during wakefulness, are reflected in differing sites of neuroregulation. Hypothalamic lesions in experimental studies inhibit the nocturnal rise in GH and prolactin, but leave the circadian rhythm of ACTH unaffected. Conversely, lesions which alter human cortisol production do not change the hormonal periodicity of GH/prolactin or ACTH.[24] In a double-blind study of postmenopausal females, Schiff et al. found that estrogen administration selectively blunted LH and prolactin changes during sleep, but did not affect the rise in cortisol.[25] To summarize, there is much

indication that the alterations in hormonal levels and sleep during the menopause are connected, but elucidating the exact causal connections requires more than these correlative observations.

Hormonal Effects on Menopausal Symptoms

Another important adjunct in studying sleep disorders is that of psychometric testing for mood disturbance and other psychopathology.[26,27] It is known that menopausal patients are more prone to mood depression and suicidal tendencies.[28,51] High dose estrogens have been reported to have psychostimulatory and antidepressive effects in both menopausal and/or depressed patients.[44] Nevertheless, in double-blind studies of hormonal therapy vs. placebo and their effects on a variety of menopausal symptoms, a marked placebo effect is obtained on a short-term basis.[30,31] In fact, estrogens in short-term studies when compared to placebo have also been shown not to benefit a menopausal individual's overall sense of well being, as determined by a battery of psychometric tests.[32] It must be emphasized that due to this marked placebo effect, double-blind, long-term studies with crossover comparisons are imperative.[11,33]

When double-blind studies of the effects of estrogens or progesterone on vasomotor flushes are conducted, the placebo effect observed is significant. There is a marked therapeutic effect when placebo is given initially, but further improvement occurs when the active drug is then given. In contrast, when estrogen is first introduced, symptoms significantly worsen at the crossover from drug to placebo. Albrecht et al. showed a significant decrease in the amount of objectively recorded vasomotor flushes when placebo and medroxyprogesterone acetate were studied, the latter causing greater suppression.[11]

The fact that placebo had such a large effect in menopausal studies bears additional discussion in regard to recent literature on endorphins. These are peptide fragments of the pituitary hormone β-lipoprotein. Endorphins appear to have a stimulatory effect on growth hormone and prolactin secretion. They also effect gonadotropin secretion. Morphine, an opioid agonist, decreased serum LH levels in ovariectomized rats, but this effect varies with the dose of morphine and the stage of the estrus cycle. Opioids interfere with dopaminergic systems in the brain—decreasing both the storage and turnover of brain dopamine in the median eminence.[34] By this effect they may modulate LH and prolactin secretion.[35] Since the effects of endorphins on behavior and mental illness are currently being investigated, it is theoretically possible that the placebo effect may actually be endorphin-related. We may conclude that although estrogen probably lessens menopausal vasomotor symptoms through its suppression of gonadotrophin secretion, its lessening of menopausal psychological symptoms may stem from improvement of sleep, fewer vasomotor symptoms, and some direct stimulation of neural function on a placebo effect.

Biogenic Amines

Biogenic amines are specific substances that are found in various regions of the central nervous system and are causally related to sleep–waking cycles. Among the biogenic amines involved in regulating sleep are the catecholamines, norepinephrine and dopamine, and the indoleamine serotonin. Outside the CNS the catecholamines are produced in sympathetic ganglia, sympathetic nerve endings, and chromaffin cells. Serotonin is found also in the gastrointestinal tract and circulating platelets. The biogenic amines, norepinephrine and serotonin, affect both mood and sleep, with each regulating a different type of sleep. Norepinephrine is the predominant neurotransmitter in the nuclei of the upper pons, which control REM sleep. Serotonin is the predominant neurotransmitter in the midline brain stem nuclei, which control deep sleep. When these biogenic amines are depleted, a patient is more likely to become depressed. Menopausal patients do sleep less, possibly as a result of the same biogenic amine depletion (see Fig. 12–7 for review of synthesis).

Norepinephrine was the first biogenic amine implicated in regulating the sleep–wake cycle. Evidence suggests that if norepinephrine or dopamine-containing sites are lesioned, there

is a decreae in REM sleep. If serotonin-containing sites are lesioned, NREM sleep activity diminishes. However, partial norepinephrine depletion, e.g., via reserpine use, can cause an increase in REM sleep; therefore, there is probably a critical ratio of these neurotransmitters that is necessary. For instance, the ratio of norepinephrine to serotonin in the brain produces proportional levels of REM and NREM sleep; higher ratios are associated with REM sleep.[36]

The relationship between pituitary hormonal secretion and these higher monoaminergic neuronal systems as they affect sleep and mood is a fascinating area of research. It was first proposed by Pare in 1959 that depleted catecholamines cause affective disorders.[37] The hypothesis has since been unable to explain some effects, like the therapeutic effect of lithium and the lag period before antidepressants exert clinical effects.[39] The basis for antidepressant drug action is to slow destruction of biogenic amine neurotransmitters, either by inhibiting their reuptake from the synaptic cleft between pre- and postsynaptic neurons into the presynaptic neuron, or by inhibiting monoamine oxidase in the presynaptic neuron. This increases local concentrations of the amine in the synaptic cleft, and thus facilitates neurotransmission. Von Praag and de Haan[39] showed that certain endogenously depressed patients had lower serotonin levels.

There is also a growing body of knowledge concerning the effects of age and estrogen deficiency on tyrosine hydroxylase, monoamine oxidase, and catechol-o-methyl transferase (COMT) levels—the enzymes that critically control the levels of these bioamines.

Monoamine oxidase (MAO) (which inactivates norepinephrine, tryptophan, and serotonin) levels are elevated and plasma tryptophan levels are lowered with increasing age,[40] depressive syndromes,[41] amenorrheic disorders, and menopause.[42] Aging also decreases levels of the biosynthetic enzymes tyrosine hydroxylase and dopa decarboxylase.[43] Estrogens may have a MAO inhibitor effect.[44] During the menstrual cyle, when estrogens reach peak levels, and during therapy with oral contraceptives, which are higher in estrogen dosage, there is lowering of MAO activity.[45,46]

Estrogens interfere with certain vitamin B_6 enzyme systems in tryptophan metabolism—

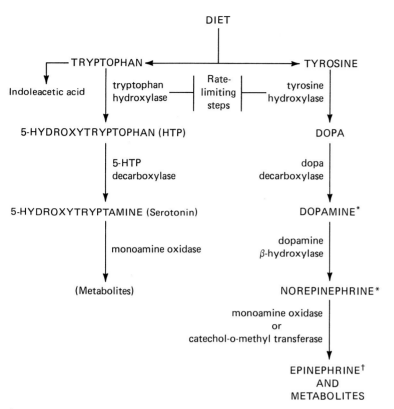

Fig. 12–7. Synthesis of biogenic amines. *, central nervous system neurotransmitter; †, peripheral nervous system neurotransmitter.

*Central nervous system neurotransmitter

†Peripheral nervous system neurotransmitter

specifically, they induce 5-hydroxytryptophan decarboxylase in vitro.[47] This in turn lowers the levels of centrally secreted serotonin. Dopa-decarboxylase is also vitamin B_6 dependent; the concentration of dopamine could similarly be affected. The turnover rate of

norepinephrine is also found to increase after ovariectomy; therefore, this appears to increase the ratio of norepinephrine to dopamine in the brain. The ratio is reversed when estrogens are restored.[48,49]

Moreover, mediators of central estrogen ef-

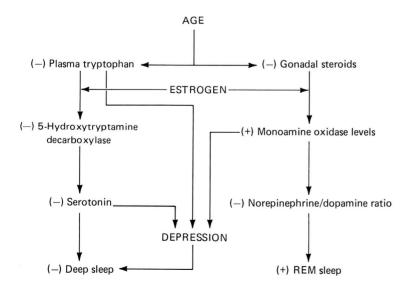

Fig. 12–8. Proposed scheme for the interplay of central amines and sleep in menopause.

fect—the catecholestrogens—may potentiate the action of catecholamines centrally. Catecholestrogens competitively inhibit the enzymatic methylation and biologic inactivation of norepinephrine by COMT.[50] The effect of estrogen on COMT may potentiate the action of norepinephrine. The complexity of these interactions highlights the difficulty in separating the effects of biogenic amines on sleep centers in the brain stem from their effects on depression and behavior symptoms which in turn alter sleep behavior.

Figure 12–8 attempts to summarize the interplay between the biogenic amines, their enzyme systems, and sleep and depression.

In attempting to correlate peripheral plasma norepinephrine, epinephrine, and dopamine levels with LH spikes in objectively recorded hot flushes, no significant increase was found.[1] However, peripheral concentrations of these amines may not reflect central changes.

In summary, the presence of estrogen increases nervous system levels of those neurotransmitters which regulate both sleep and mood. This may, in part, mediate their therapeutic effects.

Treatment of Menopausal Symptoms

Since there is a high rate of anxiety and mood depression in the menopause, and since suicide and mental illness peak in the menopause,[51] Klaiber[43] treated ambulatory depressed patients with pharmacologic doses of estrogens which lowered MAO levels and had some effect on psychiatric symptoms. Aylward,[52] in a double-blind crossover study, showed that estrogens increased plasma free tryptophan, a precursor of CNS serotonin, and decreased mental depression. Campbell and Whitehead,[53] comparing 1.25 mg Premarin with placebo, found a significant improvement in well being, both psychologic and symptomatic, in patients with moderate or severe menopausal symptoms.

Recently, Paterson[54] reported a randomized double-blind crossover study concerning the effect of mestranol and norethisterone concentrations on climacteric symptoms. This study detected only a slight improvement in insomnia, lack of energy, and confidence. Furthermore, Dennerstein et al.[55] postulate that ad-

junctive replacement with progesterone may negate the beneficial estrogen effect. Progesterone was hypothesized to produce a dysphoric effect. This suggestion is important since we now frequently add periodic progestins to menopausal estrogen replacement therapy to prevent endometrial hyperplasia.

To test the assumption that estrogens have a central tonic effect in improving the sleep of the menopausal patient, several studies have been done. Thomson and Oswald,[56] in a double-blind controlled study, determined the effects of placebo vs. piperazine estrone sulfate in a group of perimenopausal females undergoing EEG recording of sleep. The individuals receiving estrogen definitely had less arousals during the night and more REM sleep but this was not statistically significant when compared to placebo. However, a marked placebo effect was seen with respect to the occurrence of hot flushes, depression, and anxiety.

Schiff et al.[57] used a double-blind crossover study with conjugated estrogens 0.625 mg vs. placebo in 16 hypogonadal females. After 1 month of estrogen therapy, gonadotropins fell (FSH, 31%; LH, 19%), vasomotor flushes decreased, sleep latency decreased, and REM sleep increased. Of all the symptoms measured, hot flushes showed the greatest decrease. The latter finding was also observed by Thomson and Oswald.[56] However, they did not find any change in sleep latency. Furthermore, on the basis of objective psychometric testing, Regestein et al.[58] concluded that this beneficial effect of estrogen on sleep was correlated with psychologic intactness.

Whether the improved sleep after estrogen administration is due to a decrease in hot flushes was addressed by Erlik et al.[59] In a single-blind study, nine subjects (aged 30 to 55) with severe hot flushes were studied with EEG recordings and measurements of peripheral skin temperature and resistance. Four of the subjects were then studied a second time after administration of 0.05 mg ethinyl estradiol for 30 days, all were subsequently compared to five premenopausal women in the follicular stage of the menstrual cycle. The results demonstrated a beneficial effect of estrogens on sleep and hot flushes. Moreover, 45 of the 47 hot flushes were accompanied by waking episodes measured by EEG. A curious finding was that the waking episodes preceded any measurable changes in skin temperature or skin resistance. The authors speculate that the initiation of the waking episodes may occur with the downward setting of the thermoregulatory centers in the rostral preoptic area. That event is followed by a rise in skin temperature and a decrease in skin resistance—the objective markers.

Phylogenetically, the presence of REM sleep parallels the development of thermoregulation.[60] Therefore, we might speculate that the frequent nocturnal awakening in menopausal patients is somehow directly correlated with thermoregulatory dysfunction as evidenced by vasomotor flushing episodes.

Summary

In conclusion, estrogens decrease night wakenings and increase REM sleep. Current research demonstrates the close relationships among the abatement of vasomotor symptoms via estrogen therapy, the improvement of sleep, thermoregulatory stability, and releasing hormone LH pulses;[20] thus estrogens may definitely have a "central tonic effect." This effect may be mediated through catecholamines or endogenous opioids. The lessening of depression with estrogens also supports this hypothesis. Finally, it is difficult to separate the effects of aging and the effects of hormonal deprivation. Nevertheless, menopausal women do manifest a complex of gonadal hypofunction, vasomotor flushes, and difficulty sleeping. More research in this area of psychoneuroendocrinology is needed to interrelate the central changes in endogenous opioids and biogenic amines with these peripheral manifestations.

REFERENCES

1. Casper RF, Yen SSC, Wilkes MM. Menopausal flushes: neuroendocrine link with pulsatile LH release. Science 1980; 205:823–5.
2. Meldrum DR, Tataryn IV, Frumar AM, et al. Gonadotropins, estrogens, and adrenal steroids during menopausal hot flash. J Clin Endocrinol Metab. 1980; 50:585–9.
3. Tataryn IV, Meldrum DR, Lu KH. LH, FSH, and skin temperature during menopausal hot flash. J Clin Endocrinol Metab. 1979; 49: 152–4.
4. Altman N, Sachar EJ, Gruen PH, et al. Reduced plasma LH concentrations in postmenopausal depressed women. Psychosom Med. 1975; 37:274–6.
5. Ballinger S. A comparison of possible effects of acute and chronic stress on postmenopausal urinary estrogen levels. Maturitas 1981; 2: 107–13.
6. Dement WC, Kleitman N. Cyclic variations in EEG during sleep and their relationship to eye movement, body motility, and dreaming electroencephalogram. Clin Neurophysiol. 1975; 9:673.
7. Rechtschaffen A, Kales A, eds. A manual for standardized terminology, techniques and scoring system for sleep stages of human subjects. National Institute of Health Publication No. 204. Washington D.C.: U.S. Government Printing Office, 1968.
8. Molnar GW. Body temperatures during menopausal hot flushes. J Appl Physiol. 1975; 38:499–503.
9. Meldrum DR, Shamoke IM, Frumar AN, et al. Elevations of skin temperature of the finger as an objective index of postmenopausal hot flushes: Standardization of the technique. Am J Obstet Gynecol. 1979; 135:713–7.
10. Sturdee DW, Wilson KA, Pipili E, et al. Physiologic aspects of the menopausal hot flush. Br Med J. 1978; 2:79–81.
11. Albrecht B, Schiff I, Tulchinsky D, et al. Objective evidence that placebo and oral medroxyprogesterone acetate diminishes menopausal hot flushes. Am J Obstet Gynecol. 1981; 139:631–5.
12. Schiff I. The effect of conjugated estrogens on gonadotropin. Fertil Steril. 1980; 33:333–4.
13. Takayaski Y, Kaysnes DM, Daughaday WH. Growth hormone secretion during sleep. J Clin Endocrinol Metab. 1968; 47:2079–90.
14. Gruen P, Sachar EJ, Altman N, et al. Growth hormone responses to hypoglycemia in postmenopausal depressed women. Arch Gen Psychiatr. 1975; 32:31–3.
15. Sassin J, Frantz A, Wietzman E, et al. Human prolactin 24-hour pattern with increased release during cycles. Science 1972; 177:1205–7.
16. Kapen S, Boyar RB, Hellman L, et al. Episodic release of luteinizing hormone at mid-menstrual cycle in normal adult women. J Clin Endocrinol Metab. 1973; 36:724–9.
17. Boyar RB, Finkelstein J, Roffworg H, et al. Synchronization of augmented lutenizing hormone secretion with sleep during puberty. N Engl J Med. 1972; 287:582–6.
18. Kapen S, Boyar RB, Finkelstein J, et al. Effect of sleep-wake cycle reversal on luteinizing hormone secretion pattern in puberty. J Clin Endocrinol Metab. 1974; 39:293–9.

19. Meldrum DR, Erlik Y, Lu JKH, et al. Objectively recorded hot flushes in patients with pituitary insufficiency. J Clin Endocrinol Metab. 1981; 52:684–7.

20. Ravnikar V, Elkind-Hirsch K, Schiff I, et al. The association between LHRH, LH, and vasomotor flushes. Presented at the 63rd Annual Meeting of The Endocrine Society, June 17–19, 1981. Abstract #310.

21. Hellman L, Nakada F, Curte J, et al. Cortisol is secreted episodically in normal men. J Clin Endocrinol Metab. 1970; 30:411–422.

22. Orth DN, Island DP. Light synchronization of the circadian rhythm in plasma cortisol (17-OHCS) concentration in man. J Clin Endo. 1969; 29:479–486.

23. Evans JI, McLean AM. Circulating levels of plasma testosterone during sleep. Proc Roy Soc Med. 1971; 64:841–4.

24. Schaub C, Betti O, Bluet-Pajot MI, et al. Circadian patterns of growth hormone, prolactin, and corticotrophin secretion in hypothalamic and extrahypothalamic lesions localized by stereotactic neuroradiology in humans. Acta Psychiatr Belg. 1980; 80:376–80.

25. Schiff I, Regestein Q, Schinfeld J, et al. Interactions of oestrogens and hours of sleep on cortisol, FSH, LH, prolactin in hypogonadal women. Maturitas 1980; 2:179–83.

26. Hathaway SR, McKinley JC. Minnesota Multiphasic Personality Inventory. New York: Psychology Corp., 1951.

27. Hamilton M.: A rating scale for depression. J Neurol Neurosurg Psychiatr. 1980; 23:56–62.

28. Ballinger CB. Psychiatric morbidity and the menopause: Survey of gynecologic outpatient clinic. Br J Psychiatr. 1977; 131:83–9.

29. Campbell S. Double blind psychometric studies on the effects of a natural estrogen on postmenopausal women. Chapter 13 in: The Management of the Menopause and Postmenopausal Years. London: University Park Press, 1975: 149–58.

30. Donovan JC. The menopausal syndrome: A study of case histories. Am J Obstet Gynecol. 1951; 62:1281–91.

31. Pratt JP, Thomas WL. The endocrine treatment of menopausal phenomena. JAMA. 1939; 109:1975–7.

32. Campbell S, Whitehead M. Estrogen therapy in the menopausal syndrome. Clin Obstet Gynecol. 1977; 4:31–47.

33. Strickler RC, Borth R, Cecutti A, et al. The role of oestrogen replacement in the climacteric syndrome. Psychol Med. 1977; 7:631–9.

34. Meites J, Bruni JF, Van Vugt A, et al. Relation of endogenous opioid peptides and morphine to neuroendocrine functions. Life Sci. 1979; 24:1325–36.

35. Van Loon GR, Ho D, Kim C. β-Endorphin-induced decrease in hypothalamic turnover. Endocrinology. 1980; 106:76–80.

36. Webb WB. Partial and differential sleep deprivation. In: Kayes A, ed. Sleep physiology and pathology. Philadelphia: Lippincott, 1969: 221–44.

37. Pare CMB, Sandler M. A clinical and biochemical study of a trial of iproniazid in the treatment of depression. J Neurol Neurosurg Psychiatr. 1959; 22:247–51.

38. Baldessarini RJ. The basis for the amine hypothesis in affective disorders. Arch Gen Psychiatr. 1975; 32:1087–93.

39. Van Praag HM, DeHaan S. Central serotonin deficiency—A factor which increases depression vulnerability? Acta Psychiatr Scand. 1980; 61(Suppl. 280):89–96.

40. Tryding N, Tufeessom G, Nilsson S, et al. Aging, monoamines and monoamine oxidase levels. Lancet 1972; 1:489.

41. Nies A, Robinson AS, Rovares CL, et al. Amine and monoamine oxidase levels in relation to aging and depression in man. Psychosom Med. 1971; 33:470.

42. Klaiber EL, Kobayashi Y, Boverman D, et al. Plasma monoamine oxidase activity in regularly cycling women and in amenorrheic women receiving cyclic therapy with estrogen and progesterone. J Clin Endocrinol Metab. 1971; 33:630–8.

43. McGeer E, McGeer PL. Neurotransmitter metabolism in the aging brain. In: Terry RD, Gerkson S, eds. Neurobiology of aging. New York: Raven Press, 1976:389–403.

44. Klaiber EI, Broverman DM, Vogel W, et al. Effects of estrogen therapy on plasma MAO activity and EEG during responses in depressed women. Am J Psychiatr. 1972; 128:1492–8.

45. Holzbauer, M, Yondim MBH. The estrous cycle and monoamine oxidase levels. Br J Pharmacol. 1973; 48:600–8.

46. Luhby AL, Davis P, Murphy M, et al. Pyridoxine and oral contraceptives. Lancet. 1970; 2:1083.

47. Mason M, Schirch L. Inhibition of vitamin B$_6$ enzymes by free and conjugated estrogens. Fed Proc. 1961; 20:200.

48. Beattie CW, Rodgers CH, Soyka LF. Influence of ovariectomy and ovarian steroids on hypothalamic tyrosine hydroxylase activity in the rat. Endocrinology. 1972; 91:276–9.

49. Bapna J, Neff NH, Costa E. A method for studying the norepinephrine and serotonin metabolism of rat brain: Effect of ovariectomy

on amine metabolism in anterior and posterior hypothalamus. Endocrinology. 1971; 89: 1345–9.

50. Bare P, Knuppen R, Haupt E, et al. Interactions between estrogens and catecholamines. III. Studies on the methylation of catecholestrogens, catecholamines, and other catechols by the catechol-*o*-methyltransferase of human liver. J Clin Endocrinol Metab. 1972; 736–46.

51. Hagnell O: The incidence and duration of episodes of mental illness in a total population. In: Hare EH, Wing JK, eds. Psychiatric epidemiology. London: Oxford University Press, 1970:213–24.

52. Aylward M. Estrogens, plasma tryptophan levels in perimenopausal patients. Chapter 12 in: Campbell S (ed.). The Management of the Menopause and Post-Menopausal Years. London, University Part Press, 1975, pp 135–147.

53. Campbell S, Whitehead M. Oestrogen withdrawal therapy and the menopausal syndrome. Clin Obstet Gynecol. 1977; 31–47.

54. Paterson MEL. A randomised, double-blind cross-over study into the effect of sequential mestranol and norethisterone on climacteric symptoms and biochemical parameters. Maturitas 1982; 2:83–4.

55. Dennerstein L, Burrows G, Woods C, et al. Hormones and sexuality: Effects of estrogen and progesterone. Obstet Gynecol. 1980; 56:316–22.

56. Thomson J, Oswald J. The effect of estrogen on the sleep, mood, and anxiety of postmenopausal women. Br Med J. 1977; 2:1317–9.

57. Schiff I, Regestein Q, Tulchinsky D, et al. Effects of estrogens on sleep and the psychologic state of hypogonadal women. JAMA 1979; 242:2405–7.

58. Regestein QR, Schiff I, Tulchinsky D, et al. Relationships among estrogen-induced psychophysiological changes in hypogonadal women. Psychosom Med. 1981; 43:147–55.

59. Erlik Y, Tartaryn I, Meldrum D, et al. Association of waking episodes with menopausal hot flushes. JAMA, 1981; 245:1741–1747.

60. Allison J, Van Twyer H. The evolution of sleep. Natural History, 1979; 79,57.

Sexuality 13

James P. Semmens

General Considerations

Sexuality is that dimension of personality that reflects one's comfort with one's role as a male or female and the need to share one's emotional, intellectual, and physical self with other human beings, both socially and privately. Sexual intercourse is a significant part, but not all, of sexuality. Sexuality includes the emotional, somatic, intellectual, social, and ethical dimensions of existence. Ideally, throughout life, sexuality should involve a process of growth and development leading to (1) enhancement of personality, (2) commitment and healthy relationships, and (3) a capacity for pleasure, intimacy, and love.[1]

How a menopausal woman feels about herself as an acceptable sexual partner is influenced by physical, psychologic, and physiologic changes associated with aging. These directly affect her sexual capability and her interest level. The health and well being of her partner, his sexual interest level, and his functional capabilities also play a role. Neurovascular changes of aging which affect the erectile, ejaculatory, and lubricative functions frequently dictate the degree of involvement for older couples.

A menopausal woman may be understandably confused by the multiple roles she is required to assume during this period. She frequently finds herself as someone's daughter, wife, mistress, mother, and even grandmother. Being a mistress to a husband who equates his sexual performance with his hold on youth, while appearing as a tender, loving grandmother to her children's children, can be a significant challenge. The single, widowed, or divorced menopausal woman, on the other hand, functions in a social environment characterized by a paucity of acceptable male partners. Her opportunities for social contact may be limited by the moral code of her generation, which creates guilt and frustration if she seeks acceptable outlets for her emotional and physical needs.[2]

Even so, menopause need not be a time of loss and despair. It can be a time of sexual renewal for the woman who abhorred contraceptive pills or a dependence on condoms, foam, and jelly to control her fertility. Liberated from the fear of pregnancy, many menopausal women more openly express their needs for greater sexual frequency and variety.

Causes of Sexual Dysfunction: An Overview

Problems of sexual dysfunction can occur at any age; however, both medical professionals and society at large find it easier to accept diminished sexual interest, erectile and ejaculatory dysfunction, dyspareunia, and secondary nonorgasmia in persons who are over 50 years of age. The tragedy is that sexual dysfunction is seldom experienced to the same degree or at the same time by both partners, and its impact depends on whether their previous sexual relationship has been satisfactory. For many couples, advancing age becomes an excuse to escape from sexual commitments that have always been a painful part of their lives, and society supports that decision. Many professional counselors (including physicians) automatically attribute sexual difficulties to the physiologic changes of middle age and do not take the time to obtain a problem-oriented sexual history or to provide information and counsel to the middle-aged couple. Because of this lack of interest in the sexual problems of the older population, there has been only limited research concerning alterations in sexual response during the postmenopausal years. Better research would either support or refute these assumptions which are so deeply ingrained in our culture.

Sexual stimulation is essentially a neurovascular response which can be quite sensitive to the arteriosclerotic and neurologic changes of aging. Approximately 40% of episodes of erectile failure in middle-aged men are now thought to be due at least in part to vascular changes. Women fail to achieve sufficient perivaginal congestion to permit an adequate transudation of vaginal fluids for lubrication. The result for both partners is increased physical discomfort during coitus. Couples who have been sexually well adjusted in the past respond with a range of emotions that vary from acceptance to fear to panic. Unfortunately, most couples do not seek medical advice because they assume that the problem is due to age. When professional consultation is sought, the physician may be personally uncomfortable with the subject of sexuality. Rather than dealing with it as any other medical complaint, he or she may flippantly dismiss it as age related. Physicians must be introspective enough to recognize that such reactions are directly related to their own lack of information or their inhibitions. At all times, their role should be to make a diagnosis and offer treatment.

In practice, a physician will also encounter couples whose sexual relationships have been free of dysfunction and who are unwilling to accept aging itself as the cause of their difficulties. Loss of sexual capability may be due to the side-effects of medication the patient is taking for hypertension, anxiety, or depression. The incidence of disabling and debilitating disease also increases in the fifth and sixth decades of life, and the alert physician realizes that sexual dysfunction may be an important medical clue. When diabetes has its onset later in life, sexual capability does not always return with metabolic regulation, as it frequently does in those whose disease is diagnosed before the age of 30. Similarly, the incidence of sexual dysfunction following gynecologic surgery and other treatments for neoplastic disease is five times greater in women confronted with these crises after middle age. Surgical correction for pelvic relaxation (cystocele, rectocele, and descensus uteri) denudes the submucosa and vaginal epithelium, leaving areas of anesthesia, particularly in the lower third of the vagina. This is the site of the tactile nerve endings which are important in sexual arousal and make up the orgasmic platform described by Masters and Johnson. Patients undergoing total hysterectomy (abdominal or vaginal) may end up with a shortened vagina which is sexually incapacitating. Dysfunction following gynecologic or breast surgery can be partially avoided with effective preparation and counseling of both partners.

Physical limitations which affect sexual performance or response force couples to consider other sexual options, a choice which is usually more difficult for couples over 50 years of age. Often they choose abstinence rather than compromise a code of "moral sexual behavior." Some may not even be aware of sexual options because the physician, psychologist, social worker, nurse, or rehabilitative counselor is too uncomfortable with his or her own sexuality to discuss the matter.

Sexual dysfunction occurring during the pre- and postclimacteric years may be (1) physiologic, where circulatory and neurologic changes due to aging affect the capacity of the male to achieve erection or of the female to lubricate;[3] (2) psychologic, brought about by stress and tension resulting from deteriorating communication, in which one or both partners fail to achieve their expectations within the relationship; (3) sociologic, created by the loss of or separation from a spouse or by a lack of opportunity to secure sexual partners within the peer group; (4) medical, caused by diseases that directly affect the patient's physical capability or self-image, possibly necessitating behavioral modification; (5) due to gynecologic or urologic problems directly related to genitourinary function; (6) due to side-effects of medication, including those of over-the-counter drugs; or (7) due to estrogen deprivation related to ovarian failure, or decreasing testosterone levels in male partners.

Physiologic Causes of Sexual Dysfunction

The effects of aging on the neurovascular mechanism responsible for male penile tumescence and erection are well documented in the literature.[4] Much has also been written about atrophic vaginitis, which causes thinning of the vaginal mucosa, shortening and narrowing of the vaginal canal, and dyspareunia. Both the systemic and topical routes of estrogen replacement therapy have now been shown to produce comparable blood levels.[5] Most gynecologists recommend replacement therapy in patients with atrophic vaginitis. Unfortunately, they frequently withhold such treatment until the clinical manifestations are well advanced. Emphasis on the carcinogenic effect (endometrial carcinoma) of estrogen replacement therapy has confused the lay public even when clinical and laboratory evidence supports such treatment. Many patients still reject their physician's advice that with proper monitoring the risk of endometrial cancer is minimal.

In 1978 the author conducted a study of the effects of menopause on vaginal physiologic function; i.e., the quantity, chemical composition, and acidity of the vaginal secretions, alterations in vaginal circulation, and the ability of vaginal tissues to transudate electrolytes during the secretory process.[6] Studies of subjects between the ages of 50 and 70, who had not taken estrogen 3 months to 12 years before entering the study, showed a decrease in circulatory response, an increase in vaginal pH, and decreases in quantity and electrolyte content of the vaginal secretions in the estrogen-depleted state. Following baseline studies, the subjects were given Premarin 0.625 mg (if their uteri were intact) or 1.25 mg daily for the first 25 days of each month. The response to replacement therapy was a 30% improvement in vaginal circulation, a drop in pH to near premenopausal levels, and an increase in quantity of vaginal fluids. The response to estrogen therapy was most remarkable during the first 30 days (actually an overshoot), and a leveling off of the response was noted at 3- and 6-month follow-up examinations (Table 13–1).[6] Patients who discontinued estrogen therapy returned to the pretreatment state.

Current studies at the Medical University of South Carolina utilizing the same techniques confirm the findings of the pilot study and demonstrate continuing improvement (as evidenced by a return to the norm for younger individuals) at 6-, 12-, and 18-month follow-up examinations. Increased gonadotropin levels and cytologic changes have occurred within the first 30 days after initiation of exogenous estrogen therapy. Physiologic changes (functional improvements) are progressive and require a much longer period of time, perhaps 12, 18, or 24 months. In the current study (24

TABLE 13–1. Baseline Data (Pilot Study): Physiologic Changes in Vaginal Function Due to Menopause and Response to Exogenous Estrogen.

PHYSIOLOGIC EVALUATION	BASELINE: ESTROGEN-DEPRIVED STATE	EXOGENOUS ESTROGEN			
		1 month	3 months	6 months	*p*
Vaginal blood flow (mW) 212*	208	236	244	225	0.004
Vaginal secretions (g) 0.20*	0.08	0.11	0.14	0.10	0.001
Vaginal pH 4.0*	5.4	4.8	4.6	4.7	0.006
Transvaginal electropotential difference 44*	22.7	28.8	36.0	27.0	0.001

* Normal values for women under 40.

individuals), pH and the capability of the vaginal tissues to transudate electrolytes (potassium) have shown significant improvement at the 6- and 12-month evaluations. An increase in quantity of vaginal secretions has again been documented. No effort was made in the preceding studies to determine the effect of estrogen replacement on sexual arousal, but laboratory studies carried out in Copenhagen, Denmark, by Dr. Gorm Wagner and the author showed increased circulatory response as documented by increased heat requirement to maintain the vaginal epithelium at 43°C.

The effect of aging on vaginal tumescence (congestive buildup of the orgasmic platform) and lubrication is estrogen-related, as determined by both the pilot study in Copenhagen and the current studies at the Medical University of South Carolina. Any deficiency in estrogen directly affects vaginal blood flow and the transudative vaginal secretory process. Menopause, however, is not an instantaneous state, and many women experience lubricative difficulties early (at 40 to 50 years of age), with a progressive increase in the incidence of dyspareunia during the fifth and sixth decades of life. After age 55, the incidence of dyspareunia is twice that experienced by women under 40 years of age, in whom the primary causes are more likely to be organic or psychologic. During the fifth and sixth decades of life, dyspareunia may occur as frequently as every or every other sexual encounter, whereas in patients in their thirties and forties it may be only an occasional experience. When dyspareunia becomes frequent and severe, the uninformed often choose sexual abstinence as their only relief.

Psychologic Causes of Sexual Dysfunction

The psychologic causes of sexual dysfunction in the menopausal female are directly related to poor sexual communication. Neither partner feels free to express needs, desires, and feelings. A reference to a partner as being "like an old shoe" with whom one is comfortable in the nonsexual phases of one's life may imply deep discomfort arising from behavioral patterns that are dull and repetitive. Nash reported the case of a woman who said that her husband made love the same way during the entire 30 years of their marriage.[7] She likened the experience to a trip to the supermarket. She knew his every move and what was next. She said that she could knit by his movements; with a few passionate pants, his ego was satisfied. What the female partner obtained from such a relationship is obvious. This is a sad commentary on the degree to which sexual communication can degenerate over a period of time.

Equally important during a couple's middle years are their individual concerns about future social, economic, and physical well being. Such concerns create varying degrees of tension and stress. The woman may have an increased tendency toward hypochondria at this time, as she wonders whether she will be the one among her peer group to experience cancer of the breast or uterus. There is a sudden increase in awareness of even minimal discomfort or changes in body function. The male partner, on the other hand, is concerned about urinary tract obstruction and possible prostatic disorders, problems which are frequently discussed by his peers. These concerns are compounded by anxieties about cardiac disease, and by the fear that a sexual encounter may even precipitate myocardial infarction or stroke. Many couples subconsciously or consciously avoid total sexual encounter for this reason. The wife finds herself alone, with the family out of the home, and with a need for more sexual communication to identify her role within the relationship. Her new goals may cause conflict or feelings of rejection and result in sexual dysfunction. Many women fix the blame for failing sexual communication on their partners and hold that it is the male's responsibility to initiate and create the proper degree of interest and arousal necessary for a satisfactory response. This is a time in life when the male partner can no longer take responsibility to initiate touching and coitus, and it is extremely important for the female partner to share.

The middle-aged couple also faces depression brought about by the realization that certain goals for themselves and their families may be beyond their capability. The financial position they had hoped to achieve or the secure retirement they had looked forward to has for one reason or another eluded them. A significant clue to depression is a sudden loss of sexual interest by one or both partners. It becomes difficult to feel good about oneself and one's relationship, or even to enjoy living, in the face of bitter disappointment. A physician seeing a couple for a sexual complaint should be aware of this important implication that psychiatric help may be indicated. The depressed female may suddenly find herself nonorgasmic. Her partner, in turn, may experience erectile difficulty. The couple present themselves as individuals who have lost interest in intimacy, including the desire to express their sexuality within their marriage. Counseling for such couples should assist them to recognize and accept reality. Sexual difficulties will frequently resolve themselves when social values, communicative adjustments, and realistic goals are accepted.

Sociologic Factors

Middle-aged couples may lose the opportunity to participate in intercourse not only through the death or infirmity of one partner, but also through a prolonged period of abstinence. Sexual abstinence over a long interval decreases the individual's assurance of sexual capability and may lead to complete denial of sexual needs. Often, such denial becomes a coping mechanism for widows or divorced women over 50, who have a limited number of available partners owing to the disproportionate ratio of women to men in the older population. The problem is less acute for older males, because society accepts sexual outlets for older men with younger partners, professional escorts, or prostitutes. In larger urban areas it is becoming more acceptable for middle-aged women to make similar contacts with male partners; but the moral code for the majority of the current menopausal population remains psychologically restrictive.

Another frequent cause for sexual dysfunction in older couples is excessive intake of food and alcohol. The combination of aging, excessive eating, and heavy drinking dulls the senses to the point where sexual response and performance may be seriously compromised. Fatigue brought about by physical or mental exertion may also interfere with sexual function. Older couples would do well to change their sexual patterns and attempt intercourse during the morning or early evening, rather than late at night. In our clinic, we suggest that male testosterone levels are higher in the morning and that intercourse may therefore be more successful early in the day. Although such suggestions are not based totally on fact, they do reinforce positive expectations by encouraging a couple to abandon a pattern which has been ineffective in favor of a fresh approach. Changing sexual behavior patterns is easier for couples of all ages than altering other forms of human response.

Medical Disorders

Forty percent of the patients we see with sexual dysfunction have some form of concurrent medical illness. In some patients, the illness does not have a direct effect on the neurovascular system, whereas in others sexual function is directly affected by the disease process. Medical illness which interferes with the individual's positive self-concept (such as extensive skin lesions of chronic psoriasis) may cause her to feel that she is an unacceptable sexual partner. Associated pain and discomfort may also limit physical capabilities.

The primary diseases which contribute to sexual dysfunction are those which cause chronic fatigue. In the past, tuberculosis headed the list. Today, the most common debilitating conditions are neoplastic diseases and severe anemias. In the advanced stages of any chronic disease, the individual has barely enough energy to maintain essential daily functions, let alone to consider sexual intercourse. Patients in this category also include those undergoing dialysis or awaiting a renal transplant. The dialysis patient functions best immediately after treatment and becomes quite aware of a loss of sexual capability as the need for dialysis recurs. The diabetic whose illness begins after age 50 has more pronounced sexual problems than the individual who had the onset of disease in the twenties or thirties. Normally, after metabolic control, younger patients experience a return of sexual function. It is difficult to offer patients over age 50 the same reassurance, since both the vascular and neurologic complications may be well advanced at the time of diagnosis. The response following metabolic control is much more limited. It has been reported that the neurologic changes affect not only male erectile capability but female lubricative capacity and clitoral response as well. Patients with rheumatoid arthritis may find that sexual activity causes increased joint pain, particularly in the lower back. Support of the affected part of the body with pillows and the use of a hot bath prior to engaging in sexual activity may be helpful. The Arthritis Foundation publishes informational material and diagrams of sexual positions helpful to individuals so affected.

Occasionally, the treatment of a medical illness in itself may cause the loss of sexual function. For example, during renal transplantation the sympathetic and parasympathetric nerve plexuses in the retroperitoneal area of the pelvis may be compromised by the seating of the donor kidney. The internal sphincter of the bladder may also be affected, causing retrograde ejaculatory and erectile problems in the male. If these possible complications are not properly explained, the woman may feel that her partner's failure to ejaculate is a form of rejection.

Genitourinary Pathology

Middle-aged individuals are prone to genitourinary problems which can directly affect sexual capability. Urologists now employ topical estrogen cream as effective therapy in combating the female urethral syndrome and find it helpful as an adjunct to antibiotic therapy in treating urethritis, trigonitis, and cystitis in menopausal women.

The treatment of gynecologic cancer, especially cancer of the cervix, frequently involves radiation therapy and/or radical surgery. Either form of treatment mitigates against a normal lubricative function and may cause severe dyspareunia. Without counseling and planning to preserve and support continuing coital communication, these individuals have little choice except eventual abstinence. Males should be counseled concerning future sexual relations with their partners. They may be concerned that the cancer could be contagious or that the radiation could affect them directly. They may feel that sexual activity will cause a recurrence of the disease. Many cancer treatment centers now incorporate pretreatment counseling regarding sexual communication for the couple; and where extensive surgery is contemplated, an artificial vaginal tract may be included in the surgical reconstruction and rehabilitative program. Many centers even permit weekend leaves of absence when radiation and chemotherapy are carried out over a long period of time. This allows the couple an opportunity for privacy and communication at whatever level they are comfortable with, and it helps to prepare them for the transition following treatment.

Continued sexual communication is extremely important for the self-image of individuals with genital, urinary, or breast malignancy because of the sexual implications of these conditions. We recommend the use of "Transi-Lube"* as a sexual lubricant to enhance coital activity for the female following irradiation and for the male partner who fails to achieve full erectile tumescence. It is also of benefit for those who are unable to tolerate exogenous estrogen and who are suffering from atrophic vaginitis. Those with psychologic problems benefit from its use as an adjunct to counseling until they develop sufficient self-assurance to allow a return of function.

When discussing vulvectomy, radical or simple, or pelvic exenteration for gynecologic cancer, it is appropriate to obtain a sexual history from the couple. For those who have enjoyed a warm, close relationship, assurance that a functional vaginal tract can be created to enable them to continue intercourse is important. This type of counseling, as well as helping the couple to explore other sexual options, is part of total patient care.

The Effects of Medication

The more liberal use of anticholinergics, adrenergics, and beta blockers to treat hypertension, vascular disease, peptic ulcer, dyskinesia, and glaucoma has focused new interest on the effect of these drugs on sexual performance. In combination with narcotics, sedatives, and alcohol, such drugs are capable of causing even greater difficulties in sexual function. The

---

* Transi-Lube, Young's Drug Products, Piscataway, N.J. 08854.

phenothiazines and monoamine oxidase inhibitors used in treating neurosis and psychosis may also interfere with sexual function, even though these are prescribed to decrease anxiety. Mellaril causes retrograde ejaculation by relaxing the internal vesical sphincter.

Therefore, it is extremely important to obtain a complete history of all prescription and over-the-counter medications that the patient is presently taking. If there is indeed a relationship between the initiation of a new drug therapy and the onset of sexual dysfunction, one needs to consult with those who prescribed the medication before discontinuing it or recommending an alternative. Many times the side-effects of drugs do not manifest themselves initially, and the adverse effects on sexuality occur only when it becomes necessary to increase the dosage to overcome an established tolerance. Most drugs which contribute to lubricative dysfunction in the female in all probability contribute to erectile dysfunction in the male and a low sexual interest level in both partners.

Although alcohol is not specifically considered a drug, an accurate evaluation of alcohol intake is an important part of any sexual history because of its implications in both erectile and lubricative dysfunction.[3,8] Early writings regarding cirrhosis of the liver mentioned sexual dysfunction as an early sign of the disease. It has been demonstrated that excess alcohol intake has a direct effect on testosterone levels, spermatogenesis, and male sexual interest level. The depressed woman who is experiencing sexual disability for psychologic reasons may resort to alcohol as a crutch, further compromising her functional capability.

Hormonal Causes of Sexual Dysfunction

Menopause for the female does not always result in a total loss of estrogen, but in our current study subjects' estradiol (E_2) levels could not be detected using radioimmunoassay (see Chapter 1). Greenblatt and coworkers evaluated the effects of estrogen, androgen, and estrogen-androgen combinations as well as placebos in the treatment of menopause.[9] Their 1950 report indicated a 12.3% increase in libido for patients receiving diethylstilbestrol 0.25 mg in combination with 5.0 mg of methyltestosterone, and a 42% increase in libido for patients receiving methyltestosterone 0.5 mg. Greenblatt's most recent report indicated that the estrogen-androgen preparation was preferred by the majority of his patients because of improved well being and marked increase in libido.[10] He currently recommends conjugated estrogen or estrone sulfate 0.625–1.25 mg and methyltestosterone 2.5 mg or fluroxymesterone daily for 21 days each month, or Monday through Friday each week.

Dennerstein and associates studied 33 patients who had undergone hysterectomy and oophorectomy and found that 30% complained of deterioration of their sexual relationships, which they attributed to the surgery.[11] There was a definite loss of desire for sexual intercourse. Estrogen administration, while not affecting overall sexual behavior, was specifically associated with a lower incidence of dyspareunia. Like Greenblatt, Dennerstein now advocates the administration of an oral estrogen-androgen preparation, reporting it to be highly effective in overcoming loss of libido. Greenblatt also reported that progesterone alone had a dampening effect on sexual desire when used during menopause.

Exogenous estrogen may improve sexual desire, but only because of physical improvement in vaginal turgor, vaginal circulation, and the quantity of vaginal secretions, which decrease coital discomfort. Estrogen is not recommended for purely psychologic support or to increase libido. Androgens in combination with estrogen are not universally recommended to enhance libido. The androgen may cause virilization (acne, hirsutism, voice changes) over a period of time. An anabolic effect on libido has also been suggested.

Summary

We have identified the physiologic role of estrogen as it relates to the sexual capability of the female. Estrogen replacement therapy instituted early has the advantage of preserving the turgor of the vaginal mucosa and its lubricative capabilities. When replacement therapy has been delayed and atrophic changes occur, months are required to achieve a response at both the cellular and functional levels.

In conclusion, sexual activity in the older female patient requires further evaluation. In our current clinical sample (N = 24), 40% of subjects were limited to two or three sexual encounters per year and demonstrated lower baseline readings and more limited response to estrogen replacement therapy than the sexually active menopausal women previously studies in Denmark. Any form of sexual arousal which contributes to tumescence and congestion in the pelvic area, whether fantasy, masturbation, intercourse, or even reading or films, will have varying degrees of beneficial results, making absence of an available partner academic.

REFERENCES

1. Lief HI, ed. Sexual problems in medical practice. Chicago: American Medical Association, 1981.
2. Renshaw DC: Sex and the older woman. Female Patient. 1978; 3(November):83.
3. Masters WH, Johnson VE. Human sexual inadequacy. Boston: Little, Brown, 1970:274–276, 316–350.
4. Wagner G, Green R. Impotence. New York: Plenum Press, 1981:25, 51, 81.
5. Rigg LA, Hermann H, Yen SSC: Absorption of estrogens from vaginal creams. N Engl J Med. 1978; 298:195–197.
6. Semmens JP, Wagner G: Estrogen deprivation and vaginal function in postmenopausal women. JAMA. 1982; 248:445.
7. Nash EM, Jessner L, Abse DW. Marriage counseling in medical practice. Chapel Hill, N.C.: University of North Carolina Press, 1964.
8. Kaplan HS. The new sex therapy. New York: Brunner/Mazel, 1974:86–104.
9. Greenblatt RB, Barfield WE, Garner JF, et al. Evaluation of estrogen, androgen, estrogen-androgen combination, and a placebo on the treatment of menopause. J Clin Endocrinol. 1950; 10:1547.
10. Greenblatt R: An endocrinologist comments on hormones for sexual dysfunction. Female Patient. 1979; 4:43–46.
11. Dennerstein L, Wood C, Burrows GD: Sexual response following hysterectomy and oophorectomy. Obstet Gynecol. 1977; 49:92–96.

The Breast 14

Douglas J. Marchant

Recent surveys have indicated that American women are more concerned about breast cancer than any other disease. The American Cancer Society predicted that there would be approximately 110,000 new cases in the United States, and 36,800 deaths per year. Breast cancer represents 28% of the estimated cancer incidence in females and 19% of the cancer deaths. One in 11 newborn infants is destined to develop breast cancer.[1]

The obstetrician-gynecologist is considered by many the primary physician to women. Careful breast examination should be part of every examination. It is especially important in the evaluation of the pregnant patient. Since 80% of the cancers are discovered in women over age 40, breast examination is mandatory in the perimenopausal and menopausal patient.

History and Physical Examination

Complete evaluation of the breast begins with an accurate history. Age, menstrual history, date of the last menstrual period, family history, use of medications, date of birth of the first child, and surgery, including treatment of previous breast disease, must be recorded. For specific symptoms such as nipple discharge it is important to note the date of onset, the character, and whether it is spontaneous or produced by manipulation. It is also important to note the association of the discharge with menstrual irregularities and the use of medications, particularly tranquilizers. Nipple discharge may be associated with elevated serum prolactin levels. At least one study has demonstrated that breast examination does not significantly affect serum prolactin levels, although the frequency of basal hyperprolactinemia was noted to be much higher than had generally been accepted.[2] Oral contraceptives and phenothiazines produce nipple discharge and, more recently, bilateral discharge has been associated with the nipple stimulation occurring during jogging.

The history should be recorded in a legible and logical sequence with particular emphasis on the date and whether the patient discovered the lesion. The exact location of the lesion in the breast and the disposition of the patient must be recorded. A review of physicians' records for medicolegal purposes often reveals a striking lack of detail concerning these points.

A good physical examination of the breast requires about 4 min if it includes instruction in breast self-examination. The breasts are first examined in the sitting or standing position (Fig. 14–1). Contour, symmetry, and skin changes are noted. The vascular pattern is observed and the condition of the areola and nipple recorded. These changes may be exaggerated by asking the patient to elevate the arm or by asking her to place her hands on the hips and contract the pectoralis major muscles (Fig. 14–2). While the patient is in this position the axilla is palpated, being careful to support the arm with the opposite hand (Fig. 14–3). This examination, even if well performed, is inaccurate. On the other hand, it is important to detect *clinically* evident metastasis prior to any

Fig. 14–1. Examination in the sitting position.

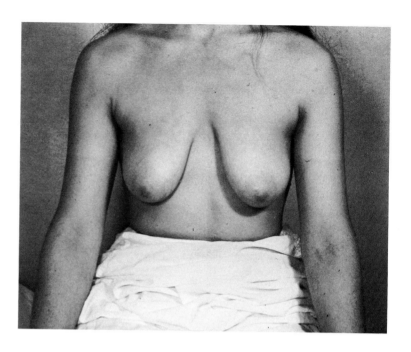

recommended treatment. While in the sitting or standing position the breasts are carefully palpated in a systematic fashion, using the flat of the hand and noting any irregularities. The patient is then placed in the supine position and a wedge or towel inserted under the patient to elevate the breast. The breast is palpated in a systematic manner, again using the flat of the hand (Fig. 14–4). The use of pHiso-

Hex or talcum powder permits the identification of even minor alterations. Approximately 80% of American women discover their own lesions, many when taking a shower. The use of this so-called "wet" technique permits the identification of very subtle changes in breast texture. The areola and finally the nipple should be carefully examined and palpated.

Certain physical findings are helpful in the

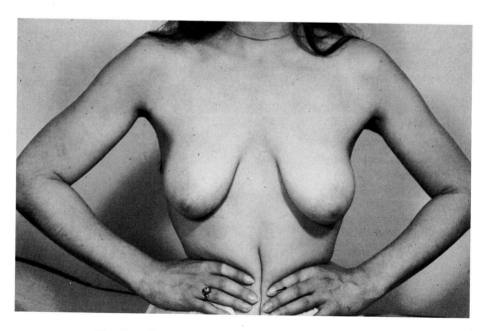

Fig. 14–2. Contraction of the pectoral muscles by placing hands on the hips.

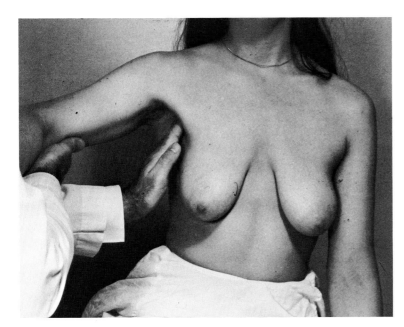

Fig. 14–3. Palpation of the axilla.

differential diagnosis. Multiple indistinct lesions suggest a benign condition, whereas a single hard dominant mass suggests malignancy. Venous engorgement, particularly in the young patient, suggests cystosarcoma phyllodes. Bilateral venous engorgement, nipple discharge, or areolar excoriation suggests a benign lesion. Unilateral alterations are more common in malignancy. Excoriation of the nipple may suggest Paget's disease. Skin dimpling suggests cancer, although such entities as

Mondor's disease may simulate this condition. Obviously, chest wall fixation, edema, and regional involvement are characteristic findings of late-stage disease.

Several aspects of the history, when evaluated together with the physical findings, are helpful. Pain and tenderness usually are absent in breast cancer and frequently present in benign disease. These symptoms may vary with the menstrual cycle. Rarely is there any change in a malignant lesion with menses. Unilateral,

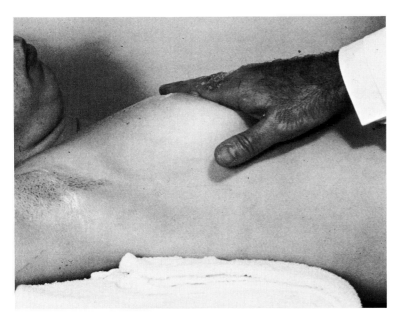

Fig. 14–4. Palpation in the supine position.

bloody, or serosanguineous discharge suggests a benign intraductal papilloma, although malignancy cannot be ruled out. Watery, milky, or greenish discharge suggests physiologic alterations, possibly associated with medication and elevated serum prolactin levels. Prior history of trauma is of little help, although a firm, tender area may be associated with fat necrosis and easily confused with cancer.

The discovery of a palpable lesion does not indicate early breast cancer. According to cellular kinetics and an estimation of doubling times, a palpable lesion 1 cm in diameter has already gone through approximately 30 doublings or three-quarters of its life span as a tumor. Using a conservative estimate of growth rate, approximately 8 years are required to achieve this diameter of 1 cm. Thus the earliest palpable lesion has undergone considerable subclinical growth.

As previously mentioned, the physical findings and history should be carefully documented. A diagram is most helpful. It clearly indicates the breast involved, the location and size of the lesion, and associated conditions such as skin dimpling and regional involvement. Increasing litigation in this area demands careful documentation of the history, physical findings, and most importantly, the disposition of the case. If biopsy has been recommended, this should be carefully noted. If aspiration has been performed, the amount and character of the fluid must be recorded; and if a mammogram or xeromammogram has been recommended, the findings and the recommendations to the patient, including the date, should be recorded.

Breast Self-examination

A survey by the National Cancer Institute entitled "Breast Cancer: A Measure of Progress in Public Understanding" examines three broad areas: women's knowledge, attitudes, and practices related to breast cancer.[3] The survey noted that (1) women fear breast cancer more than any other disease; (2) they underestimate the number of cases of breast cancer; (3) blacks and Hispanics are more concerned than white females about changes breast cancer will bring to their lives; and (4) women who practice breast self-examination monthly have received instruction from a physician or a nurse.[3]

The practice of breast self-examination is not without controversy. Haagensen has said, "From the point of view of the greatest possible gains and early diagnosis, teaching women how to examine their own breast is more important than teaching the technique of breast examination to physicians."[4] Moore, in an editorial in *The New England Journal of Medicine,* noted that "intentional self-examination has proved to be unreliable and a nonproductive method for case finding. It is asking too much of the average woman to indulge in this sort of examination."[5]

In spite of advances in screening, most breast cancers continue to be self-detected. Women who practice monthly breast self-examination present with more favorable clinical-pathologic stages than do women who never practice breast self-examination. If early detection is possible through breast self-examination, this technique could affect mortality. However, the true impact of breast self-examination on mortality will remain unanswered until a well-designed prospective study can be completed. Opponents of breast self-examination argue that a monthly self-examination is anxiety producing, uncomfortable, and potentially falsely reassuring. On the other hand, proponents often exaggerate its benefits. Evidence to support the claim that it is life-saving has yet to be produced, and health education studies dispute the assumption that it is easily learned or reassuring. Most importantly, there is no evidence that the lesion actually discovered is palpated during the deliberate monthly act of breast self-examination. It may be discovered accidentally during the interval between examinations.

To be successful, breast self-examination must be properly taught, utilized, and reinforced by health professionals. It requires careful instruction of the individual by the health care provider, and must include practice, palpation techniques, and a review of the learned behavior. A Gallop poll taken in 1973 revealed that the method of instruction was the most important factor in promoting confidence in the woman's ability to detect a lump. The poll also indicated that two-thirds of the women never had breast self-examination discussed by their physicians. Even when breast self-examination was suggested by the physician, discussion was not always accompanied by a demonstration. Even those physicians who discussed and demonstrated the technique of self-examination rarely reexamined their patients' capacity to perform the examination in subsequent visits. Most disturbing of all, the poll indicated that two-thirds of obstetricians and gynecologists failed to demonstrate breast self-examination to their patients.[3] Instruction should begin with women who are at high risk for developing the disease and those who already have been diagnosed and treated for breast cancer. There is no unanimity of opinion concerning the best time to begin teaching breast self-examination. Many junior and senior high schools have programs for teaching and promoting breast self-examination. Since risk increases with age, certainly every woman over age 30 should be familiar with breast self-examination.

The relative merits of physical examination, mammography, and breast self-examination continue to be debated. One study has suggested that the annual clinical examination is the best available screening test, although it was noted that approximately 90% of women studied were performing breast self-examination competently and confidently, suggesting that this screening method "may be as useful as annual clinical breast examination by a competent physician."[6] Physical examination and mammography are not competing techniques. In fact, they are complementary. Every woman should be taught the importance of breast self-examination. This should be reinforced by the physician as he or she performs a careful breast examination. A suspicious lesion, except in rare circumstances, requires mammography. A negative mammogram associated with a three-dimensional mass should not deter the surgeon from performing a biopsy. Conversely, suspicious findings noted on a mammogram but not palpable require appropriate localization techniques and biopsy.

Screening

It seems logical to assume that if a cancer is found early enough, it can be cured. It has been noted that improved survival through screening does not mean that the duration of the natural history of the disease has been shortened. To be effective, screening must increase the time from detection to the onset of symptoms, the usual time of diagnosis or death.

Some have suggested that very modest gains are to be expected from any screening program. It is possible that the long-term cost will outweigh the health benefit. For example, assuming a cost of $75 for an examination, approximately $3.6 billion would be required for a single screening of each American woman 35 years of age or older. David Eddy has noted that "every dollar spent on a mammogram, every radiologist or practitioner shifted to this activity, represents a resource that cannot be spent on other health problems, and that the net value of the screening program depends upon the value of the alternative health activities that will not be undertaken."[7]

The consumer is anxious to avoid unnecessary morbidity and mutilating surgery. Public health officials are responsive to any method that will increase case finding and lower mortality. The proponents of mammography feel that their method is the only way to find an early lesion and therefore decrease mortality. The same might be said of the proponents of thermography and ultrasonography. The question is, will screening accomplish a reduction in mortality in a cost-effective and safe manner? In addition, it must be realized that in a screening program the burden of proof of efficacy and the requirement to reduce risk is much greater than in the normal practice of medicine. In a screening program the *physician* initiates the contact with the implication that through the screening program, if a cancer is found, it will be in its earliest stages. Therefore treatment can be accomplished with much less morbidity and mutilation. In addition it is implied that the probability of death from cancer will be less than if the patient presented in the normal way. Because of this unique arrangement the requirement for proof of benefit is greater than in the physician-patient relationship established in the usual clinical practice of medicine.

In December, 1963 a program organized by the Health Insurance Plan of Greater New York (HIP) began a controlled study of screening. A report in February, 1966 stated that the results of the study were consistent with the hypothesis that "screening leads to earlier detection of breast cancer than is ordinarily experienced and that mammography contributed significantly to detection."[8]

In a report in March, 1971 it was noted that there were 52 deaths due to breast cancer in the control group as compared to 31 in the study group in the period available for follow-up. Allowing for a lead time in diagnosing breast cancer gained through screening, further publications from the study have unequivocally demonstrated the benefit from the use of screening by mammography plus physical examination, but only in women aged 50 to 59 years of age.[9]

In 1973 the National Cancer Institute (NCI) and the American Cancer Society (ACS) organized a breast cancer detection demonstration project. The basic objective was to demonstrate to the medical profession and to the public the methods of screening women for earlier detection of breast cancer. When each woman was recruited she would undergo the initial examination. The patient would then have four annual examinations, after which she would be contacted every year for an additional 5 years of follow-up. The screening methods to be utilized were clinical history, physical examination, x-ray, mammography, and thermography. In addition, each woman would be taught breast self-examination. As the program proceeded, thermography was discontinued from the screening.

A 5-year summary report released by the American Cancer Society in 1982 indicates that large numbers of women were successfully recruited into the screening program, and that these women enthusiastically returned to the program for periodic screening and education over the 5-year period.[10] Of the 4443 cancers recorded, more than 80% were detected in the 29 detection programs. Approximately one-third of the cancers detected by the centers were small cancers, either noninfiltrating or infiltrating cancers less than 1 cm in diameter. More than 80% of all cancers detected showed no evidence of nodal involvement.[10] It is clear that a high proportion of the cancers detected in the breast cancer demonstration network project were localized. These patients should have an excellent prognosis. Physical examination and mammography both contributed cases not detected by the other, but the contribution of mammography was substantially greater; in fact, it was considerably greater than in the HIP study. The relative contribution of mammography alone in the absence of positive physical findings was 41.6% compared with 8.7% for physical examination in the absence of positive mammographic findings. The relative contribution of mammography was impressively high in the detection of smaller cancers—59% of noninfiltrating cancers and 52.6% for infiltrating cancers of less than 1 cm. The relative contribution of mammography was also impressively higher than in the HIP study for breast cancer detection in younger women. When mammography was removed as the routine screening modality for women under 50 years of age, the minimal cancer detection rates in this age group decreased.[10]

In spite of increasing enthusiasm for the accuracy and safety of screening programs, there continues to be a concern among the general population regarding the risks attributed to mammography. These risks include the induction of anxiety, unnecessary surgery, false security, and the induction of cancer. Procedures of low specificity that result in false-positive errors or in identification of early subclinical lesions present two serious problems. The false-positive error may result in unnecessary biopsies and, in some cases, unnecessary definitive treatment, and in the particular case of breast screening programs, identification of a lesion on a mammogram may result in a number of unnecessary biopsies simply because mammography cannot distinguish between benign and small malignant lesions. Most authorities believe that a ratio of 5 : 1 is clinically acceptable; i.e., five biopsies to detect one cancer. However acceptable this is from the physician's point of view, it may not be acceptable to the patient who has been alarmed by the discovery of a lesion and rewarded with a scar or deformity as a result of the procedure.

There is always the danger of false assurance in a screening program. The patient may not understand the limitations of screening and assume that if the test results are normal, the subsequent risk for developing cancer is low. She may, therefore, ignore warning signs and symptoms.

Most of the information concerning radiation risk has been extrapolated from follow-up studies of women exposed to radiation in the atomic bomb explosions in Japan and those exposed to roentgen rays for the treatment of acute postpartum mastitis and fluoroscopic examinations during the treatment of tuberculosis. Radiologists aware of potential dangers have reduced the radiation dose by adding appropriate filtration and by using film screen combinations. In most high-quality installations, acceptable mammography is performed with an absorbed dose to the midplane of the breast of much less than 0.5 rad per examination. Some data have suggested that sensitivity of the breast is greater in young women. This suggests that mammography be limited in this younger age group.

Finally, it is obvious that we must weigh the benefits and risks in recommending any screening program for the early detection of breast cancer. A number of epidemiologic studies have been attempted to assess the risk/benefit ratio. Most suggest that with present knowledge, the increase in lives saved over deaths caused does not appear until screening begins at age 40, and the increase is marginal at age 45. There are a number of calculations concerning the ratio of cost and benefits of screening vs. treatment for carcinoma of the breast. In all these studies it must be noted that the estimates are based upon assumptions that in themselves are not absolute.

Wolfe suggested that mammography can be used for more than early detection of breast cancer and that, in fact, it might be utilized to assess the risk for developing this disease. He has described four mammographic categories according to the relative amounts of fat, epithelial and connective tissue density, and the presence or absence of prominent ducts.[11] A number of investigators have been critical of this approach. A recent study from Sweden concludes, "Any predictive value that mammographic patterns may have in younger women is short-lived as all pattern groups have a high cancer frequency in the older age groups. We do not believe that the mammographic parenchymal pattern should be used to influence the planning of screening programs since most cancers can be expected to occur in the so-called low risk groups."[12]

There is evidence that postmenopausal estrogen replacement therapy may produce changes in the breast suggestive of cystic or dysplastic alterations. When the hormone is discontinued these changes regress. It is therefore suggested that in an attempt to reverse these dysplastic changes, estrogen replacement therapy be discontinued if mammograms show any abnormality.[13]

The following are American Cancer Society guidelines for asymptomatic women[10]:

1. Women 20 years of age and older should perform breast self-examination every month.
2. Women aged 20–40 should have a physical examination of the breast every 3 years, and women over age 40 should have a physical examination of the breast every year.
3. Women between the ages of 35 and 40 should have a baseline mammogram.
4. Women under age 50 should consult their personal physicians about the need for mammography.
5. Women over age 50 should have a mammogram every year when feasible.
6. Women with personal or family histories of breast cancer should consult their physicians about the need for more frequent examinations or about beginning periodic mammography before the age of 50.

It should be emphasized that these guidelines refer to asymptomatic women. As mentioned earlier, breast examination should be an essential part of every prenatal evaluation. Most would agree that careful breast examination is part of the routine physical examination for women and should be performed on an annual basis. Advancing age is the most important risk factor. Most breast cancers occur in women over age 50, and in this group there is definite proof that screening for breast cancer lowers the death rate by 30% and that mammography and physical examination of the breast accounted for this reduction. All would agree that screening using both modalities should become a routine part of an annual medical examination of women over age 50 (Figs. 14–5 to 14–8).

Physicians must be aware of the limitations of mammography and should remember that x-ray study of the breast is a complementary procedure. If physical examination reveals findings sufficient to advise biopsy, a biopsy must be performed even in the presence of a mammogram described as normal.

The role of thermography in screening is difficult to assess.[14] The medical interest in thermography was initiated more than 20 years ago when Lawson noted that the temperature of the skin over a breast cancer was greater than that of the normal tissue. Essentially thermography measures infrared radiation by the skin and this is converted directly into temperature values. The radiation can be

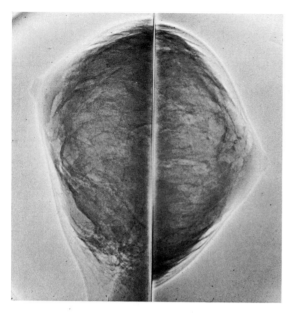

Fig. 14–5. Xeromammogram showing dense breasts in a young patient.

detected either by contact thermography or te-lethermography. Contact thermography uti-lizes liquid cholesterol crystals that change col-ors under the influence of infrared rays. Telethermography uses optics to capture in-frared rays which are then converted to elec-tricity and displayed on a photographic plate or an oscilloscope screen. The proper use of

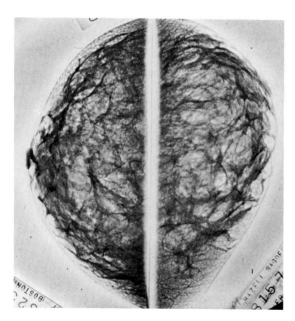

Fig. 14–6. Xeromammogram showing "dyplastic" pattern.

thermography involves measurement of the temperature difference (Δt) between one or more areas of the thermogram. Equipment is available that permits a display of the tempera-ture difference in color that enhances the rec-ognition of any thermic alterations. The cor-rect use of thermography requires, in addition to modern equipment, a draft-free and tem-perature- and humidity-controlled room where a temperature of approximately 20°C is maintained during the period of examination. The breast must be exposed for approximately 10 min prior to the examination to permit equilibration of the skin and the environmen-tal temperature. Following equilibration the examination takes about 5 min. Any palpation of the breast should follow thermography since it may disturb the heat pattern.

Although all agree that thermography is harmless, its specificity is quite low. Most data suggest that in approximately 30% of cases of early carcinoma, no thermopathologic signs are produced. Thermography should not be used alone as a method of screening for breast cancer but must be considered as an extension of the physical examination, preferably in con-junction with mammography. This is the posi-tion adopted by the American College of Radi-ology and the American Thermographic Society.

It is possible that thermography may be used as a risk and prognostic indicator. Abnormal thermographic findings added to the historical and clinical items may help to indicate those at higher risk for breast cancer. Some investiga-tors have reported differences in survival cor-related with thermographic findings. Survival rate was higher in patients with carcinoma of the breast in whom the thermogram was nor-mal than in those in whom the thermogram was abnormal. It is suggested that the thermo-gram indicates the biologic activity of the tu-mor, a greater Δt indicating increased biologic activity and, perhaps, increased virulence.[15] There are many unanswered questions. Until these have been addressed by means of a care-fully constructed clinical protocol, the role of thermography remains difficult to define. It should not be advertised as a screening device in the absence of physical examination and mammography.

Several reports have indicated promising results with the use of ultrasound. Clinical

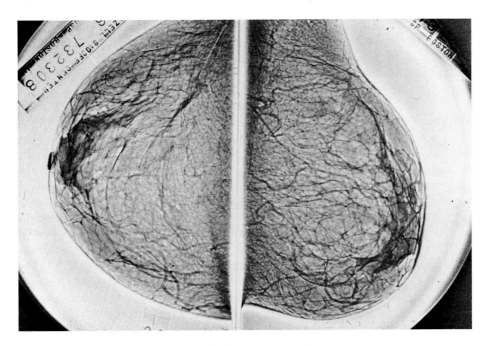

Fig. 14–7. Xeromammogram showing typical postmenopausal pattern.

sonography of the breast is increasingly being used because of high diagnostic accuracy and improved image quality. Breast tissue, fat layers, Cooper's ligaments, and the chest wall with muscle layers can now be well visualized in routine echograms. New developments in instrumentation utilize the simple arc and sector scanning motion simultaneously to overcome geometric and amplitude distortion and physical scanning limitations. The automated scanning device with remote focus arc scanning can be used for the examination of large breasts.

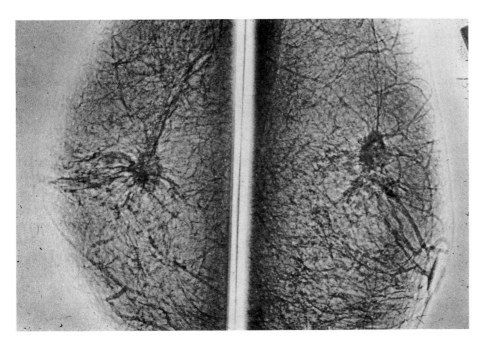

Fig. 14–8. Xeromammogram showing obvious carcinoma.

According to Kobayashi the application of combined telethermography and echography has enabled the detection of breast cancer in 91.8% of patients and benign tumors in 86.4%, with 13.6% false-positive findings in the latter group.[16]

Ultrasonographic examination is particularly useful when there is discordance between mammographic and clinical findings. Most authorities agree that ultrasonography, at least in its present state, is unsuited for screening, specifically because of the lack of sophisticated equipment and operators trained in its use. The equipment available for the physician's office is totally unsuitable for screening and large installations utilizing water-coupling techniques are available only in specialized institutions. Further investigation should focus on the establishment of screening equipment and the studies of ultrasonic tissue characterizations. This would provide a solid basis for developing more refined equipment that would improve diagnostic accuracy and clinical reliability in detecting early breast cancer.

Epidemiology of Breast Cancer

Progress in understanding the etiology of human breast cancer has been slow. However, a number of specific hypotheses have appeared. With the development of refined methods to determine serum levels of the three estrogens—estradiol, estriol, and estrone—and the sensitive assays for peptide hormones, there has been renewed interest in the carcinogenic potential of these hormones.

A number of factors have been associated with increased risk for breast cancer including demographic, anthropometric, dietary, menstrual, reproductive, hormonal, genetic, and others including a history of benign breast disease.

There is general agreement that there is a marked racial preference for breast cancer in whites contrasted with Orientals living in the Orient. The highest incidence of breast cancer in the United States is found in the northeastern part of the country.

The incidence of breast cancer also quite closely parallels meat consumption. That is, those countries with the lowest consumption of meat have the lowest incidence of breast cancer. It should be noted that key risk factors such as age at menarche and weight are determined by the diet, and thus diet must be considered a fundamental risk factor. It is not known, however, whether dietary differences that do not influence either the age at menarche or the weight will have any effect on breast cancer risk. Other studies, however, point to dietary *total* fat as possibly increasing the risk. Epidemiologic studies have shown that breast cancer mortality rates in various regions of Japan are highly correlated with fat consumption. It is interesting to note that with the "westernization" of young Japanese, breast cancer incidence is approaching that of the white population.[17]

Key risk factors include (1) previous cancer of one breast; (2) age; (3) age at menarche; (4) age at first full-term pregnancy; (5) age at menopause; and (6) weight.

Women with previous cancer of one breast are at risk for cancer in the opposite breast. The risk is approximately 1% per year. Thus a woman at age 30 with breast cancer has a greatly increased risk for eventually developing cancer in the opposite breast. The factor(s) responsible for breast cancer must act in both breasts. It is unknown why one breast expresses the disease earlier than the other. Women who have breast cancer in the late postmenopausal years do not live long enough to develop cancer in the opposite breast.

A significantly higher risk of developing breast cancer occurs in women with early menarche. It is the hormonal event associated with menarche that provides for the growth and development of both ductal epithelium and alveoli. This may explain the rather steep rise in age-specific incidence of breast cancer until age 40, at which point it begins to level off but increases gradually through old age. There is a critical ratio of body weight and height that is necessary for the menarche to occur. Obviously chronic malnutrition and disease during childhood may delay the age of menarche, whereas improved nutrition and the control of infectious disease may have combined to lower the age.

For a number of years epidemiologists have noted a decreased risk associated with increased parity. MacMahon et al. have clearly demonstrated that the protective effect of parity is due to early age of first birth.[18] The woman with the first birth under age 20 has about one-half the risk of a nulliparous woman. Clearly, abortions before the first full-term pregnancy do not have any protective effect. Whatever the reason, the mechanism producing this protective effect is not brought into play until the pregnancy has proceeded beyond the first trimester.

The relationship between menopause and breast cancer has been known for a number of years. Women whose natural menopause occurs before the age of 45 have only one-half the breast cancer risk of those whose menopause occurs after the age of 55. Age at menarche is not correlated with age at menopause. Thus women with 40 or more years of active menstruation have twice the risk of those with less than 30 years of menstrual activity. It has been shown that artificial menopause, either by bilateral oophorectomy or pelvic irradiation, markedly reduces breast cancer risk. Women who have their ovaries removed before the age of 35 have a 70% reduction in the incidence of breast cancer.

There is a strong relationship between weight and breast cancer, particularly in postmenopausal women. For women under age 50 there is little or no increased risk, but in the 60- to 69-year-old age group an increase in weight from 60 to 70 kg or greater increases the risk by approximately 80%. It is not known whether the effect is one of excess weight or body fat or sheer body mass. The effect shown for weight in postmenopausal women is independent of the effect of menarche, first birth, and menopause.[19]

POSSIBLE CAUSES OF BREAST CANCER. Several causal hypotheses have been proposed including genetic, viral, and endocrine.

There is an undeniable familial aggregation of breast cancer in female relatives of premenopausal patients, particularly with bilateral breast cancer. However, when examined carefully there is no recognizable pattern of inheritance for the majority of patients, and high risk families are extremely rare. Obviously, familial aggregation is consistent with an environmental cause.

For a number of years it has been suspected that at least in some women a virus is associated with the development of breast cancer. Epidemiologic studies, however, are inconclusive.

The most attractive hypotheses dealing with breast cancer concern those related to endocrine factors, particularly prolactin and estrogen. As noted previously, early menarche and late menopause are related to increased risk for breast cancer. When ovulation ceases in the perimenopausal woman, it is associated with 2, 3, or more years of anovulary bleeding. Thus at each end of the reproductive cycle the patient with early menarche and late menopause may have prolonged periods of anovulary bleeding.

There has been intense interest in the role of prolactin in human breast cancer. Prolactin is released or inhibitied by hypothalamic neurohormones. Serum concentrations of prolactin are increased by interfering with the inhibitory control. A number of factors are known to alter serum prolactin concentration—hypothalamic lesions, tranquilizers such as phenothiazines, and the anesthetic agent Innovar. Reserpine also increases serum prolactin. A decrease in serum prolactin is produced by L-dopa derivatives such as ergonovine and 2-bromo-alpha-ergocryptine. One study has shown that daughters of patients with cancer have a consistent elevation of plasma prolactin levels. There is a suggestion that the values of serum prolactin are elevated in breast cancer patients. However, other studies have not confirmed this and one must conclude that at the present time probably no difference exists.[19]

THE ROLE OF ESTROGENS. With the development of refined assays to determine serum levels of the three estrogens, there has been renewed interest in the investigation of the carcinogenic potential of estrone, estradiol, and estriol. Some evidence suggests that estrogens play an important part in determining the hormonal milieu that favors the development of human breast cancer. The previously described risk factors noted in epidemiologic studies are associated with increased risk and diminished production with decreased risk. Height and weight factors that contribute to increased risk in postmenopausal women can be explained by increased peripheral conversion of androgen to estrogen (see Chapter 1). The administration of estrogen to postmenopausal women may result in a small increase in the risk of mammary cancer. Finally, therapeutic strategies that are effective in the treatment of breast cancer in premenopausal women can be explained on the basis of reduction or elimination of endogenous estrogens.

How does one explain the occurrence of carcinoma of the breast in postmenopausal women when ovarian function and therefore estrogen levels are declining? Recent evidence suggests that there is considerable peripheral conversion of adrenal androgen to estrogen.[20] Androstenedione is converted in adipose tissue, including the breast, to estrone. Some of the estrone is converted to the liver to estriol. Since estradiol and progesterone are not produced by the ovaries in the postmenopausal woman, the two estrogens competing for cytoplasmic binding sites are estrone and estriol. A number of years ago it was suggested that the estriol ratio—i.e., the ratio of estriol to estrone and estradiol—predicted the risk of development of breast cancer. An increased ratio was said to be protective. Recent data do not support this, however. A decreased estriol ratio in the urine often is caused by decreased estradiol plus estrone excretion, rather than by increased estriol excretion. Urinary excretion levels of estriol are increased in women with breast cancer, but in the same women there is increased peripheral metabolism of estradiol to estriol. Finally, estriol given orally does not inhibit estradiol uptake by a tumor. Some studies on the mechanism of action of estriol indicate that it is neither an impeded estrogen nor an estrogen antagonist when present in a continuous or chronic fashion. Finally, the validity of this hypothesis becomes totally unlikely with the finding that estriol itself is as carcinogenic as the other estrogens in experimental rodent cancers.[21]

The other hypothesis is the so-called estrone hypothesis: this suggests that estrone quantitatively is the most important estrogen after menopause and has an effect on estrogen-specific target cells different from that of estradiol. In postmenopausal women there is considerable conversion of androstenedione to estrone, some of which is converted in the liver to estriol. Recent evidence suggests that the local concentration of estrone in target tissue is very low and that estrone from the blood is metabolized inside the cell to estradiol before binding to specific estrogen receptors. Thus the subcellular action of estrone gives no evidence for an action qualitatively or quantitatively different from that of estradiol. Estrone binds to the receptor with less affinity than estradiol, but it can induce specific estrogenic effects.[21]

What is the relationship between estrogens and cancer risk? Most investigators suggest that estrogen is preparative rather than carcinogenic. In an interesting study reported by Fechner in 1970, breast tissue was reevaluated in a blind fashion and it was determined that there was no histologic difference associated with estrogen therapy. These findings also applied when carcinoma of the breast was similarly evaluated. Fechner also noted that the frequency of breast cancer before the age of 35 remained at about 4%, suggesting that there was no association between the use of oral contraceptives and breast cancer.[22]

Studies regarding the use of postmenopausal estrogens and the development of breast cancer do not clearly show any increased risk, although some studies report that high doses for long periods may be associated with increased risk. Clearly, postmenopausal replacement therapy should be given in the lowest dose for the shortest possible period of time.

PREVIOUS HISTORY. Most epidemiologic studies support the fact that a history of benign breast disease increases the risk for breast cancer.[19] However, the term "benign breast disease" is not precise in covering a variety of clinical and pathologic entities. Since 100% of women have some form of fibrocystic change, it may not be correct to use the term "disease" when describing these alterations. It is unlikely that there is any major increase in the risk of breast cancer in patients with fibrocystic changes. Attempts to correlate the type and degree of atypia associated with fibrocystic changes suggest that the risks may be significantly increased in those patients who have dysplastic or atypical changes noted on biopsies.

In summary, a number of important factors determine the risk of breast cancer. The most important of these seem to be related to estrogen and possibly prolactin. Additional research is necessary on the role of endogenous and exogenous estrogens and the effect of diet, drugs, and other factors on the levels of estrogen and prolactin. It is unlikely that breast cancer can be prevented. We cannot alter the age of menarche, and promotion of early pregnancy to protect against breast cancer is not feasible. One risk factor that is alterable is obesity, particularly in the postmenopausal woman.

Diagnosis and Treatment of Benign Breast Disease

As mentioned earlier, 80% of breast cancers occur in women over the age of 40. However, the perimenopausal and menopausal woman may present with a number of benign conditions including nipple discharge, mastodynia, fibrocystic changes, and inflammations including Mondor's disease.

Mastodynia, although more common in the menstruating female, does occur postmenopausally, particularly in the perimenopausal patient. Frequently patients who have never had discomfort in the breast will experience pain at about the time of menstrual irregularities associated with the menopause. Pain may be cyclic or unremitting and usually is bilateral. Examination reveals tenderness most commonly in the upper outer quadrants. Diagnostic studies usually are negative. Treatment is symptomatic including well-fitting bras. The condition is self-limited. Unilateral pain may be associated with other conditions, the pain being referred to the breast. Occasionally patients in the menopausal age group will complain of pain in the breast. However, appropriate diagnostic studies will reveal angina or other cardiovascular problems. Clearly unilateral breast pain requires diagnostic studies such as mammography to rule out significant breast disease. As in the younger woman, occasional patients find relief with restriction of methylxanthines including caffeine, chocolate, and cola.[23] Vitamin E has been recommended.[23] If it is effective, the mechanism of action is unknown. Danazol, which has been recommended for some patients with significant mastodynia,[23] is not recommended for the postmenopausal patient.

Nipple discharge may be associated with the use of tranquilizers, particularly the phenothiazines. Manual stimulation, including jogging, has also been reported as a cause for clear or greenish discharge. It is important to know if the discharge is bilateral or unilateral, spontaneous or provoked, bloody or clear.

Clear or milky discharge usually is associated with physiologic alterations. Serosanguineous or bloody discharge more often indicates a benign intraductal papilloma and rarely a malignancy. Patients with unilateral serosanguineous or bloody discharge, in addition to careful palpation of the breast, should have the fluid examined by a Pap smear, and for those with grossly bloody discharge, a mammogram is indicated. Usually the quadrant involved can be identified by careful palpation. Exploration of the duct system is recommended.

Occasionally menopausal patients will palpate a mass that has been present for some time and which represents the residual of fibrocystic changes. A benign fibroadenoma may have been present for years and discovered only on a routine examination many years later. This may be related to a change in breast size due to weight reduction or weight gain, or the atrophy that normally accompanies the menopause. Cystic changes or gross cystic disease are unusual following the menopause. However, long-term use of estrogen replacement therapy may be associated with symptoms of the lumpy, painful breast and the occasional appearance of macrocysts.

Apparent inflammation may be associated with trauma and subsequent fat necrosis or Mondor's disease, a superficial thrombophlebitis, or a subcutaneous angiitis. The patient usually complains of the sudden onset of breast pain and appearance of a hard, tender cord in the outer quadrant of the breast. This appears to be a superficial phlebitis of the veins of the chest wall. No etiology has been discovered.[24] Treatment with analgesics usually will cause the phlebitis to resolve within a few weeks. The major problem is the diagnosis. It clearly can be confused with breast cancer, particularly inflammatory cancer. Mammography and excisional biopsy often are required.

Occasional menopausal patients will have duct ectasia or plasma cell mastitis manifested by a multicolored sticky nipple discharge occurring from multiple ducts. A firm mass is palpated beneath the areola. This can easily be confused with carcinoma. Mammography is mandatory and, if there is any question, an excisional biopsy should be performed.

Sebaceous cysts are common, particularly in menopausal patients. They may occur in the skin over the breast, on the sternum, or in the inframammary fold. Occasional inflammation may be confused with inflammatory carcinoma. These lesions are superficial and circumscribed, and contain a dilated sebaceous duct in the overlying skin. Treatment is local excision.

When the patient notes a mass, or a lesion is discovered on physical examination, the lesion may be cystic or solid, benign or malignant. If the lesion appears to be solid, mammography and excisional biopsy are recommended. If the mass appears to be cystic, an attempt should be made to aspirate the lesion with a 20- or 21-gauge needle. If the fluid is clear or cloudy and no residual mass is palpated immediately following the aspiration, follow-up examination in 1 month with reassurance and monthly breast self-examination are recommended. If the mass remains immediately following aspiration or if the fluid is bloody, the patient should have a mammogram and a biopsy. If there is a residual mass on the first follow-up examination, mammography and biopsy are mandatory.

Outpatient biopsy is becoming increasingly popular. With properly selected cases it is uncomplicated and cost effective. The lesion should be small and relatively superficial. Occult lesions as noted on the mammogram are difficult to biopsy under local anesthesia. The surgery is best performed in a regular operat-

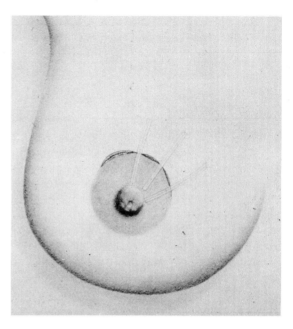

Fig. 14–10. Closure of incision with subcuticular suture.

ing room setting with assistance, but it may be performed in a properly equipped office. Local anesthesia is employed and, if possible, a circumareolar incision that follows the lines of Langer is utilized (Fig. 14–9). Rarely is an inframammary incision justified, and a radial incision never. Meticulous hemostasis must be employed. A minimum number of sutures should be utilized to reconstruct the breast tissue. Most surgeons allow the breast tissue to be approximated without sutures, once hemostasis has been achieved. The incision can be closed with fine nylon sutures, a subcuticular suture, polyglycolic material, or steristrips (Fig. 14–10). As a general rule, a minimal amount of suture material should be left in the breast. A pressure dressing is employed for 24 h to reduce ecchymosis and discomfort. When this is removed the incision is covered with a small sterile dressing until the sutures are removed.

Diagnosis and Treatment of Breast Cancer

Breast cancer is a disease of postmenopausal women. Guidelines published by the American Cancer Society, the American College of Radiology, and the American College of Obstetricians and Gynecologists suggest that screening mammography be performed on women over

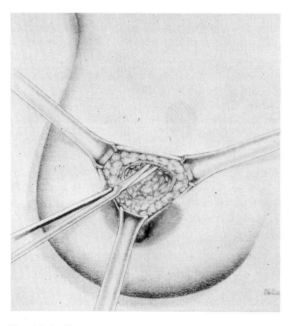

Fig. 14–9. Circumareolar incision following the Lines of Langer.

age 50. A majority of patients, however, will present with a mass discovered either by breast self-examination or by the health care provider at the time of a routine examination. As noted previously, a careful history must be obtained and the information from the history and physical examination carefully documented in the record. Aspiration biopsy using the "skinny needle" technique is becoming more popular. This, however, requires an understanding of the technique involved and a cytopathologist capable of interpreting the smear. A standard disposable syringe can be used with a 21- to 25-gauge needle. Local anesthesia is not required. The needle is plunged into the mass and approximately 5 cc of suction applied. Several passes are made through the tissue. The needle and syringe are withdrawn and the contents of the needle placed on a slide for evaluation. Results are available in 15–20 min and, in capable hands, are quite accurate. Obviously, before treatment is recommended, appropriate preoperative studies, including mammography, are mandatory.

Outpatient biopsy and definitive diagnosis are becoming more popular for lesions that appear to be clinically malignant. Available data suggest that the delay of definitive treatment for 1 or 2 weeks does not adversely influence survival. However, it is absolutely essential that this surgery be carefully performed with minimal manipulation of breast tissue. Sharp dissection, meticulous hemostasis, and absolute asepsis are required. Infection or marked ecchymosis greatly interfere with the definitive surgical treatment. Biopsy and delay of treatment can be justified only under ideal conditions. This means careful biopsy technique and immediate consultation with the surgeon responsible for definitive treatment. If the lesion is suspicious, at least 500 mg of tissue should be sent to the pathologist with a note that estrogen and progesterone receptor studies should be performed. This will require a frozen section to determine whether the lesion is benign or malignant. It is therefore advisable for all but the most obvious lesions to request frozen section to determine whether estrogen and progesterone binding studies should be performed.

Once the diagnosis of breast cancer has been established, a number of preoperative studies should be obtained. As mentioned before, mammography is absolutely essential to rule out carcinoma in the opposite breast. Synchronous carcinoma has been noted in 4% of patients. Also, multicentric disease may be noted in the involved breast. All patients should have a chest x-ray, routine blood studies, and liver function tests; for invasive lesions most surgeons recommend a bone scan and appropriate x-ray films. Clinical staging should be noted using the T-N-M classification where T represents the tumor; N, nodal involvement; and M, metastatic disease. Pathologic staging is supplied by the pathologist following removal of the specimen and includes the status of the regional lymph nodes and the information obtained from the preoperative evaluation including the bone scan and appropriate skeletal x-rays.

OVERVIEW OF TREATMENT. A number of reports support the concept that cancer of the breast often is a systemic disease with 50% or more of patients presenting with metastases. Thus it is entirely proper that previously held concepts for therapeutic approaches be reassessed and placed in proper perspective.

For most patients a two-step diagnostic and therapeutic program is recommended. Biopsy performed either on an outpatient or inpatient basis or by aspiration needle biopsy is essential. If cancer is present, appropriate estrogen and progesterone binding studies are performed. For those patients who have an excisional or incisional biopsy, permanent sections are obtained, and upon review of these sections treatment options are discussed with the patient. There is no evidence that a delay of 1 to 2 weeks between diagnosis and definitive treatment affects prognosis. In at least two states—Massachusetts and California—state law mandates that the physician must discuss alternative treatments with the patient.[25] Obviously this leads to second and even third opinions, further delaying the diagnosis. However, as noted above, a delay of 1 to 2 weeks does not affect prognosis.

SURGERY. About 10 years ago radical mastectomy was the most widely performed operation in the United States for the primary treatment of breast cancer. At present it remains the standard in terms of results against which all other procedures must be judged. When a radical mastectomy is performed, the pectoralis muscles—pectoralis major and minor—are removed and a complete axillary dissection is done. In about 20% of the cases, significant morbidity or functional impairment is associated with this type of mastectomy.

Total mastectomy with axillary dissection (modified radical mastectomy) has largely supplanted the radical operation and is the operation of choice of most surgeons for T-1 and T-2 curable breast cancer. The total removal of the breast and axillary dissection are common to both procedures, although it is recognized that a complete axillary dissection is technically more difficult when the chest wall muscles are not removed. In the Madden modification the pectoralis major and minor muscles both are preserved, thus making a complete dissection of level 1 and 2 nodes more difficult. The Patey modification, favored by most surgeons, removes the pectoralis minor muscle, thus facilitating exposure in the axilla. Cosmetically, the preservation of the bulk of the pectoralis major muscle leads to a less deformed chest wall. Functionally, arm strength and mobility may be preserved more fully and there is less swelling and edema. Psychologically, preservation of the chest wall musculature permits better plastic reconstructive procedures later if desired by the patient. The modified mastectomy appears to be about as effective as the more radical procedure in the surgical treatment of curable breast cancer.

RADIATION THERAPY. Radiation therapy as an alternative to surgery has the chief advantage of a better functional cosmetic result with equal or less morbidity.[26,27] Complete tumor excision is important for good local control and cosmesis. High doses of radiation are necessary for control of gross tumor, and these doses occasionally are associated with unacceptable cosmetic and functional results. Following gross removal of the tumor a modest dose of radiation of 5000 rad will control microscopic disease. Boost therapy to the area of excision can be done with the electron beam or with interstitial implantation of radionucleotides. If primary radiotherapy is recommended, it should be restricted to patients with lesions that are relatively small in comparison to the size of the breast. In premenopausal patients it is important to have an axillary sampling to determine those women with positive nodes who may benefit from adjuvant therapy.

ADJUVANT THERAPY. It is clear that a significant increase in survival in curable breast cancer will depend upon earlier diagnosis prior to the occurrence of metastasis or the treatment of such micrometastasis immediately following local therapy. Recent studies have indicated that adjuvant chemotherapy is most effective in premenopausal patients with significant axillary involvement.[28] No single form of adjuvant therapy may be considered as an established form of therapy. At present patients with T-1 and T-2 lesions with no histologic evidence of nodal involvement should not be treated with adjuvant therapy. Adjuvant regimens designed for individual patients significantly different from published programs are discouraged. It has been suggested that postmenopausal patients may benefit from appropriate adjuvant therapy if the therapy can be given in adequate doses. Published reports indicate that many postmenopausal patients cannot tolerate the dosage schedule recommended for appropriate adjuvant therapy. The dose for these patients has been reduced and for this reason the results may not be comparable.[29] Regardless of the use of adjuvant chemotherapy, axillary sampling is important to determine prognosis and should be performed on most patients.

It is now well established that estrogen-positive tumors are associated with clinical response to therapeutic hormone manipulation and a prolonged interval between diagnosis of breast cancer and recurrence.[30] If the estrogen receptor is positive (greater than 10 femtomoles/mg protein), the likelihood of response is greater than 50%. If the estrogen response is negative (less than 10 femtomoles/mg protein), the response is less than 80%. Furthermore, a high content greater than 100 femtomoles/mg protein is associated with an increased response of greater than 80%. The estrogen assay should be utilized along with other clinical factors that predict response to select patients for hormone treatment. These clinical factors include a tumor-free interval of greater than 2 years, postmenopausal status, prior response to hormone treatment, and metastatic or recurrent disease predominantly in skin or lymph nodes. The relationship of the estrogen receptor assay to the clinical response to cytotoxic chemotherapy remains controversial. However, current opinion supports the fact that no such predictive relationship exists for chemotherapy response.[31]

RECURRENT OR METASTATIC DISEASE. Treatment of recurrent or metastatic disease consists of hormone manipulation based upon endocrine receptor values, the menopausal status of the patient, and the location of the metastatic disease. If the estrogen receptor value is negative or if there is rapidly advancing visceral disease, chemotherapy should be started immediately. In a postmenopausal patient who is estrogen positive, estrogens or Tamoxifen may be employed followed by adrenalectomy. If there is failure, the patient is treated with chemotherapy. Combination chemotherapy given either weekly or cyclically seems to achieve the highest response rate, greatest complete response, longest remission duration, and the greatest increase in survival. Tamoxifen may be the best choice of therapy for patients with metastatic breast cancer after conventional endocrine therapy and combination chemotherapy have failed.

RECONSTRUCTION. For properly selected patients, reconstruction after mastectomy is an important part of their complete rehabilitation. Although anatomic results are imperfect, the psychologic benefits are significant. In discussing alternatives in treatment the possibility of breast reconstruction should be mentioned. This attitude on the part of the surgeon, plus the realization by the patient that she need not have a deformity, may encourage more women to perform breast self-examination and to consult their physicians earlier in the course of disease.

Following a properly performed modified radical mastectomy, a satisfactory reconstruction can be performed by placing an implant beneath the pectoral muscles. Appropriate techniques are available to improve cosmesis by providing a nipple and areola. Patients with radical mastectomy or with radiotherapy and considerable fibrosis will require additional surgical procedures, including the rotation of a flap to provide the necessary skin for the reconstruction. Most surgeons favor an interval of from 6 months to 1 year following mastectomy before reconstruction is attempted. However, in some cases it may be done immediately following the cancer operation.

Summary

The obstetrician-gynecologist often is referred to as the primary physician to women, and as such has an extraordinary opportunity to diagnose early breast lesions. Careful breast examination should be part of every gynecologic and obstetric examination. Cancer of the breast is rare during pregnancy. However, delay in diagnosis often has resulted in the treatment of late stage disease. The diagnosis and treatment of breast cancer is a team effort requiring the expertise of the surgeon or gynecologist, radiologist, medical oncologist, radiotherapist, and plastic surgeon, and most importantly, appropriate psychosocial support provided either by trained oncology nurses, social workers, or a psychiatrist. Selective treatment must be the goal. Few patients are willing to participate in a screening program that results in the loss of their breast.

REFERENCES

1. American Cancer Society. Facts and figures. 1981.
2. Jarrell J, et al. Breast examination does not elevate serum prolactin. Fertil Steril. 1980; 33:49.
3. National Survey on Breast Cancer. A measure of progress in public understanding. Washington, D.C.: U.S. Dept. of Public Health and Human Services, Public Health Service, National Institutes of Health, 1980.
4. Haagensen CD. Diseases of the breast. Philadelphia: Saunders, 1971.
5. Moore FD. Editorial: breast self-examination. N Engl J Med 1978; 299:304.
6. Mahoney LJ, Byrd BL, Cook GM. Annual clinical examination, the best available screening test for breast cancer. N Engl J Med 1979; 301:315.
7. Eddy DM. Personal communication.
8. Shapiro S, Strax P, Venet L. Evaluation of periodic breast cancer screening with mammography. JAMA. 1966; 195:111.
9. Shapiro S, Strax P, Venet L. Periodic breast cancer screening in reducing mortality in breast cancer. JAMA. 1971; 215:1777.
10. Baker LH. Breast cancer detection demonstration project: five-year summary report. Ca. 1982; 32:194–225.

11. Wolfe JN. Breast patterns as an index of risk for developing breast cancer. Am J Roentgenol. 1976; 126:1130.

12. Tabar L, Dean PB. Mammographic parenchymal patterns: Risk indicator for breast cancer? JAMA. 1982; 247:185–189.

13. Peck DR, Lowman RM. Estrogen and the postmenopausal breast. JAMA. 1978; 240:1733.

14. Nyirjesy I, Abernathy ME, Billingsley FS, et al. Thermography and detection of breast carcinoma: A review and comments. J Reprod Med. 1977; 18:165.

15. Libshitz HI. Thermography of the breast: Current status and future expectations. JAMA. 1977; 238:1953.

16. Kobayashi T. Current status of breast echography. In: Kurjak A, ed. Progress in medical ultrasound, Vol. 2. Amsterdam: Excerpta Medica, 1981:123–125.

17. Yonemoto RH. Breast cancer in Japan and the United States. Arch Surg. 1980; 115:1056.

18. MacMahon B, Cole P, Brown JP, et al. Urine estrogen profiles of Asian and North American women. Int J Cancer. 1974; 14:161.

19. Henderson BE, Pike MC, Gray GE. The epidemiology of breast cancer. In: Hoogstraten B, McDivitt RW, eds. Breast cancer. Boca Raton, Fla.: CRC Press, 1981:7.

20. Siiteri PK, Williams JE, Takaki NK. Steroid abnormalities in endometrial and breast carcinoma: A unifying hypothesis. J Steroid Biochem; 1976; 897–903.

21. Poortman J. Role of steroid hormones in the genesis of human mammary cancer. In: Stoll BL, ed. Reviews on endocrine related cancer, No. 6. 1980.

22. Marchant DJ. Epidemiology of breast cancer. In: Marchant DJ, Nyirjesy I, eds. Breast disease. New York: Grune & Stratton, 1979:53–61.

23. Marchant DJ. Screening evaluation and management of breast lesions. In: Osofsky H, ed. Advances in clinical obstetrics and gynecology. Philadelphia: Williams & Wilkins (in press).

24. Dutt P. Mondor's disease. Obstet Gynecol. 1981; 58:118.

25. Massachusetts Patients' Bill of Rights. Aug. 23, 1797.

26. Harris JR, Levene MB, Hellmen S. The role of radiation therapy in the primary treatment of carcinoma of the breast. Semin Oncol. 1978; 5:403–16.

27. Prosnitz LR, Goldenberg IS, Packard RA, et al. Radiation therapy as initial treatment for early stage cancer of the breast without mastectomy. Cancer. 1977; 39:917–23.

28. Adjuvant chemotherapy of breast cancer. National Institute of Health Consensus Development. Conference summary 3, No. 3. U.S. Dept. of Health & Human Services, P.H.S., N.I.H., Office of Medical Applications of Research.

29. Bonadonna G, Valagussa P. Dose response effect of adjuvant chemotherapy in breast cancer. N Engl J Med. 1981; 304:10–15.

30. Lippman ME, Allegra JC. Current concepts in cancer: Receptors in breast cancer. N Engl J Med. 1978; 299:930–32.

31. Kiang DT, et al. Estrogen receptors and responses to chemotherapy and hormonal therapy in advanced breast cancer. N Engl J Med. 1978; 299:1330–34.

Sports and Exercise 15

Mona M. Shangold

Few peri- and postmenopausal women learned the benefits of exercise when they were young, and most acquired sedentary lifestyles as a result. In providing primary care to senior citizens, gynecologists should inform their patients about how exercise can prevent or relieve several common problems and should offer guidelines for initiating and continuing such a program.

The most prevalent peri- and postmenopausal disorders are vasomotor symptoms, osteoporosis, cardiovascular and thromboembolic disease, atrophic vaginitis, depression and other psychiatric disturbances, abnormal uterine bleeding, and obesity. Several of these are apparently related to estrogen deficiency and are optimally treated with estrogen replacement therapy. Some of these can be prevented or alleviated with a prescription for exercise.

Vasomotor Symptoms

Vasomotor symptoms are experienced by as many as 75% of postmenopausal women, in 80% of whom they persist longer than 1 year and in 33% longer than 5 years. The sequence of symptoms in the vasomotor flush has been described,[1] although the initiating etiologic neurotransmitter remains to be identified. Significant sleep deprivation can result from frequent vasomotor symptoms, and this can lead to a variety of psychiatric and behavioral disorders. Estrogen[2,3] or progestin[4] therapy can reduce the frequency and severity of flushes, and can thus alleviate the related psychiatric distur-

bances. Estrogen and progestin also may modify mood and behavior by their known effects on neurotransmission (Chapters 6 and 7). Estrogen reduces monoamine oxidase (MAO) activity, whereas progesterone raises it.[5–7] Thus, estrogen raises levels of catecholamines and serotonin, whereas progesterone lowers them. The enhancing effects of catecholamines on alertness and of serotonin on mood often may be seen in response to estrogen therapy. Wallace[8] has observed no consistent effects of exercise on the frequency or severity of vasomotor symptoms in peri- and postmenopausal women.

Depression and Other Psychiatric Disturbances

Although some behavioral and psychiatric disturbances can result from the chronic sleep deprivation that occurs in women who have frequent vasomotor symptoms, other dysfunction may be due to aging itself. With increasing age, tyrosine hydroxylase and DOPA decarboxylase decrease,[9] as a result of which less catecholamine synthesis takes place. There is also an increase in monoamine oxidase activity, resulting in elevated catecholamine metabolism.[10,11] Thus, older people tend to have lower brain levels of catecholamines, which have been associated with depression.[11,12] By preventing norepinephrine catabolism, MAO inhibitors increase norepinephrine concentrations and thus prevent or relieve depression.

Reduced serotonin also has been associated

with depression,[12] and aging is associated with reduced serotonin synthesis and increased serotonin metabolism.[10] Exercise is associated with higher brain concentrations of both norepinephrine and serotonin in rats.[13] This may explain the success of exercise in prevention and treatment of depression.

Osteoporosis

Osteoporosis remains the most serious postmenopausal problem and is thoroughly discussed in Chapter 4. Exercise can lead to an increase in bone density, but only when dietary calcium intake is adequate.[14] Albanese has observed greater bone densities in a group of heavily exercised males, compared to a group of moderately exercised males who had greater bone densities than a group of sedentary controls.[14] He noted lower bone densities in women ingesting only 400 mg of calcium daily than in average women the same age; and he observed that bone density in this low-calcium group did not correlate with exercise.[14] Aloia has associated decreased total body calcium and bone mineral content with bed rest and increased total body calcium and bone mineral content with exercise.[15] With 99% of total body calcium distributed in bones and teeth, this suggests significant loss of bone density with bed rest and enhancement of bone density with exercise. Smith has observed maintenance of bone density in association with either physical exercise or supplemental calcium (750 mg/day) and vitamin D (400 IU/day), in comparison with sedentary controls.[16] These data strongly suggest that exercise preserves bone density and provide compelling evidence for encouragement of activity among the elderly.

Cardiovascular and Thromboembolic Disease

Cardiovascular and thromboembolic disease increase in prevalence with increasing age in both sexes. Although more common among men than women, coronary artery disease and myocardial infarction have not been proven to be related to estrogen deficiency. The Framingham study noted that heart disease increased in frequency after the menopause,[17,18] but oophorectomized women have a similar prevalence of arteriosclerotic heart disease when compared to nonoophorectomized, hysterectomized controls.[19] These data are unchanged by estrogen administration.[19]

High density lipoprotein (HDL) cholesterol concentrations in marathon runners are greater than in controls.[20] HDL levels increase with physical activity[21] and are associated with a protective effect against ischemic heart disease.[22] The beneficial effects of exercise in prevention of cardiovascular disease extend beyond this propitious lipoprotein change. Williams has noted that the augmentation of fibrinolytic activity that occurs in response to venous occlusion is enhanced with physical conditioning.[23] This effect was most marked in women, in individuals with low initial levels of stimulated fibrinolysis, and in those with low initial levels of cardiovascular fitness. These data demonstrate reduced cardiovascular and thromboembolic risks in women by more than one mechanism.

Atrophic Vaginitis

The association of atrophic vaginitis and urethritis with estrogen deficiency is well documented. Estrogen treatment by any route restores estrogen-dependent tissues of the genitourinary tract to normal and relieves symptoms promptly. Other treatments remain to be identified and are not expected to offer comparable results.

Obesity

Obesity is associated with an increased risk of cardiovascular disease, diabetes mellitus, gallbladder disease, gout, and several cancers. The tendency of many older women toward obesity is due to lifestyle, education, and estrogen effect. Serotonin affects appetite as well as mood. Midbrain depletion of serotonin leads to hyperphagia in rats,[24] and it has been suggested that serotonin suppresses appetite.[25,26] Exercised rats have higher concentrations of serotonin,[13] suggesting that exercise may promote reduced caloric intake, as well as increased caloric expenditure. The beneficial effects of exercise on weight loss and fat reduction warrant encouragement and endorsement. The increased caloric expenditure promoted by exercise persists for several hours after exercise has ceased.[27] Thus, more calories will be utilized even while resting in those who exercise regularly.

Recommendations

Previously sedentary women need guidelines for regular activity. For cardiovascular benefits, they should exercise three to five times per week, at a sustained heart rate of at least 110–120 beats/min, maintained for 15–60 continuous min.[28] This target heart rate represents 60% of the maximum heart rate reserve, which is the percentage difference between resting and maximum heart rate, added to the resting heart rate. Exercising for a longer interval will burn more calories but will not improve cardiovascular fitness significantly. Exercising more frequently also will burn more calories but may lead to injury, as a result of providing inadequate postexercise healing time for muscles.

Maximum oxygen uptake ($\dot{V}_{O_2max}$) is the maximum amount of oxygen that can be taken up, transported, and utilized per unit time. Its level depends upon both conditioning and the size of the muscle group employed in the exercise (i.e., a higher maximum oxygen uptake will be recorded during running, which uses large leg muscles, than during piano playing, which uses small finger muscles). The role of specific conditioning is demonstrated by the fact that a trained runner will record a higher maximum oxygen uptake when tested in running rather than in cycling, whereas a trained cyclist will record a higher value when tested in cycling rather than in running, since the athlete's muscles are trained to utilize oxygen in the specific sport. Maximum oxygen uptake is generally expressed in liters per minute or in milliliters per kilogram body weight per minute.

In order to increase maximum oxygen uptake (i.e., aerobic capacity), at least 60% of the maximum heart rate reserve or at least 50% of the maximum oxygen uptake must be attained and sustained.[29,30] "Fitness" is achieved when heart rate decreases by at least 30 beats/min within the first 60 s after cessation of maximum exercise sustained for at least 2 min. A woman can raise her maximum oxygen uptake by regular endurance training, as outlined above.

Anaerobic threshold is the point above which significant amounts of lactic acid begin to accumulate in the blood, as the result of incurring an oxygen debt. A woman can raise her anaerobic threshold by incurring an oxygen debt during exercise one to two times each week. This induces oxidative muscle enzymes, which permit faster clearance of lactate from exercising muscles, and also induces toleration of higher lactate levels without impairment of performance.

Interval training is the most effective method by which an athlete can raise her anaerobic threshold. This term refers to alternating fast and slow intervals. The fast intervals consist of exercising in the specific sport as fast as possible; these are alternated with slow periods of recovery, during which the oxygen debt of the fast interval is repaid. Fast intervals may last for a 30-s maximum or for a 2-min minimum. Short intervals permit neuromuscular training at a very fast pace; since less lactic acid accumulates during each interval, many short intervals may be repeated during each exercise session. Long intervals (lasting at least 2 min each) induce oxidative muscle enzymes and tolerance of higher lactate levels in the exercising muscles; since a great deal of lactic acid accumulates during each long interval, fewer long intervals may be repeated during each exercise session. Interval training (speed work) should be practiced only once or twice each week for most individuals.

The usefulness and accuracy of cardiac stress tests in screening asymptomatic women remain controversial because false positives and false negatives occur with a high degree of frequency. At present it appears unnecessary to test asymptomatic women unless they have hypertension, hypercholesterolemia, a family history of myocardial infarction, chest pain with exercise, diabetes mellitus, a resting heart rate greater than 80 beats/min, a heart rate after exercise that remains more than 20 beats/min above the resting heart rate after 30 min of rest, or dyspnea with mild exertion.

Although jogging has become fashionable and popular, and although it offers efficient and relatively prompt weight loss and fitness, it is not the best exercise for those who have been sedentary for a long time. New joggers usually incur too many injuries to allow continued training, and activity often ceases permanently following such injuries. Better choices are brisk walking, stationary bicycling, and swimming. The latter two require no weight bearing, thus further decreasing the risks of injury. Aerobic dancing offers an opportunity for excellent cardiovascular conditioning, as well as the comfort of a class that is both socially and culturally acceptable to many women who were not previously oriented toward sports. The other well-known, socially acceptable sports, such as tennis, racquetball, or badminton, do not require enough sustained exertion to provide cardiovascular fitness. (Most casual tennis players spend most time chasing balls at a comfortable pace, rather than exercising vigorously.)

It is advisable for older women to "warm-up" gradually before each exercise session by using the same muscles that will be exercised in the activity (i.e., slow jogging to warm-up for jogging, slow cycling to warm-up for cycling, and so on). Such specific warming-up is the only appropriate type of warm-up, and it serves several functions. It permits the muscles to contract faster and decreases the risk of cardiac arrhythmias and muscle injuries during exercise.[31,32] Women should be encouraged to "cool-down" gradually after exercising, in order to prevent venous pooling and the concomitant increase in cardiac load, as well as to diminish the postexercise hyperthermic response.[33]

Although many athletes at all levels stretch their muscles prior to exercise, the advisability of such stretching remains controversial. Muscles lose elasticity with aging, as a result of which many older individuals incur injuries when they stretch cold muscles. Most older athletes would benefit more and risk less by stretching only when their muscles are warm (i.e., following exercise). Many sustain injuries when stretching at any time and consequently should not attempt stretching at all.

Summary

In conclusion, regular physical exercise offers many benefits to older women, who generally need greater encouragement to initiate such a program of activity. The likelihood of developing osteoporosis, cardiovascular disease, psychiatric disturbances, and obesity and its related problems can be diminished, and an overall feeling of well being can be anticipated, in addition. Gynecologists should encourage nearly all of their aging patients, friends, and colleagues to initiate and/or maintain a regular exercise program, in view of these rewards.

REFERENCES

1. Tataryn I, Lomax P, Meldrum D, et al. Objective techniques for the assessment of postmenopausal hot flashes. Obstet Gynecol. 1981; 57:340–344.
2. Meldrum D, Shamonki I, Frumar M, et al. Elevations in skin temperature of the finger as an objective index of post-menopausal hot flashes: Standardization of the technique. Am J Obstet Gynecol. 1979; 135:713–717.
3. Campbell S, Whitehead M. Estrogen therapy and the postmenopausal syndrome. Clin Obstet Gynecol. 1977; 4:31.
4. Morrison JC, Martin DC, Blair RA, et al. The use of medroxyprogesterone acetate for relief of climacteric symptoms. Am J Obstet Gynecol. 1980; 138:99–104.
5. Briggs M, Briggs M. Relationship between monoamine oxidase activity and sex hormone concentration in human blood plasma. J Reprod Fertil. 1972; 29:447–450.
6. Holzbauer M, Youdim M. The estrous cycle and monoamine oxidase activity. Br J Pharmacol. 1973; 48:600–608.
7. Klaiber E, Kobayashi Y, Broverman D, et al. Plasma monoamine oxidase activity in regularly menstruating women and in amenorrheic women receiving cyclic treatment with estrogens and a progestin. J Clin Endocrinol. 1971; 33:630–638.
8. Wallace J. Serum concentrations of sex hormones during exercise in pre-, peri-, and postmenopausal women. Doctoral thesis. Pennsylvania State University, 1981.
9. McGeer E, McGeer P. Neurotransmitter metabolism in the aging brain. In: Terry RD, Gershon S, eds. Neurobiology of Aging, Vol. 3. New York: Raven Press, 1976:389.
10. Robinson D, et al. Aging, monoamines and monoamine oxidase levels. Lancet. 1972; 1:290–291.
11. Robinson D. Changes in monoamine oxidase and monoamines with human development and aging. Fed Proc. 1975; 34:103–107.
12. von Praag HM, Korf J. Monoamine metabolism

in depression: Clinical application of the probenecid test. In: Barchas J, Usdin E, eds. Serotonin and behavior. New York: Academic Press, 1973.

13. Brown B, Payne T, Kim C, et al. Chronic response of rat brain norepinephrine and serotonin levels to endurance training. J Appl Physiol. 1979; 46:19–23.
14. Albanese A. Personal communication.
15. Aloia J, Cohn S, Ostuni J, et al. Prevention of involutional bone loss by exercise. Ann Intern Med. 1978; 89:356–358.
16. Smith E, Reddan W, Smith P. Physical activity and calcium modalities for bone mineral increase in aged women. Med Sci Sports 1981; 13:60–64.
17. Kannel W, Hjortland M, McNamara P, et al. Menopause and coronary heart disease. Ann Intern Med. 1976; 85:447–452.
18. Gordon T, Kannel W, Hjortland M, et al. Menopause and coronary heart disease. Ann Intern Med. 1978; 89:157–161.
19. Ritterband A, Jaffe I, Densen P, et al. Gonadal function and the development of coronary heart disease. Circulation. 1963; 27:237–251.
20. Wood P, Klein H, Lewis S, et al. Plasma lipoprotein concentrations in middle-aged male runners. Circulation. 1974; 50(Suppl. 3):115.
21. Lopez A, Vial R, Balart L, et al. Effect of exercise and physical fitness on serum lipids and lipoproteins. Atherosclerosis. 1974; 20:1–9.
22. Gordon T, Castelli W, Hjortland M, et al. High density lipoprotein as a protective factor against coronary heart disease: The Framingham study. Am. J Med. 1977; 62:707–714.
23. Williams R, Logue E, Lewis J, et al. Physical conditioning augments the fibrinolytic response

to venous occlusion in healthy adults. N Engl J Med. 1980; 302:987–991.
24. Coscina D, Stancer H. Selective blockade of hypothalamic hyperphagia and obesity in rats by serotonin-depleting midbrain lesions. Science. 1977; 195:416–419.
25. Blundell JE, Latham CJ. Serotoninergic influences on food intake. Pharm Biochem Behav. 1979; 11:431–437.
26. Latham CJ, Blundell JE. Evidence for the effect of tryptophan on the pattern of food consumption in free-feeding and deprived rats. Life Sci. 1979; 24:1971–1978.
27. deVries HA, Gray De. After effects of exercise upon resting metabolic rate. Res Q. 1963; 34:314–321.
28. American College of Sports Medicine, Position statement on the recommended quantity and quality of exercise for developing and maintaining fitness in healthy adults. Med Sci Sports. 1978; 10(3):vii–x.
29. Karvonen J, Kentala K, Mustala O. The effects of training heart rate: a longitudinal study. Ann Med Exp Biol Fenn. 1957; 35:307.
30. Davis J, Convertino V. A comparison of heart rate methods for predicting endurance training intensity. Med Sci Sports. 1975; 7:295–298.
31. Barnard R, Gardner G, Diaco N, et al. Cardiovascular responses to sudden strenuous exercise—heart rate, blood pressure, and ECG. J Appl Physiol. 1973; 34:833–837.
32. Martin B, Robinson S, Wiegman D, et al. Effect of warm-up on metabolic responses to strenuous exercise. Med Sci Sports. 1975; 7:146–149.
33. deVries H. Physiology of exercise for physical education and athletics. Dubuque, Iowa: Brown, 1974:138.

The Perimenopausal Woman in Literature 16

Marie DuMont Low

General Trends

Sensitive treatment of the aging woman and her problems is not a dominant theme in Anglo-American literature. Throughout much of our cultural history, the youthful heroine, not her older sister, has captivated writers and painters of both sexes. The English novel repeatedly chronicles the tale of the young virgin who passes from innocence to experience—preferably through marriage—and as a result of her relationship with a man assumes her proper place in society. Individual self-development is traded for security; the self is subordinated to the broader social good—the need to bear children to insure the continuity of the race. One readily recalls variants of this archetype: Emily Bronte's Catherine, who loves Heathcliffe but marries socially stable Edgar Linton and dies while still in her youth; Thomas Hardy's Tess, whose surrender to sex outside marriage is the source of her tragedy because it violates social mores still sacrosanct in the late nineteenth century.

Several influences combined to limit artistic focus on the postmenopausal woman. First and foremost, the older female was an uncommon figure in society until the mid-nineteenth century. Between 10,000 B.C. and 1640 A.D., average female life expectancy increased only about 4 years: from 28 to 32. Infectious diseases (plague, tuberculosis, smallpox) of course took their toll of both sexes. Women, however, bore the additional risk of disorders directly related to child-bearing: puerperal fever, postpartum hemorrhage, and atypical presentation. By 1800 (a significant date because it marks the beginning of the Golden Age of the English novel) a woman's life expectancy was still just 50 years: the age typically marking her passage through menopause.

In such a world, exercise of the capacity to bear children became a social imperative. The Judeo-Christian religious tradition gave the social imperative the added force of moral sanction. The single or widowed woman became an object of pity or satire. The children borne to a married woman were a divine gift, but the process by which she conceived them was not openly discussed. This exaggerated sense of propriety continued throughout the nineteenth century, even after a significant number of women (the Brontes, George Eliot, Harriet Martineau, Elizabeth Gaskell, and a host of minor novelists) began to earn a living from writing. The private lives of these novelists may have been often unconventional, but in their art they deviated only slightly from the traditional concepts of woman's role. Most heroines remained youthful; their trials were confined to selection of the right husband; their success was intricately tied to marriage; and their stories ended before they made the crucial passage into their post-childbearing years.

The twentieth century has brought a dramatic turnabout in the literary and artistic conceptualization of women. Medical advances have extended life expectancy well beyond the menopause, and changing social mores have legitimized woman's participation in the world of work. No longer must the woman writer feel a tension between her life and her art. The number of successful female novelists has increased exponentially, especially in the last 25 years, and they are tackling subjects beyond the scope of their nineteenth century counterparts: sexual desire, marital discord, the single life as a legitimate choice, the rewards and costs of a career. Realistic portrayal of the perimenopausal woman has become an important aspect of the increased realism of the modern novel.

Although generalizations are as dangerous in literature as they are in medicine, it is largely true that throughout our literary history, interest in the problems of the aging female has come predominantly from women writers. Even as the majority developed, refined, and maintained the stereotype of the young woman's passage from youth to experience, a brave minority espoused more realistic portrayal of women of all ages. The remainder of this chapter will consider these important pre–twentieth century exceptions, relate them to the prevailing ethos of their times, and show their ultimate vindication in several popular works of the past decade.

Biblical Origins

At least eight biblical heroines are specifically stated to live to an advanced age. The best known of these are Eve and Sarah from the Book of Genesis, and Elizabeth and Anna from the Gospel of St. Luke.

In the vast majority of stories of women in both the Old and New Testaments, motherhood is celebrated as the highest calling for a woman, and faith as her greatest virtue. In the tales of postmenopausal women, these themes are often linked: through trust in God, a woman is able to conceive well past her normal time for childbearing. At a very advanced age, long after her expulsion from Eden, Eve gives birth to her last son, Seth. In his first epistle to Timothy (2:13–15), Paul recalls this event as an act of faith that partly mitigates Eve's earlier transgression.

A much closer look at the link between faith and later-life conception is provided in the story of Sarah, wife of Abraham and mother of Isaac. Early in her marriage, God promised Sarah that she would become the Mother of Nations and Founder of the House of Israel. Throughout these years, however, she was unable to conceive. In her frustration, she performed what must surely be one of the first recorded tests of male fertility: she encouraged Abraham to sleep with her maid Hagar, whose subsequent pregnancy confirmed that Abraham was not the source of the difficulty.

After the birth of Hagar's child, Sarah is visited by three divine messengers who indicate that at long last she will conceive and bear a son. Showing a sound knowledge of physiology (but a temporary mistrust of the divine origin of the visitors), Sarah replies: "After I am waxed old shall I have pleasure, my lord being old also?" (Genesis 18:2).

The advanced age of the couple at the time of Sarah's conception is later confirmed in Paul's Epistle to the Romans: "And being not weak in faith, [Abraham] considered not his own body now dead, when he was about an hundred years old, neither yet the deadness of Sarah's womb" (Romans 4:19). The messengers had predicted accurately, and Isaac is born, only to be almost snatched away from his distraught parents when Abraham's faith is further tested on the holy mountain. Sarah dies at the very advanced age of 127—the only woman in the Bible whose age at death is explicitly given.[1]

Two New Testament analogs for Sarah are Elizabeth, the mother of John the Baptist, and Anna, the aging widow and prophetess who lives in the Temple of Jerusalem. The latter's story is allotted only a few verses in Luke's gospel, yet we are explicitly told that she has been denied the joys of motherhood. Of Elizabeth, we learn much more. Her pregnancy with John occurs in her later years and is an obvious contrast to that of her cousin Mary, who is consistently portrayed both in the Bible itself and in medieval and Renaissance art as in the flower of youth at the time of Christ's birth. Elizabeth, like Sarah, is rewarded with a miraculous postmenopausal conception through her consistent goodness and faith.

The Middle Ages

The biblical stories of Sarah and Elizabeth reveal a sensitive understanding of human disappointment and joy. This flesh-and-blood dimension is often lacking, however, in the English and continental literature of the twelfth to fifteenth centuries. Many heroines of the Bible reappear in medieval allegory and romance, but they are transformed into mere representations of psychologic and philosophic issues influencing the world of men. "Good" biblical women (such as Judith, Esther, or Ruth) are symbols of beauty, reason, righteousness, or even the Christian church; "bad" biblical women (such as Delilah or Potiphar's wife) are emblematic of the passions, especially of sexual desire. The wandering hero who is the focus of much medieval romance is torn between these extreme claims upon his personality. If he overcomes his weaker impulses, he is rewarded with marriage to the woman he loves. Marriage, then, becomes in medieval literature more than a means of continuing the human race. It represents unity in the individual and his universe—a theme that will assume great importance in later literature.

What is the role of the postmenopausal woman in medieval romance, with its almost cloying emphasis on feminine youth and beauty? The older woman does have her place, but she is usually a sorceress or a temptress. Unlike her biblical antecedents, she is allowed no interest in sexual fulfillment or procreation. Rather, she serves as a constant reminder to the young woman of the transience of physical beauty. As John Gower, a contemporary of Chaucer, wrote in *The Mirror of Man*, "More than all of them I despise/The old woman who is flirtatious/When her breasts are withered."[2]

Paradoxically, however, the very physical decline that made the older medieval woman an object of satire also freed her from the bounds of pure symbolism and permitted her to make use of her intelligence. Several romances and histories suggest that medieval women (and especially older women) were knowledgeable about childbirth, contraception, and abortion, and even treated battlefield injuries. They "seem to have been tolerated in medical practice as in no other profession,"[2] perhaps because it was considered unseemly for men to perform physical examinations on women. Indeed, the early fifteenth century *Sloane Manuscript 2463*, the first textbook of gynecology published in English, demonstrates a surprising understanding of menarche, menstruation, and menopause, despite its reliance on the theory of the Four Humors:

Therefore, you must understand that women have less heat in their bodies than men and have more moisture because of lack of heat that would dry their moisture and their humors, but nevertheless they have bleeding which makes their bodies clean and whole from sickness. And they have such purgations from the age of twelve to fifty. Even so, some women have purgations for a longer time because they are of a high complexion and are nourished with hot food and drink and live in much ease.[2]

It is speculated, although not proven, that the Sloane manuscript was written by a woman.

Shakespeare and the Renaissance

The literature of the English Renaissance (roughly mid-sixteenth to mid-seventeenth centuries) is of course dominated by the plays of William Shakespeare. Shakespeare, in turn, was much influenced by the social, political, and religious ideas of his day, as well as by the classical and Anglo-Saxon legends that formed the basis for his plots. He wrote many of his plays during the long reign of Queen Elizabeth, who ruled from 1558 to 1603. As the focus of both political policy and cultural taste in her day, Elizabeth called into question the stereotypes of women that pervaded medieval literature. Significantly, she was not only the first English queen actively to formulate policy; she was also unmarried and continued to rule to an advanced age. Although earlier literary historians emphasized her vanity and love of flattery, more recent work has suggested a synergy between Elizabeth and the philosophy of the Renaissance humanists, who underscored the individuality of women rather than their symbolism.[3] Elizabeth demonstrated to her subjects that options other than marriage or the religious life were possible for women, and that women could grow old with dignity.

The tension between a more humanistic concept of women and the medieval view of the aging woman as a sorceress or object of satire is very evident in Shakespeare's dramas, e.g., the witches in *Macbeth*. Several lines in *The Taming of the Shrew* make the attack on the aging woman more explicit: she is described as "an old trot, with ne'er a tooth in her head although she may have as many diseases as two and fifty horses" (I.ii.89). And then there is Gertrude, Hamlet's mother, who marries the infamous Claudius after he murders Hamlet's father to obtain the Danish throne. In describing Gertrude's duplicity to Hamlet in Act I, the Ghost seems to find her resurgent sexuality especially contemptible because it occurs in one who is old enough to have had a previous marriage:

> O Hamlet, what a falling-off was there!
> From me, whose love was of that dignity
> That it went hand in hand even with the vow
> I made to her in marriage, and to decline
> Upon a wretch whose natural gifts were poor
> To these of mine! . . .
> So lust, though to a radiant angel link'd,
> Will sate itself in a celestial bed,
> And prey on garbage.
>
> (I.v.47–52, 55–57)

It is a concept that owes much to the Middle Ages.

Juliet's aging nurse in *Romeo and Juliet* takes what both Shakespeare and his medieval forbears would find to be a more appropriate approach to her sexuality. The nurse has lived through the deaths of both a husband and a daughter, and she has learned to cope with her environment through a self-preserving cynicism:

> There's no trust,
> No faith, no honesty in men; all perjured,
> All forsworn, all naught, all dissemblers.
>
> (III.ii.84–86)

She eschews further romantic involvements for herself and instead is content to sponsor trysts between the young lovers and to warn them when others are approaching. Her interest in the relationship leads directly to its tragic conclusion. It is the nurse who first finds Juliet after she takes the sleeping potion, assumes she is dead, and precipitates Romeo's suicide.

The nurse's age is, of course, a counterpoint to Juliet's youth. Many of Shakespeare's women are at one pole or the other of the youth-age continuum, so that female characters approaching the time of menopause are unusual in his plays. A well-known exception is Lady Macbeth. We know that Lady Macbeth has already borne children. In Act I, she tells us: "I have given suck, and know/How tender 'tis to love the babe that milks me" (I.ii.54–55). She has not, however, reached the point where

her family is complete, for later in Act I Macbeth admonishes her to "bring forth men children only" (I.vii.73). Given her husband's influential position—his possibility of obtaining the crown by assassinating Duncan—we can imagine that Lady Macbeth may be in her early forties. If that is indeed the case, her self-control and single-minded determination are a sharp contrast to the mood swings that are characteristic of the years preceding menopause. Although the assassination is not initially her idea, she is the one who keeps Macbeth on course with the plan: "Screw your courage to the sticking point, and we'll not fail."

The Golden Age of the Novel (Eighteenth and Nineteenth Centuries)

Lady Macbeth possesses tremendous energy, which she expends in the service of her husband's evil ambitions. The words "husband" and "evil" are significant. The same energy imbues many women in the eighteenth century English novel, but its purpose is the more positive one of self-preservation in a world that is often harsh and inhospitable. Beginning with Daniel Defoe's *Moll Flanders,* the heroine of the early novel is typically single (at least at the outset), intelligent, independent, and above all a survivor. Although she may establish relationships with men, she does not do so because she believes her life is worthless in the absence of marriage; rather, men can be used to preserve her security and freedom.[4] Indeed, with the exception of such excessively sentimental works as Richardson's *Pamela, or Virtue Rewarded,* the early novel did not essentially discriminate between the "picaresque" hero and the self-sufficient heroine. Men and women alike must triumph over their environment—a sharp contrast to the situation in the medieval romance (the picaresque novel's forebear), where men undertake the quest and women wait at home. *Moll Flanders* is an especially important example of this genre because it allows us to follow the heroine from youth into middle age.

The American novel, like the British, was concerned in its early phases with the interaction between the individual and the environment. This environment, however, is not the civilized world of social intercourse but the harsher, male-dominated world of the new frontier. There are few heroines in James Fennimore Cooper's primeval forest or aboard Herman Melville's *Pequod* as it sails in pursuit of Moby Dick. Still, one important exception, Nathaniel Hawthorne's *The Scarlet Letter,* affords an intriguing variation upon our theme of female aging.

Hester Prynne's later years are not the focus of *The Scarlet Letter*; indeed, Hawthorne covers them hastily in a short epilogue in which Hester returns to New England, the scene of her sexual transgression, because mere geographic separation cannot free her from her past. Earlier in the story, however, he gives us a fascinating description of the physical and emotional transformation which Hester undergoes after she is separated from her lover and forced to live the life of isolation and shame symbolized by the scarlet A:

> All the light and graceful foliage of her character had been withered up by this red-hot brand [the Scarlet Letter], and had long ago fallen away, leaving a bare and harsh outline. . . . Even the attractiveness of her person had undergone a similar change. . . . Some attribute had departed from her, the permanence of which had been essential to keep her a woman. . . . Much of the marble coldness of Hester's impression was to be attributed to the circumstance that her life had turned, in a great measure, from passion and feeling, to thought. (Chap. 13)

The changes in Hester's appearance bear a remarkable resemblance to some of the physical changes accompanying menopause. Indeed, Hester may be seen as undergoing a form of psychologic menopause through the suppression of her emotional responses. Many years would pass before American fiction provided an equally sophisticated analysis.

While Hester attempted to cope with separation and loneliness, the women of the early British Victorian novel—women of all ages—faced a very different destiny. The early Victorians were preoccupied with the concepts of duty and sacrifice. A woman's duties (not unlike the duties of the women of the Bible) were first and foremost to serve her husband and children. Numerous male philosophers and social theorists underscored this point, and thus

it was easy to assume that women actually disliked sexual intercourse and submitted to it only out of their great desire to be mothers.* To be unmarried, especially in middle age, was once again an embarrassment; Agress notes that it was customary for single women to assume the title of "Mrs." when they reached their forties.[5] The life of the single, middle-aged woman was at its best austere and lonely, and at its worst impoverished as well. There was little compensation for failing to fit the ideal of the perfect mother and wife, for many of the professions were still closed to women. "Career" choices were limited to servant, governess, factory worker, or (increasingly) prostitute.

Middle-aged women were depicted by simplified, symbolic characterizations in many Victorian novels. The vigor of Moll Flanders gave way to the satirical stereotypes of Charles Dickens. Dickens was especially harsh on the older woman, whom he used to symbolize the emptiness of a life lived without husband or children. Mrs. Pipchin, head of a boarding school attended by Paul Dombey in *Dombey and Son,* is one such figure. She is described as a "marvelous ill-favoured, ill-conditioned old lady, a stooping figure [osteoporosis?], with a hook nose, and a hard grey eye." Miss Murdstone, one of the jailers of David's mother in *David Copperfield,* seems to have developed arthritis as she has grown older: she has "cold stiff fingers." And who can forget Miss Havisham of *Great Expectations,* the ultimate caricature as she sits in her cobweb-filled parlor, with the windows shut and the curtains drawn, wearing her wedding dress, and with the clock stopped at the precise time when she was jilted by her fiancé on her wedding day?

While Dickens portrayed middle-aged spinsterhood strictly from the perspective of satire, other Victorian novelists (many of them women) chose to examine critically the belief that a woman's sole responsibilities were submissiveness and procreation. Indeed, the issue of what a woman did during her reproductive life—and by extension, the self-worth she

---

* See, for example, William Acton's *The Functions and Disorders of the Reproductive Organs* (1857). Although Acton had been elected to the Royal Medical and Chirurgical Society in 1842, his work contained little discussion of the menarche or menopause. In relation to its time, it was far more reactionary than the medieval Sloane manuscript.

maintained after her childbearing years were over—was examined with such frequency after 1850 that it came to be known as "the woman question."

Charlotte Bronte's complex portrayals of schoolmistresses and governesses are one approach to "the woman question." Through her own employment as a teacher, Bronte was acutely conscious of the harsh existence lived by many women who practiced her profession. But she also recognized that teaching was one of the better occupations available to women of her day. Her struggle to reconcile this ambivalence is especially poignant in *Villette,* a novel which has never achieved the popularity of *Jane Eyre,* but which is considered by many to be her masterpiece. *Villette* quickly establishes a counterpoint between Lucy Snowe, a young Englishwoman who accepts a position at a boarding school in France, and Madame Beck, the French school's headmistress. The contrast is not simply one between inexperience and experience; it is also fundamentally one between youth and approaching middle age. Madame Beck, who is in her early forties, is now what Lucy may become. Hence Lucy analyzes her meticulously and struggles hard to find value in her independence. The price that Madame Beck has paid, however, is overwhelming:

> She was a charitable woman, and did a great deal of good. There never was a mistress whose rule was milder. . . . Very good sense she often showed; very sound opinions she often broached. . . . [But] to attempt to touch her heart was the surest way to rouse her antipathy, and to make of her a secret foe. It proved to her that she had no heart to be touched. . . . (Chap. 8)

Later in the novel, Bronte underscores the limited choices facing the Victorian woman through a series of paintings, entitled "The Life of a Woman," which Lucy views at an art museum. The artist has reduced woman's history to four stages. The first painting shows a young girl, the second a bride in a long white veil, and the third a new mother holding a baby in her arms. The final painting, entitled "Widow," reveals the isolation of a woman in middle age, even when she has chosen the accepted path of wife and mother. Bronte has deflated the ideal espoused by the early Victorians, but despite her sympathy, she cannot provide her characters with a successful alternative.

Whereas *Villette* addresses "the woman question" by juxtaposing a character of relative youth with one of middle age, Thackeray's *Vanity Fair* and George Eliot's *Middlemarch* reveal the progression from naivete to disenchantment in a single character. Thackeray's Becky Sharpe is a direct descendent of *Moll Flanders*: energetic and enterprising, she pursues a husband not for the accepted Victorian reasons, but rather to secure a superior position for herself in society. Security, however, brings her in middle age to a humdrum life of "good works" in a small provincial town—a fate which does small justice to her talents. Eliot's Dorothea Brooke is no more successful. Equally anxious to escape banality, she too finds herself in "the prison of womanhood" in her twilight years.[6]

Only much later would women begin to escape the prison.

Popular American Novels of the 1970s and 1980s

Charles Dickens (who wrote for the general reader rather than for the scholarly few) perhaps most accurately fictionalized the image of women held by his fellow Victorians. The permutation of that concept which has come with the twentieth century is also best documented in works of popular fiction. And since art may influence life as much as life imitates art, it is instructive for the clinician to sample some of the recent novels by and about women which now populate his patients' bookshelves. All of the novels discussed in this section have been best-sellers—and their sensitivity to the needs and conflicts of modern women more than compensates for their occasional absence of literary sophistication.

The heroine of the post-1970 novel does not completely escape the confines of small-town existence. But another alternative is opening up for her: the choice of a fulltime professional career. No longer is she either an ingenue or an aged crone; rather, we now often see her in the difficult years of approaching middle age. Her growth is not a simple passage from innocence to experience—from child-hood to marriage—but may require a confron-tation with disappointment in the years follow-ing her marriage vows. Or it may force a recognition of the costs inherent in the search for professional achievement. Especially as she approaches her forties, the contemporary woman wants fulfillment in *both* her personal and her working lives, as Gail Sheehy notes in *Passages*:

> Every woman—the caregiver, the deferred achiever, the deferred nurturer, the integra-tor—finds unanticipated questions knocking at the back door of her mind around 35, urging her to review those roles and options she has already tried against those she has set aside, and those that aging and biology will close off in the *now foreseeable* future:
> "What am I giving up for this marriage?" *or* "Is this career depriving me of personal happiness? . . .

Sheehy's comments provide a convenient framework for our discussion of the modern fictional woman in the years immediately pre-ceding and following menopause.

Erica Tate, the central character of Alison Lurie's *The War Between the Tates* (1974), is the archetypal deferred achiever. Erica is a gradu-ate of Radcliffe, and in the early years of her marriage, she wrote and illustrated several suc-cessful children's books. For some time, how-ever, she has devoted herself exclusively to car-ing for her husband (a professor of political science at a college in upstate New York) and their two teenage children. As the novel be-gins, she is about to celebrate her fortieth birthday, and she is struck by the banality of her life. She is acutely conscious of the lines and creases that she sees when she studies her face in the mirror, and at times she bursts into unexplained fits of crying. She is unable to concentrate on the household activities that govern her existence: when her husband opens his lunch at the office one day, he finds coffee grounds, crushed eggshells, and orange peels instead of the sandwich he had been ex-pecting. Her children seem rude, exasperat-ing, and inconsiderate: "How has it all come about? She is—or at least used to be—a gentle, rational, even-tempered woman, not given to violent feelings. In her whole life she cannot remember disliking anyone as much as she now sometimes dislikes Jeffrey and Matilda." Even more disconcerting is her husband's own midlife crisis. He has recently confessed to an affair with a graduate student.

Trying to extricate herself from her depres-sion, Erica vacillates between pursuing the achievement she has so long deferred and postponing the return to work by having an-other child. Preoccupied with his own passage, however, her husband shows little interest in her conflict. He thinks that she is too old to have children and that the research assistant-ship which she has been offered in the psychol-ogy department is beneath her dignity. Erica must escape from her prison alone. She sepa-rates from her husband, begins an affair with an aging bohemian who owns a student book-store, and accepts a job editing manuscripts for a professor. However, the anticipation of re-bellion is more alluring than the rather lonely reality. And so, Erica passes through her crisis and comes to the recognition that the history which she and her husband have shared consti-tutes a strong and positive bond between them. She will return to her marriage—but on a new basis which allows her to maintain her job and establish a validity outside her home. She has weathered the midlife storm, and, we sense, found a way to achieve both professional satis-faction and marital happiness.

Erica Tate is mature enough to recognize the need for change and young enough to en-joy the benefits of her changes. The premeno-pausal crisis of the deferred achiever has been documented in other novels of the 1970s, such as Marilyn French's *The Woman's Room*. Recent fiction, however, also shows us the deferred achiever who has deferred too long. She is sen-sitively portrayed in Lisa Alther's first novel, *Kinflicks*, through the character of Mrs. Bab-cock.

Kinflicks is a novel with a split personality. The flashbacks which relate the comic adven-tures of its heroine, Ginny Babcock, are defi-nitely in the picaresque tradition of *Moll Flan-ders* or *Vanity Fair*. But *Kinflicks* also has a serious side, fixed in the present rather than the past, which describes the turning points in the lives of Ginny and her mother. The con-trast is compelling indeed. Ginny, who has ex-perimented with many of the alternative life-styles of the 1960s and eventually settled down to marriage and motherhood in Vermont, has become bored with her attempt to give her life stability. Impulsively, she decides to leave her husband and 4-year-old daughter, not because she has another alternative in mind, but simply to exercise her need for change.

The freedom to make the changes is what is important, for Mrs. Babcock does not have this freedom. After dropping out of Bryn Mawr to marry her husband, she has spent all of the intervening years raising three children and following what her Tennessee upbringing has convinced her is her duty to her family. Continually deferred, but never quite forgotten, are her ambitions to complete her college education and begin a career in teaching. She passes through menopause, the departure of her children, and the death of her husband—still waiting.

But it is too late. Mrs. Babcock has contracted a bleeding disorder, and now she lies in a hospital bed, becoming progressively weaker as the blood vessels throughout her body slowly disintegrate. The disorder progresses to her reproductive tract, and the bleeding becomes a mockery of the menstrual bleeding which is no longer possible: "As she dried herself, she realized that blood was oozing from her vagina, which was theoretically impossible because she'd reached menopause several years ago" (p. 155). The role of midlife as a precursor of death becomes tragically apparent to her:

> A leaf . . . began dying in midsummer, when the days were long and hot. The vivid green leaves on the elm outside, for instance, had already begun dying. In midsummer, in response to genes and hormones and environmental influences, the delicate balance in a leaf—between growth and decay, between order and chaos, between elaboration and disintegration—tipped in favor of decay. (p. 425)

Although Ginny, at 28, is some distance from her own menopause, her mother's predicament (emphasized by the continual ticking of a clock by her hospital bedside) reinforces Ginny's conviction that experiences must be seized rather than long postponed.

In the age contrast between Ginny and Mrs. Babcock, we recognize a restatement of the young woman/older woman theme of Charlotte Bronte's *Villette*. A more complex variant of this theme is seen in Anne Tolstoi Wallach's novel, *Women's Work* (1981). Here the heroine, as she approaches 40, finds her life intertwined with the lives of three women of ages different from her own: a young woman of 20 just starting her career, a woman in her seventies whose career is nearing its conclusion, and most importantly, a close friend just past 40 whose feelings strongly influence the heroine's own.

Whereas *Kinflicks* and *The War Between the Tates* showed us the frustrations of middle-aged women in small towns, *Women's Work* takes us to the glamorous, fast-paced, and highly competitive world of big-city advertising. Its women, without exception, are paying the price exacted by success achieved or sought. They are not deferred achievers but deferred nurturers. Belle Rosner, who established her own business as a consultant to the fashion industry after her husband died early in their marriage, has worked long hours for so much of her life that retirement is an impossible boredom. On the other hand, M. J. Kent, a 20-year-old art assistant in a large advertising agency, already has learned to regard her sexuality as strictly an instrument for advancing her career. And Maran Slade's exacting career as a fashion model has left her little time to establish a fulfilling marital relationship.

In *Women's Work*, the years just preceding menopause are a time for reassessment, for coming to terms with the price of success. The modeling world's obsession with youth has forced Maran to change careers and has made her fear the signs of aging:

> She bought pink lightbulbs for the apartment, altered her passport age by ten years by changing one digit, worked out a system of dressing that kept her from mirrors. Age was Maran's nightmare, a nightmare that grew worse, woke her shivering in the night, gave her headaches when she caught glimpses of herself. (p. 32)

Caught between careers, she searches for an occupation that will calm her apprehension and make age an asset rather than a liability. Managing promotional campaigns for the fashion industry "could be a stepping-stone to a special place, a world where it was good for you to be experienced, to be old. . . . She wanted this job so her years could be an asset instead of a hideous, disfiguring, shameful thing" (p. 32).

Like Maran, Domina Drexler (the central character of *Women's Work*) finds her midlife reassessment precipitated by an obstacle in the path of her career. After more than 15 years of experience in advertising, many of them managing major national accounts, she believes it is time that her agency recognize her contributions by offering her a senior vice-presidency. The obstacle is virtually immovable, however, for the Potter Jackson Agency has never accorded such high status to a woman. With her professional future uncertain, and aware of Maran's and Belle Rosner's situations, Domina subjects her own life to new scrutiny. Although her salary has passed $70,000, she has divorced her husband and sent her two children away to school. No one has filled the place vacated by her husband: "[She] had no need of anybody. Well, maybe she had a need, but one she'd decided wouldn't be met. Everything she wanted in just one man? No. The best she could hope for was different pieces of what she wanted from several men" (p. 8). The worlds of personal and professional fulfillment appear to be severed irrevocably.

Women's Work has its moments of tragedy (Maran dies of heart failure during a routine operation), but ultimately it is a story of triumph. Through hard work, and some good fortune too, Domina Drexler is able to start her own advertising agency and find a man who will share both her home and her career. Those twin goals of respect and happiness, sought by perimenopausal women through so much of the history we have traced, are finally achieved in combination.

Summary

Shorter life expectancies limited the literary representation of older women until quite recently in our history. Still, the exceptions to this pattern constitute an intriguing paradigm of changing social attitudes. From the biblical heroine (who is personally reborn when she conceives at advanced age), we have moved to the sorceress of medieval romance and the misdirected sexual energy of Lady Macbeth. We have seen the suppression of this sexual energy produce physical and emotional decline in *The Scarlet Letter*. And we have examined the tension during the Victorian period between the middle-aged woman's search for fulfillment outside the traditional sphere of marriage and children, and her ultimate recognition that she is, indeed, powerless to escape well-entrenched mores. Recent popular fiction has, at last, defined and legitimized our heroine's attempt to be not only wife and mother but also professional colleague. But it has also documented the difficulty of the struggle and the fragility of the reconciliation. For the perimenopausal woman—in life as well as in art—much "woman's work" remains to be done.

REFERENCES

1. Deen E. All the Women of the Bible. New York: Harper and Brothers, 1955.
2. Rowland B. Medieval Woman's Guide to Health. Kent, Ohio: Kent State University Press, 1981:4, 6, 59.
3. Dusinberre J. Shakespeare and the Nature of Women. London: Macmillan, 1975.
4. Rogers KM. Sensitive feminism vs. conventional sympathy: Richardson and Fielding on women. Novel. 1976; 9(3):256–270.
5. Agress L. The Feminine Irony: Women in Early Nineteenth Century Literature. Rutherford, N.J.: Fairleigh Dickinson University Press, 1978.
6. Sabiston L. The prison of womanhood. Comp Lit. 1973; 25(4):336–351.
7. Sheehy G. Passages. New York: Bantam Books, 1977:377–378.

Further Reading

Basch F. Relative Creatures: Victorian Women in Society and the Novel. New York: Schocken Books, 1974.
Baym N. Women's Fiction: A Guide to Novels by and about Women in America, 1820–1870. Ithaca, N.Y.: Cornell University Press, 1978.
Beer P: Reader, I Married Him. London: Macmillan, 1974.
Ferrante JM. Woman as Image in Medieval Literature, from the 12th Century to Dante. New York: Columbia University Press, 1975.
Greenblatt RB. Search the Scriptures: A Physician Examines Medicine in the Bible. Philadelphia: Lippincott, 1963.
Millett K. Sexual Politics. New York: Doubleday and Co., 1970.

Index

Estradiol dipropionate, 62
Estradiol valerate, 62
  high density lipoproteins affected by, 91
  triglyceride concentrations affected by, 91
Estriol
  absorption, formulation, and administration of,
    62
  biliary, 66
  binding and transport of, 62
  carcinogenic potential of, 190, 191, 192
  in estrogen replacement therapy, 59, 60
  metabolism, conjugation, and excretion of, 64,
    65
  receptor binding capacity of, 67
  structure of, 57
Estriol-3-sulfate-16-glucuronide, 66
Estrogen(s)
  absorption, formulation, and administration of,
    60–62
  biliary, 66
  binding and transport of, 62–63
  bioavailability of, 62–63
  biologic effects of, 59–69
  biosynthesis of, 1–6, 58–59
    postmenopausally, 1, 2, 24
    premenopausally, 1, 23, 24
    regulation of, 2–3
  in bone cell metabolism, 37–38
  in breast cancer, 191–192
  calcium levels affected by, 90
  catecholamines affected by, 168
  in climacteric, 23–31
  coagulation affected by, 93
  conjugated, 63–67, 77, 80
    equine, 88, 91
  endometrial cancer from unopposed, 87, 103–
    105
  excretion of, 63–67
  forms of circulation of, 77
  free, 67–68, 77
  and heart disease, 30
  history of, 55–56
  insulin secretion affected by, 92
  lipoproteins affected by, 91
  mammary effect of, 95
  mechanism of action of, 85–86
  metabolism of
    progesterone in, 63–67
    stimulation of, 86, 87
  origin of, 1–6
  pharmacology of, 59, 69
  progesterone regulation of, 86
  protein-bound, 77
  receptor synthesis promotion by, 85–86
  roles of, 55
  sexual performance affected by, 170
  sleep and mood affected by, 157, 168
  structure of, 56–58

Estrogen (*Cont.*)
  synthetic, 57, 62, 67
  testosterone and, 1
  tryptophan metabolism affected by, 166–167
  vaginal development affected by, 9
  in vulva development, 9
Estrogen sulfotransferase, 86
Estrogen deficiency and deprivation
  aging and, 132
  bladder affected by, 21
  breasts affected by, 17
  calcitonin affected by, 43
  cardiovascular system affected by, 21
  cervical changes with, 14
  clinical symptomatology of, 133, 152
  endometrium affected by, 14
  fallopian tubes affected by, 14
  hot flushes from, 26
  lipid metabolism with, 91
  myometrium affected by, 14
  ovary affected by, 14–17
  and pelvic relaxation, 27–28
  and postmenopausal osteoporosis, 28–29, 41–42
  skeletal system affected by, 19, 20
  skin changes with, 17–18
  urethra affected by, 21
  urinary tract disorders secondary to, 131, 132–
    134
  uterine corpus affected by, 14
  vagina affected by, 14, 176
  vasomotor symptoms with, 153
  vulva affected by, 9
Estrogen receptors, 67–68
  in breast, 95
  clinical implications of, 68
  estrogen replacement treatment effect on, 88
  progesterone effect on, 86, 88
  in urethra, 133
Estrogen replacement therapy, 77–83
  administration of, routes for, 78–79
  by age group, 78
  for atrophic vaginitis, 200
  benefits of, 77, 79–82
  benign breast disease from, 94
  breast cancer and, 77, 83, 94, 191, 196, 197
  breast changes from, 187
  calcium levels with, 29
  contraindications to, 78
  disadvantages of, 85
  dosages in, 78
  duration of, 79
  endometrial biopsy prior to, 79
  endometrial cancer from, 77, 82, 87, 103, 137
  glucose metabolism altered by, 83
  for headaches, 28
  for hot flushes, 199
  hypertension exacerbated by, 77, 82
  for hypogonadal individuals, 78